Clinical Topics in Cardiology

Clinical Topics in Cardiology

Edited by Harrison Cox

hayle
medical

New York

Hayle Medical,
750 Third Avenue, 9th Floor,
New York, NY 10017, USA

Visit us on the World Wide Web at:
www.haylemedical.com

ISBN: 978-1-63241-560-8

Cataloging-in-Publication Data

Clinical topics in cardiology / edited by Harrison Cox.
    p. cm.
Includes bibliographical references and index.
ISBN 978-1-63241-560-8
1. Cardiology. 2. Heart--Diseases. 3. Heart--Diseases--Treatment.
4. Clinical medicine. I. Cox, Harrison.
RC667 .C55 2019
616.1--dc23

Table of Contents

Preface

Over the recent decade, advancements and applications have progressed exponentially. This has led to the increased interest in this field and projects are being conducted to enhance knowledge. The main objective of this book is to present some of the critical challenges and provide insights into possible solutions. This book will answer the varied questions that arise in the field and also provide an increased scope for furthering studies.

Cardiology is a sub-field of medicine concerned with the conditions of the heart and the circulatory system. This field encompasses the diagnosis and treatment of coronary artery disease, congenital heart defects, valvular heart disease and heart failure, among others. The chief specializations in cardiology fall within the two domains of adult cardiology and pediatric cardiology. Within these specific fields, there exist sub-specialties such as cardiac electrophysiology, echocardiography, cardiogeriatrics, pulmonary atresia, Ebstein anomaly, tetralogy of Fallot, etc. The heart is the center of focus in cardiology. Any patient with chest pain or any symptom suggestive of cardiovascular pathology will undergo a cardiac examination, which follows the stages of inspection, palpation and auscultation. This book covers in detail some existing theories and innovative concepts revolving around cardiology. The various sub-fields along with technological progress that have future implications are glanced at herein. For someone with an interest and eye for detail, this book covers the most significant topics in the field of cardiology.

I hope that this book, with its visionary approach, will be a valuable addition and will promote interest among readers. Each of the authors has provided their extraordinary competence in their specific fields by providing different perspectives as they come from diverse nations and regions. I thank them for their contributions.

Editor

Depression and Anxiety following Coronary Artery Bypass Graft: Current Indian Scenario

Suprakash Chaudhury,[1] **Rajiv Saini,**[2] **Ajay Kumar Bakhla,**[3] **and Jaswinder Singh**[4]

[1]*Department of Psychiatry, Pravara Institute of Medical Sciences (Deemed University), Loni, Maharashtra 413736, India*
[2]*Department of Psychiatry, AFMC, Pune, Maharashtra 411040, India*
[3]*Department of Psychiatry, Rajendra Institute of Medical Sciences, Ranchi, Jharkhand 834009, India*
[4]*Department of Cardiothoracic Surgery, MH CTC, Pune, Maharashtra 411040, India*

Correspondence should be addressed to Suprakash Chaudhury; suprakashch@gmail.com

Academic Editor: Terrence D. Ruddy

Epidemiological studies have shown a high prevalence of coronary artery disease among the Indian Population. Due to increasing availability and affordability of tertiary care in many parts of India, carefully selected patients undergo coronary artery bypass surgery to improve cardiac function. However, the procedure is commonly associated with depression and anxiety which can adversely affect overall prognosis. The objective of this review is to highlight early identifiable symptoms of depression and anxiety following coronary artery bypass graft (CABG) in Indian context so as to facilitate prompt intervention for better outcome. The current review was able to establish firm evidence in support of screening for depression and anxiety following CABG. Management of depression and anxiety following CABG is briefly reviewed.

1. Introduction

World Health Organization (WHO) describes health as a state of complete physical, mental, and social well-being and not merely an absence of disease or infirmity. Psychosomatic medicine acts as a bridge between psychiatry and other medical disciplines. Conceptually, the mind-body link has always fascinated medical man as ultimate acknowledgement of good treatment will eventually be appreciated by the mind and not the body.

However, psychiatric care has always been looked down upon as being meant for those who are inferior or mentally weak [1]. The situation is prevalent in all societies owing to stigma and discrimination towards mental illness and the mentally ill [2]. The practice often leads to denial of essential medical care with adverse outcomes. Psychiatrists, practicing on the interface of medicine and psychiatry, often find themselves creating new models of care to cater to local needs based on available resources. The issue has been discussed in detail wherein authors describe benefits of holistic medical care with active collaboration of psychiatrist and the primary care physician [3].

Vascular psychiatry is a newly emerging concept highlighting the need for psychiatric intervention in patients suffering from diseases of blood vessels [4]. It is well known that cardiovascular and cerebrovascular syndromes yield highest psychiatric morbidity and mortality. In daily practice, psychiatrists commonly encounter vascular syndromes, such as vascular depression, vascular cognitive impairment, and depression in heart disease. More often than not, psychiatric and vascular disorders occur together indicating common underlying etiopathological mechanisms [5]. Further, their association extends well into the immediate and long term care. These examples serve as innovative ways to collaborate and integrate comprehensive health care.

2. Coronary Artery Disease and Psychopathology

Coronary artery disease is the leading cause of morbidity and mortality worldwide. For more than 15 years, WHO has been sounding an alarm on the rapidly rising burden of cardiovascular disorders. The reported prevalence of coronary artery disease (CAD) in adult surveys has risen 4-fold over the last 40 years to a present level of around 10% [6, 7]. It is the leading cause of death and disability worldwide. The incidence and prevalence in Indian population may be higher because of sociodemographic reasons. The recent past has been witness to some exciting advancements in cardiac care with emphasis on prevention, early detection, and therapeutic procedures [8].

During early stages, management of CAD includes dietary and life style modification, lipid lowering agents, blood pressure monitoring, glycemic control, and antiplatelet agents. As the disease progresses, these measures are not sufficient to maintain a satisfactory quality of life. Coronary angioplasty and coronary artery bypass graft surgery (CABG) offer promise of improved quality of life in such cases though their indications undergo revision in pace with latest recommendations. CABG is the commonest surgical method of management of CAD in India [9]. Over the years, refinement of surgical and anesthetic procedures has led to significant reduction in mortality and morbidity [10]. However, still a significant number of patients do have associated psychological morbidity which is disabling and distressing. Relationship of psychological symptoms with coronary heart disease has been well known since a long time [11]. It is important to note that psychological illness when comorbid with cardiac illness generally leads to poorer outcomes [12]. Depression has been found to be an independent prognostic factor for mortality, readmission, cardiac events, and lack of functional benefits 6 months to 5 years after CABG [13–16]. These observations highlight the need for integrating psychosocial interventions to provide holistic and effective management after CABG.

3. Cardiology, Neurology, and Psychiatry Interface

The interface between heart and the mind is too strong to be negated. For reasoning to exist, a fine balance between the mind and the heart is needed for rational decision-making. When we speak of the mind we refer to the software of the hardware that we call brain. The integrity and the functionality of this software (mind) are based on optimal functioning of the underlying hardware (brain). Any insult to the structural integrity of the brain often gets translated into cognitive, emotional, motor, or sensory symptoms [17]. Motor, sensory, and neurocognitive domains are not under consideration in this paper though technically it is difficult to segregate them. The purpose of this review study is to highlight the role of early identification and management of emotional disorders that are encountered while caring for the patients undergoing CABG. We reviewed the literature for associations of CABG with negative emotions of depression or anxiety and their relationships with positive health related activities like regular drug adherence, healthy eating habits, regular exercise, and yoga.

4. Concept of Depression and Anxiety

According to the International Classification for Diseases-tenth edition (ICD-10), depression is characterized by low mood and/or anhedonia (loss of interest in activities that once were pleasurable) that lasts for two weeks or more and is accompanied by significant functional impairment and somatic complaints of disturbed sleep, fatigue, body aches, digestive or sexual problems, and negative thoughts. Anxiety on the other hand refers to feeling of apprehension and unease. Anxiety has somatic, physiological, and cognitive components. Somatic component refers to digital tremors, palpitations, and sweaty palms. The physiological component refers to tachycardia, hyperventilation, muscular tension, and an irritable bladder. The cognitive component is that of worry which refers to undue fear of something untoward happening [18].

It is not uncommon to find both depression and anxiety to coexist on a continuum so much so that they are considered together as both impair one's quality of life and interfere significantly with the ability to think rationally. In fact, anxiety has often been described to be an integral component of depressive disorder and they respond to similar drugs to a large extent [19].

Researchers have tried to pinpoint the etiological basis of depression in cardiac illnesses and have implicated factors like hypercortisolemia, insulin resistance and sympathetic-parasympathetic tone dysregulation, reduced heart rate variability, hypothalamic-pituitary-adrenal axis (HPA) axis, and increased inflammatory factors like platelet factor 4, fibrinogen, and C-reactive protein. Unhealthy lifestyle like cigarette smoking, excessive alcohol intake, lack of physical exercise, poor medications adherence, and unhealthy diet may also be directly or indirectly contributing to the onset and progression of depression [20–22]. The etiopathogenesis of anxiety among patients of heart disease is less well understood. Threat perception and felt need for biological integrity have been consistently shown to have sympathetic nervous system upregulation with excessive catecholamine production [23]. Patients with CAD often have abnormally high levels of catecholamines, which can result in increased myocardial oxygen demand due to elevations in heart rate, blood pressure, and the rate of ventricular contraction. Additionally, additive effects of benzodiazepines, alcohol, and smoking also must be taken into account as such patients are often found to be abusing them [24].

5. Manifestations of Depression and Anxiety in Indian Subjects

Though, the construct of Depression and anxiety is universally applicable as is the prevalence of these disorders, but cultural differences do exist as far as the description of the symptoms is concerned which may lead to underdiagnosis [25–28]. Visit to a local superspecialty hospital with more than 200 CABGs done per year revealed that only 5 cases were referred for psychiatric opinion because they had an earlier record of psychiatric treatment. To summarize, it is fair enough to accept that identification and referral pattern of patients suffering from psychiatric symptomatology are abysmally low in our population.

6. CABG: Indian Scenario

Studies on Indian immigrants and cross-sectional studies in India highlight high incidence of CAD in India [6, 7]. In absence of social security and state funding of medical care, only a fraction of them can actually afford superspecialty care like angioplasty or CABG. CABG was first performed in India in 1975 about 13 years after its advent in 1962. In the mid-1990s, some 10,000 CABG surgeries were being performed annually in India. Presently, the annual number is about 60000 according to industry sources [9, 29–31]. In the absence of a central registry, the exact numbers may not be known. There is no regularized health sector except in some metropolitan cities and health care is tightly compartmentalized. The majority of patients remain undiagnosed and those who are diagnosed have limited means of specialized care. It is also acknowledged that medical tourism is booming in this country and many tertiary care superspecialty hospitals cater to the rich who exclusively visit India for medical reasons. Many such hospitals offer medical package for a particular amount and the macro- and microeconomics determine the kind of medical care that will eventually be rendered to the patients [32]. Indian patients also have some other distinct peculiarities. These include younger age at presentation (average age 60 years), a high incidence of double (DVD) and triple vessel disease (TVD), diffuse involvement, distal disease, and significant left ventricular dysfunction at presentation [33, 34]. An angiographic study from Vellore in 1066 consecutive males admitted for CAD noted significant disease in 877 patients; of these, 55 percent were <50 yr of age, 34 percent were <45 yr of age, and 12 percent were below 40 yr of age. Although the mean age was 48 yr, TVD was more common (55%) than DVD (24%) and single vessel disease (24%) combined [30]. However, this data may not reflect true state of affairs as it comes from a tertiary care hospital. Another finding is that the majority of Indian patients also have many modifiable risk factors like high stress levels, smoking, hypertension, obesity, and diabetes [31, 35]. Such information opens a window of opportunity for collaborative intervention for long-term gains. There are several technical challenges, which cardiac surgeons in India have to face. These are chiefly related to small coronary vessels, arterial conduits, diffuse disease, and late presentation [9, 34]. In a recent study, authors noted that heart weight in Indians varied from 148 to 249 g while in the West the average weight of the heart in males is 300 g and that in females is 250 g [34]. Such smaller sized vessels pose difficulty during anastomosis and may result in early graft closure leading to higher mortality. Indians also tend to have diffuse CAD because of which vessels frequently require endarterectomy. The condition further predisposes to perioperative myocardial infarction and postoperative occlusion of bypass grafts [9, 33–38].

7. CABG and Psychopathology

Neuropsychiatric complications following CABG are well known ever since the procedure came into vogue. The range of these complications ranges from anxiety, depression, neurocognitive deficits, delirium, and cerebrovascular accident. The range varies from a conservative 2–4% to about 25–40% severe cases [39]. The scope of the current paper is restricted only to depression and anxiety and other effects like delirium; cerebrovascular and neurocognitive deficits are not being discussed here.

Depression and coronary artery disease are highly comorbid conditions with estimates of comorbidity from 14% to 47% [40, 41]. The causes of depression are no different from other causes of depression though it may appear that patient's depression is secondary to the diagnosis and will recover with surgery. The issue has been debated many times with clear finding that this is not the case. Though both depression and CAD may share same etiopathogenesis, they both need to be diagnosed and treated independently [21]. It is like a patient suffering abdominal trauma and fractured femur following an accident. Both conditions need attention for complete recovery. Preoperative depression is predictive of decreased cardiac symptom relief, quicker return of symptoms, more frequent rehospitalizations, and increased mortality in the immediate postoperative period [42–44].

Postoperative depression too is associated with delayed wound healing, higher infection rate, poor physical and emotional health, reduced pain threshold, and more adverse cardiac events like myocardial infarction and early death [45]. All these factors lead to poor overall quality of life and rising health costs.

Manifestation of anxiety in cardiac patients has been debated for some time and is often taken as a normal reaction. Some of the symptoms may closely mimic symptoms of CAD itself but an experienced clinician can easily make out the difference and understand the need to differentiate the two. Pathological anxiety manifests as a feeling of impending doom, excessive worrying thoughts of being disabled, persistent palpitations, generalized muscular tension with inability to relax, breathlessness, hyper vigilance, persistent headache, frequent urge to pass urine, butterflies in stomach, and persistent sleep disturbance. Frequently, such symptoms are either ignored or not asked/reported. However, they cause significant distress and may lead to adverse outcomes. It has been found to be unusually high for CABG patients while on the waiting list with an unknown surgery date [46]. Fear of dying before rather than during surgery has been highlighted as a pervasive and anxious preoccupation [47]. After the surgery, persistence of these symptoms is an ominous sign and may reflect poorer outcome. Incidence of anxiety was found to be more in younger than in older patients [44]. Following CABG, anxiety precipitates cardiac decompensation owing to higher autonomic arousal thus delaying healing and recovery. The most common anxiety disorders appear to be generalized anxiety disorder (GAD) and Panic Disorder with prevalence ranging from zero to 11%. Other anxiety disorders are Phobias (2.5–4.3%), Obsessive

Compulsive Disorder (0.6–9%), and posttraumatic stress disorder (PTSD) (4–11%) [40].

8. Therapeutic Implications of Depression and Anxiety in CABG

Psychological intervention with cardiac patients reduces psychological pain, severe anxiety, hostility, and depression and thus improves quality of life as well. Common therapeutic approach seems particularly important keeping in view improved outcome and reduction in overall costs [48]. Presence and persistence of depression may have direct bearing on participation in cardiac rehabilitation and lifestyle modification program among CABG surgery patients. Similarly, persisting anxiety can be disabling and may further compromise recovery. A diverse range of behavioral and psychological RCT interventions have clearly demonstrated significant improvements in overall outcome and quality of life of such patients [49]. A recent Indian study highlighted the role of structured yoga therapy in improving the outcome of patients requiring CABG. It was the first time that a structured yoga program incorporating instruments like Hospital Anxiety Depression Scale (HADS), Perceived Stress Scale (PSS-14), and Positive and Negative Affect Scale (PANAS) was used. In a single blind fashion, the study was conducted on 1026 patients and positive effects were found in terms of Left Ventricular Ejection Fraction (LVEF), Body Mass Index (BMI), blood pressure and sugar control, depression, and anxiety symptoms [50]. SSRIs have proven safety and efficacy record and are generally the preferred pharmacological agents to be used in such cases [51]. An added benefit of these drugs is that they are equally efficacious for both depression and anxiety. In selected patients, it is fair enough to start the therapy at a low dose then escalate as per the response. American Heart Association (AHA) recommends that fair trial with two SSRIs should be given before switching on to other groups of antidepressants like serotonergic noradrenergic reuptake inhibitors like Bupropion [52]. Tricyclics antidepressants are effective in treating depression and anxiety, but their use has declined owing to their potential for cardiotoxicity. Since safer options are available in today's era, role of tricyclic antidepressants is limited. The line of management of both depression and anxiety is as per the guidelines laid for these disorders. Short courses are generally of limited clinical benefit due to likelihood of relapse. No consensus exists as far as the duration of such treatment is concerned but it is prudent to follow up the patient for at least six months after surgery and then review the treatment plan. The role of lifestyle modifications and behavioral treatments like yoga cannot be underestimated here as such strategies hold promise for long-term benefits. The recommendation is keeping in view with popular sentiment in this country. In Indian settings, patients are generally hesitant in reporting emotional distress and often hesitate in seeking emotional support. Busy clinicians may also miss subtle signs of emotional distress. Therefore, sensitive instruments in the form of questionnaires must be incorporated in the workup schedule. After discharge from the hospital, an information brochure containing early warning signs of emotional disorder can be given to the patient or care giver and they must be encouraged to clarify their queries during follow-up.

9. Conclusion

Coronary artery disease is the most important cause of morbidity and mortality in Indian subcontinent. There have been rapid advances in the care of those suffering its effects. Strong biological link between emotional state and coronary artery disease is well established. The paper has attempted to contextualize the findings in Indian setting with a view towards early identification and prompt intervention with established methods. The paper ends with a broad outline towards management of such patients from psychiatrist's perspective. A collaborative approach is likely to be of benefit for the patient and cost effective in the long run. It may be prudent to screen the patients during routine workup before and after surgery. Many patients may not be able to describe their symptoms in busy outpatient set-up. Under such conditions, patient education and awareness may be a useful strategy.

References

[1] S. Jadhav, R. Littlewood, A. G. Ryder, A. Chakraborty, S. Jain, and M. Barua, "Stigmatization of severe mental illness in India: against the simple industrialization hypothesis," *Indian Journal of Psychiatry*, vol. 49, no. 3, pp. 189–194, 2007.

[2] J. Kishore, A. Gupta, R. C. Jiloha, and P. Bantman, "Myths, beliefs and perceptions about mental disorders and health-seeking behavior in Delhi, India," *Indian Journal of Psychiatry*, vol. 53, no. 4, pp. 324–329, 2011.

[3] L. A. Epstein and J. C. Huffman, "Introduction," *Harvard Review of Psychiatry*, vol. 17, no. 6, pp. 351–352, 2009.

[4] C. Ballard, M. O'Sullivan, J. Serra-Mestres, R. Stewart, and A. Thomas, "Vascular psychiatry: the interface between vascular disease and mental disorders, and its clinical relevance," in *Proceedings of the Old Age Faculty of Psychiatry Winter Meeting*, Royal College of Psychiatry, January 2013.

[5] D. E. Barnes, G. S. Alexopoulos, O. L. Lopez, J. D. Williamson, and K. Yaffe, "Depressive symptoms, vascular disease, and mild cognitive impairment. findings from the cardiovascular health study," *Journal of the American Medical Association*, vol. 63, no. 3, pp. 273–279, 2006.

[6] G. Zachariah, S. Harikrishnan, M. N. Krishnan et al., "Prevalence of coronary artery disease and coronary risk factors in Kerala, South India: a population survey—design and methods," *Indian Heart Journal*, vol. 65, no. 3, pp. 243–249, 2013.

[7] M. Rao, D. Xavier, P. Devi et al., "Prevalence, treatments and outcomes of coronary artery disease in Indians: a systematic review," *Indian Heart Journal*, vol. 67, no. 4, pp. 302–310, 2015.

[8] W. E. Cohn, "Advances in surgical treatment of acute and chronic coronary artery disease," *Texas Heart Institute Journal*, vol. 37, no. 3, pp. 328–330, 2010.

[9] U. Kaul and V. Bhatia, "Perspective on coronary interventions & cardiac surgeries in India," *Indian Journal of Medical Research*, vol. 132, no. 11, pp. 543–548, 2010.

[10] B. Erkut, O. Dag, M. A. Kaygin et al., "On-pump beating-heart versus conventional coronary artery bypass grafting for revascularization in patients with severe left ventricular dysfunction: early outcomes," *Canadian Journal of Surgery*, vol. 56, no. 6, pp. 398–404, 2013.

[11] C. Herrmann-Lingen, "Anxiety and depression in cardiology patients: how to diagnose, how to treat?" *Herz*, vol. 26, no. 5, pp. 326–334, 2001.

[12] R. Rugulies, "Depression as a predictor for coronary heart disease: a review and meta-analysis," *American Journal of Preventive Medicine*, vol. 23, no. 1, pp. 51–61, 2002.

[13] R. M. Carney, K. E. Freedland, B. Steinmeyer et al., "Depression and five year survival following acute myocardial infarction: a prospective study," *Journal of Affective Disorders*, vol. 109, no. 1-2, pp. 133–138, 2008.

[14] R. A. Mayou, D. Gill, D. R. Thompson et al., "Depression and anxiety as predictors of outcome after myocardial infarction," *Psychosomatic Medicine*, vol. 62, no. 2, pp. 212–219, 2000.

[15] H. S. Lett, J. A. Blumenthal, M. A. Babyak et al., "Depression as a risk factor for coronary artery disease: evidence, mechanisms, and treatment," *Psychosomatic Medicine*, vol. 66, no. 3, pp. 305–315, 2004.

[16] N. Frasure-Smith and F. Lespérance, "Reflections on depression as a cardiac risk factor," *Psychosomatic Medicine*, vol. 67, supplement 1, pp. S19–S25, 2005.

[17] I. Aben and F. Verhey, "Depression after a cerebrovascular accident. The importance of the integration of neurobiological and psychosocial pathogenic models," *Panminerva Medica*, vol. 48, no. 1, pp. 49–57, 2006.

[18] WHO, "ICD-10. Classification of mental and behavioural disorders," in *Clinical Descriptions and Diagnostic Guidelines*, World Health Organization, Geneva, Switzerland, 10th edition, 1992.

[19] L. A. Clark and D. Watson, "Tripartite model of anxiety and depression: psychometric evidence and taxonomic implications," *Journal of Abnormal Psychology*, vol. 100, no. 3, pp. 316–336, 1991.

[20] L. A. Pratt, D. E. Ford, R. M. Crum, H. K. Armenian, J. J. Gallo, and W. W. Eaton, "Depression, psychotropic medication, and risk of myocardial infarction: prospective data from the Baltimore ECA follow-up," *Circulation*, vol. 94, no. 12, pp. 3123–3129, 1996.

[21] S. Ravven, C. Bader, A. Azar, and J. L. Rudolph, "Depressive symptoms after CABG surgery: a meta analysis," *Harvard Review of Psychiatry*, vol. 21, no. 2, pp. 59–69, 2013.

[22] G. Hasler, "Pathophysiology of depression: do we have any solid evidence of interest to clinicians?" *World Psychiatry*, vol. 9, no. 3, pp. 155–161, 2010.

[23] M. S. Player and E. L. Peterson, "Anxiety disorders, hypertension, and cardiovascular risk: a review," *International Journal of Psychiatry in Medicine*, vol. 41, no. 4, pp. 365–377, 2011.

[24] N. Comeau, S. H. Stewart, and P. Loba, "The relations of trait anxiety, anxiety sensitivity, and sensation seeking to adolescents' motivations for alcohol, cigarette, and marijuana use," *Addictive Behaviors*, vol. 26, no. 6, pp. 803–825, 2001.

[25] S. Gautam and N. Jain, "Indian culture and psychiatry," *Indian Journal of Psychiatry*, vol. 52, no. 7, pp. 309–313, 2010.

[26] A. Avasthi, "Depression in primary care. Challenges and controversies," *Indian Journal of Medical Research*, vol. 139, pp. 188–190, 2014.

[27] S. Malhotra, S. Chakrabarti, R. Shah et al., "Development of a novel diagnostic system for a telepsychiatric application: a pilot validation study," *BMC Research Notes*, vol. 7, no. 1, article 508, 2014.

[28] M. Ganguli, S. Dube, J. M. Johnston, R. Pandav, V. Chandra, and H. H. Dodge, "Depressive symptoms, cognitive impairment and functional impairment in a rural elderly population in India: a Hindi version of the geriatric depression scale (GDS-H)," *International Journal of Geriatric Psychiatry*, vol. 14, no. 10, pp. 807–820, 1999.

[29] E. A. Enas, V. Singh, Y. P. Munjal et al., "Recommendations of the second Indo-U.S. health summit on prevention and control of cardiovascular disease among Asian Indians," *Indian Heart Journal*, vol. 61, no. 3, pp. 265–274, 2009.

[30] K. K. Saha, "Off pump coronary artery grafting in India," *Indian Heart Journal*, vol. 66, no. 2, pp. 203–207, 2014.

[31] R. R. Kasliwal, A. Kulshreshtha, S. Agrawal, M. Bansal, and N. Trehan, "Prevalence of cardiovascular risk factors in Indian patients undergoing coronary artery bypass surgery," *Journal of Association of Physicians of India*, vol. 54, pp. 371–375, 2006.

[32] Press Trust of India, *India Ranks 3rd in Medical Tourism in Asia*, Times of India, 2013.

[33] A. Indrayan, "Forecasting vascular disease cases and associated mortality in India," 2010, http://www.whoindia.org/LinkFiles.

[34] S. J. Brister, Z. Hamdulay, S. Verma, M. Maganti, and M. R. Buchanan, "Ethnic diversity: South Asian ethnicity is associated with increased coronary artery bypass grafting mortality," *Journal of Thoracic and Cardiovascular Surgery*, vol. 133, no. 1, pp. 150–154, 2007.

[35] S. Dani, N. Sinha, B. Bhargava, V. Jain, V. Y. Reddy, P. Biswas et al., "Report of the coronary cardiac interventions registry of India the cardiological society of India for the year 2006," *Indian Heart Journal*, vol. 59, pp. 528–530, 2007.

[36] J. T. Dodge Jr., B. G. Brown, E. L. Bolson, and H. T. Dodge, "Lumen diameter of normal human coronary arteries: influence of age, sex, anatomic variation, and left ventricular hypertrophy or dilation," *Circulation*, vol. 86, no. 1, pp. 232–246, 1992.

[37] F. H. Edwards, J. S. Carey, F. L. Grover, J. W. Bero, and R. S. Hartz, "Impact of gender on coronary bypass operative mortality," *Annals of Thoracic Surgery*, vol. 66, no. 1, pp. 125–131, 1998.

[38] N. J. O'Connor, J. R. Morton, J. D. Birkmeyer, E. M. Olmstead, and G. T. O'Connor, "Effect of coronary artery diameter in patients undergoing coronary bypass surgery," *Circulation*, vol. 93, no. 4, pp. 652–655, 1996.

[39] A. C. Breuer, A. J. Furlan, M. R. Hanson et al., "Central nervous system complications of coronary artery bypass graft surgery: prospective analysis of 421 patients," *Stroke*, vol. 14, no. 5, pp. 682–687, 1983.

[40] P. J. Tully and R. A. Baker, "Depression, anxiety, and cardiac morbidity outcomes after coronary artery bypass surgery: a contemporary and practical review," *Journal of Geriatric Cardiology*, vol. 9, no. 2, pp. 197–208, 2012.

[41] K. Utriyaprasit and S. Moore, "Recovery symptoms and mood states in Thai CABG patients," *Journal of Transcultural Nursing*, vol. 16, no. 2, pp. 97–106, 2005.

[42] R. Gallagher and S. McKinley, "Anxiety, depression and perceived control in patients having coronary artery bypass grafts," *Journal of Advanced Nursing*, vol. 65, no. 11, pp. 2386–2396, 2009.

[43] M. H. Nemati and B. Astaneh, "The impact of coronary artery bypass graft surgery on depression and anxiety," *Journal of Cardiovascular Medicine*, vol. 12, no. 6, pp. 401–404, 2011.

[44] J.-H. A. Krannich, P. Weyers, S. Lueger, M. Herzog, T. Bohrer, and O. Elert, "Presence of depression and anxiety before and after coronary artery bypass graft surgery and their relationship to age," *BMC Psychiatry*, vol. 7, article 47, 2007.

[45] Z. Cserép, A. Székely, and B. Merkely, "Short and long term effects of psychosocial factors on the outcome of coronary artery bypass surgery," in *Artery Bypass*, InTech, 2013.

[46] M. Koivula, M.-T. Tarkka, M. Tarkka, P. Laippala, and M. Paunonen-Ilmonen, "Fear and anxiety in patients at different time-points in the coronary artery bypass process," *International Journal of Nursing Studies*, vol. 39, no. 8, pp. 811–822, 2002.

[47] D. Fitzsimons, K. Parahoo, S. G. Richardson, and M. Stringer, "Patient anxiety while on a waiting list for coronary artery bypass surgery: a qualitative and quantitative analysis," *Heart and Lung*, vol. 32, no. 1, pp. 23–31, 2003.

[48] J. M. Donohue, B. H. Belnap, A. Men et al., "Twelve-month cost-effectiveness of telephone-delivered collaborative care for treating depression following CABG surgery: a randomized controlled trial," *General Hospital Psychiatry*, vol. 36, no. 5, pp. 453–459, 2014.

[49] B. L. Rollman, M. S. Belnap, S. Mazumdar et al., "Telephone-delivered collaborative care for treating post-CABG depression: a randomized controlled trial," *Journal of the American Medical Association*, vol. 302, no. 19, pp. 2095–2103, 2095.

[50] N. Raghuram, V. R. Parachuri, M. V. Swarnagowri et al., "Yoga based cardiac rehabilitation after coronary artery bypass surgery: one-year results on LVEF, lipid profile and psychological states. A randomized controlled study," *Indian Heart Journal*, vol. 66, no. 5, pp. 490–502, 2014.

[51] S. Chocron, P. Vandel, C. Durst et al., "Antidepressant therapy in patients undergoing coronary artery bypass grafting: the MOTIV-CABG trial," *Annals of Thoracic Surgery*, vol. 95, no. 5, pp. 1609–1618, 2013.

[52] D. L. Hillis, P. K. Smith, J. L. Anderson et al., "2011 ACCF/AHA guideline for coronary artery bypass graft surgery. A report of the American College of Cardiology Foundation/American Heart Association task force on practice guidelines," *Circulation*, vol. 124, pp. e652–e735, 2011.

2

Comparison between First- and Second-Generation Cryoballoon for Paroxysmal Atrial Fibrillation Ablation

Sergio Conti,[1] Massimo Moltrasio,[1] Gaetano Fassini,[1]
Fabrizio Tundo,[1] Stefania Riva,[1] Antonio Dello Russo,[1] Michela Casella,[1]
Benedetta Majocchi,[1] Vittoria Marino,[1] Pasquale De Iuliis,[2] Valentina Catto,[1]
Salvatore Pala,[1] and Claudio Tondo[1]

[1]*Cardiac Arrhythmia Research Centre, Centro Cardiologico Monzino IRCCS, Via Carlo Parea 4, 20138 Milan, Italy*
[2]*St. Jude Medical, Agrate Brianza, Italy*

Correspondence should be addressed to Sergio Conti; sergioconti.md@gmail.com

Academic Editor: Kai Hu

Introduction. Cryoballoon (CB) ablation has emerged as a novel treatment for pulmonary vein isolation (PVI) for patients with paroxysmal atrial fibrillation (PAF). The second-generation Arctic Front Advance (ADV) was redesigned with technical modifications aiming at procedural and outcome improvements. We aimed to compare the efficacy of the two different technologies over a long-term follow-up. *Methods.* A total of 120 patients with PAF were enrolled. Sixty patients underwent PVI using the first-generation CB and 60 patients with the ADV catheter. All patients were evaluated over a follow-up period of 2 years. *Results.* There were no significant differences between the two groups of patients. Procedures performed with the first-generation CB showed longer fluoroscopy time (36.3 ± 16.8 versus 14.2 ± 13.5 min, resp.; $p = 0.00016$) and longer procedure times as well (153.1 ± 32 versus 102 ± 24.8 min, resp.; $p = 0.019$). The overall long-term success was significantly different between the two groups (68.3 versus 86.7%, resp.; $p = 0.017$). No differences were found in the lesion areas of left and right PV between the two groups (resp., $p = 0.61$ and 0.57). There were no significant differences in procedural-related complications. *Conclusion.* The ADV catheter compared to the first-generation balloon allows obtaining a significantly higher success rate after a single PVI procedure during the long-term follow-up. Fluoroscopy and procedural times were significantly shortened using the ADV catheter.

1. Introduction

Pulmonary vein isolation (PVI) is the cornerstone of any catheter-based treatment for patients with paroxysmal atrial fibrillation (PAF) [1, 2]. Electrical isolation is commonly performed by a circumferential lesion set around the pulmonary veins [1–3]. The standard "point-by-point" technique remains challenging and time-consuming. Cryoballoon (CB) technology would theoretically allow PVI with a single application [4–8]. The first-generation CB, Arctic Front™ (Medtronic, Inc., Minneapolis, MN, USA), has been available since 2006 in Europe [7, 8]. With respect to the first-generation CB, the second-generation, Arctic Front Advance™ (ADV), version was designed with technical modifications aiming at procedural outcome improvement [9–11]. The number of injection ports has been doubled and these have been placed more distally on the catheters shaft resulting in a larger and more uniform zone of freezing on the balloons surface if compared with the previous version [12]. Aim of the study was to compare the acute and long-term success of these two different technologies.

2. Methods

2.1. Patient Population. We retrospectively analyzed 120 patients undergoing PVI using the CB technology who completed at least 2 years of follow-up. All patients had symptomatic and drug-resistant PAF according to the current ESC and HRS/EHRA/ECAS guidelines [1, 2]. Data were accurately collected for each patient from medical notes after discharge and included basic demographic, clinical information, pharmacological therapy, date of hospitalization and discharge, presence of comorbidities, and cardiovascular events during hospitalization. From June 2011 to June 2013 sixty patients underwent PVI using the Arctic Front™ CB catheter and 60 patients using the ADV ablation catheter. The 28 mm CB was used in all procedures. In addition, electroanatomical mapping using NavX Velocity 3.0 system (St. Jude Medical, Minneapolis, MN, USA) was performed in a subgroup of patients. The study protocol was approved by the local Ethics Committee.

2.2. Pulmonary Vein Isolation. All patients underwent pre-procedural transthoracic echocardiography to asses left ventricular ejection fraction and left atrial dimension. To exclude the presence of thrombi in the left atrium or in the left atrial appendage a transesophageal echocardiography was performed the day before the procedure. Moreover, a preprocedure magnetic resonance imaging or computed tomography with segmentation of the left atrium was performed to assess left atrial anatomy in detail. Procedures were performed either with continued oral anticoagulation using warfarin and therapeutic INR (2.0 to 3.0) or using low-molecular weight heparin bridging. All PVI procedures were performed by experienced operators beyond the learning curve. Briefly, all procedures were carried out in conscious sedation using propofol infusion. A deflectable decapolar catheter was inserted through right femoral vein and positioned into the coronary sinus to guide the transseptal puncture and to pace the left atrium during treatment of the left PVs and was subsequently moved to the superior vena cava where it was used to stimulate the right phrenic nerve during treatment of the right PVs. A single transseptal puncture was performed using a needle system (BRK, St. Jude Medical, St. Paul, MN, USA) and a standard transseptal sheath (SL0 8F or 8.5F, St. Jude Medical, St. Paul, MN, USA), subsequently exchanged with a steerable 15F sheath (FlexCath™, 15F, Medtronic, Inc., Minneapolis, MN, USA). Before transseptal puncture, heparin was administered intravenously as bolus (10000 U) followed by a continuous infusion (1000 U/hr) reaching ACT level >350 sec. The FlexCath was continuously irrigated with heparinized saline (2 mL/hr). An esophageal temperature probe was used in all patients (Esotherm Plus, FIAB) to monitor intraesophageal temperature increase. The probe was adjusted during the procedure to stay as close as possible to the ablation catheter. Cryotherapy was interrupted if the endoluminal esophageal temperature dropped below 18°C. Two cryotherapy applications were delivered to each PV, 240–300 seconds each, aiming for a minimum temperature of less than −40°C. After treatment of all PVs, entrance block was confirmed with high-output pacing (12 V, 2.9 ms) using the Lasso™ (Biosense Webster, Diamond Bar, CA, USA), Afocus (St. Jude Medical, Minneapolis, MN, USA), or Achieve™ mapping catheter (Medtronic, Inc., Minneapolis, MN, USA). "Far field" capture and sensing were ruled out using differential pacing maneuvers. Any residual conduction into the PVs was treated by further cryotherapy applications.

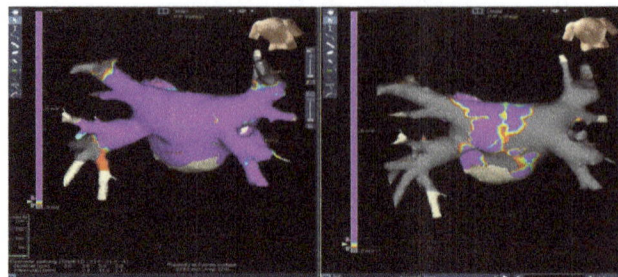

FIGURE 1: High-density voltage map of the left atrium using electroanatomic mapping, NavX Velocity 3.0, before and after the procedure.

Successful PVI was confirmed when all PV potentials were abolished or were dissociated at least 20 minutes after the last cryotherapy application to that vein.

2.3. Lesion Area Comparison. In each patient who underwent PVI using the electroanatomic mapping system NavX Velocity 3.0, a high-density voltage map of the left atrium was performed, before and after the procedure, using the mapping catheter Afocus. After cryotherapy, the border between the scar area and healthy atrial tissue was defined using a 0.1–0.5 mV as offset (0.1 mV was defined as scar or absolutely silent tissue). The border between scar and normal tissue was defined including both ipsilateral PVs. Using an implemented tool in the NavX Velocity 3.0, the lesion area (cm^2) was automatically calculated by the system (Figure 1).

2.4. Follow-Up. Patients were followed up in the outpatient clinic 3 months after the procedure and every 3 months during the first year after ablation and every 6 months thereafter. At each visit, a standard 12-lead ECG was obtained in all patients. All patients were followed up with Holter-ECG monitoring at 6 and 12 months and annually after the PVI procedure. After 90 days of blanking period, any documented episode of AF or atrial arrhythmias lasting >30 seconds was considered a recurrence. All antiarrhythmic agents were withdrawn at 3 months after ablation. Clinical events occurring during the follow-up and documentation of the events were carefully checked. Clinical success was defined as complete freedom from symptomatic arrhythmia and the absence of any atrial arrhythmia during Holter monitoring.

2.5. Statistical Analysis. This was an observational, retrospective, single-center study. Continuous variables are reported as mean ± standard deviation. Comparison of continuous variables was performed using independent sample Student's *t*-test and categorical data with Fisher's exact test. Arrhythmia-free survival curves were generated by the Kaplan-Meier method and compared with the Log Rank test. Statistical significance was considered with a *p* value of <0.05. SPSS 20.0 statistical software (SPSS Italia, Inc., Florence, Italy) was used for statistical analysis.

TABLE 1: Baseline patient characteristics.

	CB, 1st (n = 60)	CB, 2nd (n = 60)	p
Male sex, n (%)	41 (68.3)	50 (83.3)	0.14
Mean age, years (mean ± SD)	59.1 ± 12.2	57.2 ± 10.9	0.37
Body mass index, Kg/m^2 (mean ± SD)	26 ± 2	26 ± 3	0.59
Paroxysmal atrial fibrillation, n (%)	60 (100)	60 (100)	1
Left atrial diameter, mm (mean ± SD)	22.9 ± 5.1	22.5 ± 4.7	0.60
Left ventricular ejection fraction, (mean ± SD)	62.5 ± 6.1	60.9 ± 7.4	0.72
Hypertension, n (%)	25 (41.6)	23 (38.3)	0.63
Hypercholesterolemia, n (%)	12 (20)	14 (23.3)	0.61
Diabetes mellitus, n (%)	4 (6.6)	5 (8.3)	0.73
Hypertriglyceridemia, n (%)	5 (8.3)	6 (10)	0.71
Active smoking, n (%)	8 (13.3)	9 (15)	0.69
Coronary artery disease, n (%)	4 (6.6)	5 (8.3)	0.73
Dilated cardiomyopathy, n (%)	0	0	—
Valve disease, n (%)	4 (6.6)	3 (5)	0.40
Previous cardiac surgery, n (%)	3 (5)	2 (3.3)	0.46
Previous ischemic stroke, n (%)	—	1 (1.6)	0.53
Chronic renal failure, n (%)	4 (6.6)	3 (5)	0.40
Previous ablation procedures for AF, n (%)	0	0	—

TABLE 2: Fluoroscopy time and procedure time comparison between the first- and second-generation CryoBalloon catheter.

	CB, 1st	CB, 2nd	p
Procedure time, min (mean ± SD)	153.1 ± 32	102 ± 24.8	0.019
Fluoroscopy time, min (mean ± SD)	36.3 ± 16.8	14.2 ± 13.5	<0.001

3. Results

Baseline clinical characteristics of patients are reported in Table 1. There were no significant differences between the 2 study groups regarding age, gender, cardiovascular risk factors, left ventricular ejection fraction, left atrial dimension, and medical therapy. No significant differences were found between the two study groups regarding CHA2DS2-VASc and HAS-BLED scores.

No patients had evidence of left atrial thrombosis during transesophageal echocardiography. Acute success rate and procedural-related complications are reported in Table 3. Procedures performed with the first generation CB showed longer fluoroscopy time (36.3 ± 16.8 versus 14.2 ± 13.5 min, resp.; $p < 0.001$) and longer procedure times as well (153.1 ± 32 versus 102 ± 24.8 min, resp.; $p = 0.019$) compared to the second-generation ADV catheter (Table 2). Interestingly, no statistically significant differences were found in the lesion area of left and right PVc between the two groups (resp., $p = 0.61$ and 0.57, Table 4). The overall success rate after single PVI procedure including both first- and second-generation CB was 77.5%. The long-term freedom-from-AF as showed in the Kaplan-Meier survival analysis was significantly different between the two different CB (68.3% with the first-generation CB versus 86.7% with the second-generation ADV catheter, resp.; Log Rank $p = 0.017$, Figure 2).

4. Discussion

This retrospective analysis provides data on long-term efficacy of CB ablation performed in a single high-volume center. The main findings of this study are that the use of the second-generation ADV catheter significantly improved the long-term procedural success after single PVI procedure and reduced procedure duration and fluoroscopy exposure time.

Our results in terms of procedural success using the first generation CB are in line with those coming from the North American Arctic Front STOP AF Pivotal Trial (68.3% versus 69.9% resp.) [13]. Several reports have shown that CB ablation with the new ADV catheter is associated with higher success rate of PVI and better outcome. In a first report of Fürnkranz et al. comparing the first-generation CB with the ADV, single-shot PVI rate increased from 51% to 84% ($p < 0.001$) [12]. Procedure duration and fluoroscopy exposure time were also significantly decreased using the novel CB catheter. In a retrospective analysis, Aryana et al. confirmed that ADV catheter significantly reduced procedure time and fluoroscopy time. Freedom from AF at 6, 9, and 12 months was 89, 86, and 82%, respectively, during a mean follow-up of 16 ± 8 months [14]. Giovanni and coworkers recently reported a significantly higher freedom from AF at 1-year follow-up with the second-generation ADV catheter with respect to the first-generation CB. Freedom from AF

TABLE 3: Acute success and procedure-related complications.

	CB, 1st (n = 60)	CB, 2nd (n = 60)	p
PVI achieved, (%)	95	98	ns
Catheter failure, n (%)	3* (5)	1# (1.6)	ns
Need of touch-up, n (%)	3 (5)	1 (1.6)	ns
Acute PNP, n (%)	2 (3.3)	1 (1.6)	ns
Chronic PNP, n (%)	0	0	—
Cerebral embolization, n (%)	0	0	—
Pericardial effusion, n (%)	1 (1.6)	0	ns
Cardiac tamponade, n (%)	0	0	—
PV stenosis, n (%)	0	0	—
Atrioesophageal fistula, n (%)	0	0	—
Vascular injury, n (%)	3 (5)	2 (3.3)	ns

PVI: pulmonary vein isolation; PNP: phrenic nerve palsy; #: FlexCath failure; ∗: 2/3 FlexCath failure, 1/3 Cryoballoon failure.

TABLE 4: Comparison of lesion area between the first- and second-generation CryoBalloon catheter. Data obtained from electroanatomic mapping performed after cryoablation using the NavX system (St. Jude Medical, St. Paul, MN, USA).

Lesion area	CB, 1st	CB, 2nd	p
LPVs, cm^2 (mean ± SD)	68.2 ± 44	75.3 ± 26	0.61
RPVs, cm^2 (mean ± SD)	73.1 ± 33	79.4 ± 22	0.57

LPVs: left pulmonary veins; RPVs: right pulmonary veins.

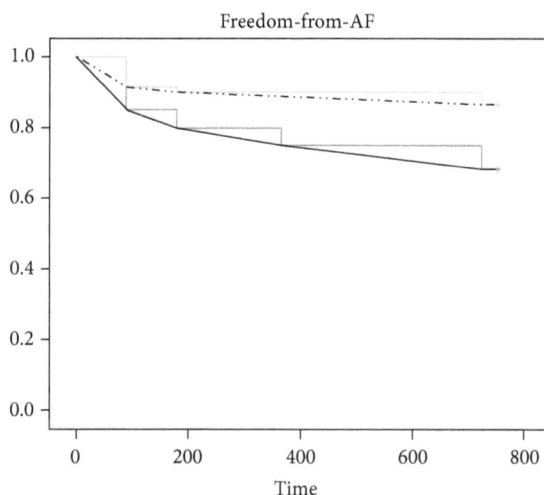

FIGURE 2: The Kaplan-Meier survival analysis shows a significant difference in freedom-from-AF recurrence between patients undergoing atrial fibrillation ablation using the first-generation Cryoballoon (CB1) and the second-generation Cryoballoon (CB2) catheter (Log Rank $p = 0.017$).

off antiarrhythmic drugs (AAD) therapy was achieved in 84% of patients treated with the ADV catheter, compared to 66% of success rate obtained with first-generation CB ($p = 0.038$). In their experience, procedural and fluoroscopy times were also significantly decreased by the use of ADV catheter [15]. Similar findings were reported by Fürnkranz et al. The authors found freedom from AF after a single procedure without AAD therapy after 1 year in 63.9% of patients treated with the first generation of CB versus 83.6% ($p = 0.008$) of patients with the ADV catheter [16]. Liu et al. during a mean follow-up of $12 ± 4$ months found an overall 76.0% of CB success rate, respectively, 89.7% with ADV catheter versus 59.7% with the first-generation CB ($p < 0.001$) [17]. In addition to previous published paper, we performed for the first time a comparison between lesion areas created by the two different CB. Despite the redesign of the ADV catheter, in our experience the improved acute and long-term procedural success seems not to be related to an increased area of lesion. The main technical limitation of the first generation CB was the temperature gradient from the equator to the distal pole of the CB. More specifically, the first-generation CB had four injection ports positioned just distal to the equator, cooling the balloon surface with a temperature gradient with relatively higher temperatures at the distal pole. As a result, continuous lesions are created if the balloon is centered in the PV antrum. Differently, eccentric CB positions may lead to incomplete lesion formation of tissue, resulting in reconnection gap. Thus, repeated freezing with different CB positions were often necessary to achieve PVI prolonging both procedural and fluoroscopy time. The ADV catheter was redesigned doubling the injection ports and placing themselves more distally on the catheters shaft creating a larger and more uniform zone of freezing on the CB surface. Together, these modifications have been shown to improve procedural and early clinical efficacy during short-term follow-up. Notably, we report a very low incidence of procedure-related complications. It could be related to the size of CB used at our center; indeed we only use the 28 mm balloon due to safety reasons. Creation of proximal lesions at the antrum of PVs should prevent or at least reduce complications such as PV stenosis and phrenic nerve palsy.

5. Study Limitations

This study has some limitations: it is a single-center retrospective analysis in a highly selected population. In order to complete at least 2 years of follow-up, we excluded patients in which the follow-up was not fully available. Finally, the follow-up was performed for the majority of patients with 12-lead ECG and Holter-ECG monitoring; unfortunately, an event recorder was not available for all patients.

6. Conclusion

On the long-term follow-up, PVI using the ADV performs significantly better when compared to the first-generation CB. Procedure duration and fluoroscopy exposure time were significantly shortened with the ADV catheter. Based on electroanatomical mapping, lesion areas created by the two CB were not statistically different.

Abbreviations

PVI: Pulmonary vein isolation
PAF: Paroxysmal atrial fibrillation
CB: Cryoballoon
ADV: Arctic front advance
PV: Pulmonary vein
AAD: Antiarrhythmic drug.

Acknowledgments

The authors thank Martina Zucchetti, M.D., Eleonora Russo, M.D., Ph.D., and Corrado Carbucicchio, M.D.

References

[1] A. J. Camm, G. Y. Lip, R. De Caterina et al., "ESC Committee for Practice Guidelines (CPG). 2012 focused update of the ESC Guidelines for the management of atrial fibrillation: an update of the 2010 ESC Guidelines for the management of atrial fibrillation. Developed with the special contribution of the European Heart Rhythm Association," *European Heart Journal*, vol. 33, pp. 2719–2747, 2012.

[2] H. Calkins, K. H. Kuck, R. Cappato et al., "2012 HRS/EHRA/ECAS expert consensus statement on catheter and surgical ablation of atrial fibrillation: recommendations for patient selection, procedural techniques, patient management and follow-up, definitions, endpoints, and research trial design," *Heart Rhythm*, vol. 9, pp. 632–696, 2012.

[3] M. Haïssaguerre, P. Jaïs, D. C. Shah et al., "Spontaneous initiation of atrial fibrillation by ectopic beats originating in the pulmonary veins," *The New England Journal of Medicine*, vol. 339, no. 10, pp. 659–666, 1998.

[4] J. G. Andrade, P. Khairy, P. G. Guerra et al., "Efficacy and safety of cryoballoon ablation for atrial fibrillation: a systematic review of published studies," *Heart Rhythm*, vol. 8, no. 9, pp. 1444–1451, 2011.

[5] Y. Van Belle, P. Janse, M. J. Rivero-Ayerza et al., "Pulmonary vein isolation using an occluding cryoballoon for circumferential ablation: feasibility, complications, and short-term outcome," *European Heart Journal*, vol. 28, no. 18, pp. 2231–2237, 2007.

[6] A. Fürnkranz, I. Köster, K. R. J. Chun et al., "Cryoballoon temperature predicts acute pulmonary vein isolation," *Heart Rhythm*, vol. 8, no. 6, pp. 821–825, 2011.

[7] K.-R. J. Chun, B. Schmidt, A. Metzner et al., "The 'single big cryoballoon' technique for acute pulmonary vein isolation in patients with paroxysmal atrial fibrillation: a prospective observational single centre study," *European Heart Journal*, vol. 30, no. 6, pp. 699–709, 2009.

[8] K.-H. Kuck and A. Fürnkranz, "Cryoballoon ablation of atrial fibrillation," *Journal of Cardiovascular Electrophysiology*, vol. 21, no. 12, pp. 1427–1431, 2010.

[9] A. Fürnkranz, K. R. J. Chun, D. Nuyens et al., "Characterization of conduction recovery after pulmonary vein isolation using the 'single big cryoballoon' technique," *Heart Rhythm*, vol. 7, no. 2, pp. 184–190, 2010.

[10] H. Ahmed, P. Neuzil, J. Skoda et al., "The permanency of pulmonary vein isolation using a balloon cryoablation catheter," *Journal of Cardiovascular Electrophysiology*, vol. 21, no. 7, pp. 731–737, 2010.

[11] C. F. Liu, "Pulmonary vein reconnection after cryoballoon ablation: back to the drawing board," *Heart Rhythm*, vol. 7, no. 2, pp. 191–192, 2010.

[12] A. Fürnkranz, S. Bordignon, B. Schmidt et al., "Improved procedural efficacy of pulmonary vein isolation using the novel second-generation cryoballoon," *Journal of Cardiovascular Electrophysiology*, vol. 24, no. 5, pp. 492–497, 2013.

[13] D. L. Packer, R. C. Kowal, K. R. Wheelan et al., "Cryoballoon ablation of pulmonary veins for paroxysmal atrial fibrillation: first results of the North American arctic front (STOP AF) pivotal trial," *Journal of the American College of Cardiology*, vol. 61, no. 16, pp. 1713–1723, 2013.

[14] A. Aryana, S. Morkoch, S. Bailey et al., "Acute procedural and cryoballoon characteristics from cryoablation of atrial fibrillation using the first- and second-generation cryoballoon: a retrospective comparative study with follow-up outcomes," *Journal of Interventional Cardiac Electrophysiology*, vol. 41, no. 2, pp. 177–186, 2014.

[15] G. D. Giovanni, K. Wauters, G.-B. Chierchia et al., "One-year follow-up after single procedure cryoballoon ablation: a comparison between the first and second generation balloon," *Journal of Cardiovascular Electrophysiology*, vol. 25, no. 8, pp. 834–839, 2014.

[16] A. Fürnkranz, S. Bordignon, D. Dugo et al., "Improved 1-year clinical success rate of pulmonary vein isolation with the second-generation cryoballoon in patients with paroxysmal atrial fibrillation," *Journal of Cardiovascular Electrophysiology*, vol. 25, no. 8, pp. 840–844, 2014.

[17] J. Liu, J. Kaufmann, C. Kriatselis, E. Fleck, and J. H. Gerds-Li, "Second generation of cryoballoons can improve efficiency of cryoablation for atrial fibrillation," *Pacing and Clinical Electrophysiology*, vol. 38, no. 1, pp. 129–135, 2015.

3

Clinical Characteristics, Management, and Outcomes of Suspected Poststroke Acute Coronary Syndrome

Sylvia Marie Biso,[1] Marvin Lu,[1] Toni Anne De Venecia,[1]
Supakanya Wongrakpanich,[1] Mary Rodriguez-Ziccardi,[1]
Sujani Yadlapati,[1] Marina Kishlyansky,[1]
Harish Seetha Rammohan,[2,3] and Vincent M. Figueredo[4,5]

[1]*Department of Medicine, Einstein Medical Center, 5401 Old York Road, Suite 363, Philadelphia, PA 19141, USA*
[2]*Bassett Medical Center, Bassett Healthcare Network, Cooperstown, NY, USA*
[3]*CUMC, College of Physicians & Surgeons, Columbia University, New York, NY, USA*
[4]*Einstein Institute for Heart and Vascular Health, Einstein Medical Center, Philadelphia, PA, USA*
[5]*Sidney Kimmel Medical College, Thomas Jefferson University, Philadelphia, PA, USA*

Correspondence should be addressed to Sylvia Marie Biso; bisosylv@einstein.edu

Academic Editor: Ilan S. Wittstein

Background. Acute coronary syndrome (ACS) can complicate acute ischemic stroke, causing significant morbidity and mortality. To date, literatures that describe poststroke acute coronary syndrome and its morbidity and mortality burden are lacking. *Methods.* This is a single center, retrospective study where clinical characteristics, cardiac evaluation, and management of patients with suspected poststroke ACS were compared and analyzed for their association with inpatient mortality and 1-year all-cause mortality. *Results.* Of the 82 patients, 32% had chest pain and 88% had ischemic ECG changes; mean peak troponin level was 18, and mean ejection fraction was 40%. The medical management group had older individuals (73 versus 67 years, $p < 0.05$), lower mean peak troponin levels (12 versus 49, $p < 0.05$), and lower mean length of stay (12 versus 25 days, $p < 0.05$) compared to those who underwent stent or CABG. Troponin levels were significantly associated with 1-year all-cause mortality. *Conclusion.* Age and troponin level appear to play a role in the current clinical decision making for patient with suspected poststroke ACS. Troponin level appears to significantly correlate with 1-year all-cause mortality. In the management of poststroke acute coronary syndrome, optimal medical therapy had similar inpatient and all-cause mortality compared to PCI and/or CABG.

1. Introduction

Acute coronary syndrome can complicate acute ischemic stroke. In the Randomized Trial of Tirilazad Mesylate in Patients with Acute Stroke (RANTTAS trial), cardiac ischemia was found to occur in 6% of patients, with 1% being life-threatening [1]. A study by Chin found that acute coronary syndrome occurred in 12.7% of patients within 3 days of an acute ischemic stroke [2]. Cardiac abnormalities also were found to be the most common cause of death after stroke. Six percent of unexpected deaths in these cases occurred in the first month [3]. Even 3.5 years after a stroke, patients were still found to have an annual 2% risk of myocardial infarction [4].

Neurologic events are known to cause myocardial injury and dysfunction. Cardiac injury after an acute stroke has been shown to occur even in the absence of underlying coronary artery disease [5]. There is a strong association between cerebrovascular disease and coronary artery disease [4]: Both stroke and coronary artery disease have the same risk factors [6] and there is high prevalence of cardiac disease among stroke patients [7]. However, the literature is scant, not only in describing patients with ischemic brain infarct and acute coronary syndrome, but also in regard to their evaluation and medical management. Current practice for myocardial infarction after a stroke is a full cardiac work-up and coronary angiography is needed to rule out significant coronary artery disease [8, 9].

Given the lack of guidelines and literature for poststroke ACS patients, the objectives of this study were to describe the demographics and comorbidities of patients with poststroke acute coronary syndrome, including their presenting symptom, peak troponin level, presence of ischemic electrocardiogram (ECG) changes, 2D-echocardiograms, and cardiac catheterization results. We compared the clinical characteristics and cardiac evaluation of patients who were medically managed and those who underwent any invasive intervention with percutaneous coronary intervention (PCI) or coronary artery bypass graft surgery (CABG). We sought to determine if there is a difference in inpatient mortality and 1-year all-cause mortality among these patients.

2. Methodology

This is a retrospective cohort study on adult patients who were admitted for acute ischemic stroke at Albert Einstein Medical Center from January 2003 to December 31, 2013, and developed acute coronary syndrome within 72 hours after ischemic stroke. Acute coronary syndrome referred to patients who fulfilled the third universal definition criteria of elevated cardiac biomarkers of at least one value above the 99th percentile upper reference limit and one of the following: symptoms of ischemia, development of pathologic Q waves in the electrocardiogram, new or presumed new significant ST-segment-T-wave (ST-T) changes or new left bundle branch block (LBBB), and imaging evidence of new loss of viable myocardium or a new regional wall motion abnormality. We excluded the patients with age < 18 years, patients with intracerebral hemorrhage, subarachnoid hemorrhage, hemorrhagic contusions, epidural hemorrhage, subdural hemorrhage, and other brain lesions, and patients with end stage renal disease on hemodialysis.

Baseline demographic data (age, gender, race, and body mass index) and comorbidities such as preexisting coronary artery disease, hypertension, hyperlipidemia, diabetes mellitus, chronic kidney disease, congestive heart failure (systolic and/or diastolic heart failure), coronary artery disease equivalents (i.e., peripheral artery disease and carotid artery disease), and smoking history were collected. Results of cardiac evaluation such as peak troponin level, ECG changes, 2D-transthoracic echocardiograms, and cardiac catheterization were also obtained. The primary outcomes of the study were inpatient mortality and 1-year all-cause mortality from the time of the acute ischemic stroke. The mortality information was acquired using social security database index (SSDI).

For data analysis, categorical data were presented as numbers and percentages and continuous data as mean ± standard deviation. The demographic characteristics, comorbidities, and cardiac evaluation results of those who were medically managed versus those who underwent cardiac catheterization and subsequent stent placement or CABG were compared using Student's t-test to test for differences between independent continuous variables and the chi-square test

TABLE 1: Demographic data of patients with poststroke acute coronary syndrome.

	Total (%)
N (%)	82
Mean age (years)	72 ± 12.5
Gender	
Female	43 (52%)
Male	39 (48%)
Race	
Caucasian	24 (30%)
African American	51 (62%)
Hispanic	5 (6%)
Asian	2 (2%)
Comorbidities	
Coronary artery disease	36 (44%)
Body mass index > 30	22 (33%)
Hypertension	79 (96%)
Hyperlipidemia	37 (45%)
Diabetes mellitus	46 (56%)
Chronic kidney disease	24 (29%)
Congestive heart failure	38 (46%)
Coronary artery disease equivalents	15 (18%)
Smoker	20 (24%)

to test for differences between categorical variables. For continuous data that are not normally distributed, a nonparametric test will be used. For example, a rank-sum test (Kruskal-Wallis test) will be used instead of t-test. In a 2 × 2 table, if one of the cells contains an expected value of less than 5, Fisher exact test will be used instead of chi-square test. To measure the association between an outcome variable (inpatient mortality and 1-year all-cause mortality) and selected exposure variable, such as peak troponin level, ischemic changes in ECG, and intervention, the relative risk will be computed. The chi-square or Fisher exact test will be used to determine the significance of the association.

3. Results

Among adult patients admitted to Albert Einstein Medical Center from 2003 to 2013, there were 82 patients who had an acute coronary syndrome after an acute ischemic stroke. The mean age was 72 years; 52% were female. Sixty-two percent of the patients in the study were African American, 30% were Caucasian, 6% were Hispanic, and 2% were Asian (Table 1).

Most of the patients in the study were found to have hypertension (96%). The next most common comorbidities were diabetes mellitus (56%), hyperlipidemia (45%), known coronary artery disease (44%), and congestive heart failure (46%). One-third of the population had a body mass index above 30 or chronic kidney disease. Around 20% were smokers or had coronary artery disease equivalents (Table 1).

Surprisingly, among patients who had acute coronary syndrome after an acute ischemic stroke, only 32% complained of chest pain. Other criteria for acute coronary

TABLE 2: Clinical data and management of patients with poststroke acute coronary syndrome.

	Total (%)
Chest pain	26 (32%)
Mean peak troponin level	18 ± 33
ECG: presence of ischemic ECG changes	72 (88%)
Echo	
Mean EF%	40 ± 20
Presence of wall motion abnormalities	35 (43%)
Corresponding to ischemic ECG changes	72 (88%)
Not corresponding to ischemic ECG changes	10 (12%)
Cardiac catheterization	
Did not undergo cardiac catheterization	55 (67%)
Underwent cardiac catheterization	27 (33%)
Cardiac catheterization results:	
No significant coronary artery disease	4 (15%)
1-vessel disease	7 (26%)
2-vessel disease	4 (15%)
3-vessel disease	12 (44%)
Management	
Medical management	69 (84%)
Stent or CABG	13 (16%)
Mean length of stay (days)	14 ± 13

syndrome occurred more frequently. Ischemic ECG changes (i.e., new T-wave inversions, new Q waves, new LBBB, ST-segment elevations, and ST-segment depressions) were found 88% of the time. The most common ischemic ECG change was new T-wave inversion (78%). Mean peak troponin level was 18. Wall motion abnormalities on 2D-echocardiograms occurred in 43% of the patients with 88% in coronary artery territories corresponding to the ischemic ECG changes. The mean ejection fraction of the patients in the study was 40% (Table 2).

Although the patients had acute coronary syndromes, 67% did not undergo cardiac catheterization and were managed conservatively. Of the 33% who underwent cardiac catheterization, 15% had no significant coronary artery disease, 26% had 1-vessel disease, 15% had 2-vessel disease, and 44% had 3-vessel disease. Overall, out of the 82 patients, only 16% underwent placement of stents or CABG. The remaining 84% were managed medically. Medical management was in accordance with the guideline-directed medical therapy for acute coronary syndromes and congestive heart failure by the American College of Cardiology/American Heart Association guidelines that include aspirin, clopidogrel, and beta-blockers. For those with reduced ejection fraction, ACE inhibitors, beta-blockers, hydralazine/nitrates, and so on (depending on patient's clinical status) were given. The mean length of stay was 14 days (Table 2).

The medical management group was significantly older (73 versus 67 years, $p < 0.05$) and had a significantly lower length of stay (12 versus 25 days, $p < 0.05$) (Table 3). In terms of comorbidities, the two groups were the same (Table 3). As for markers of cardiac injury, the mean peak troponin level

for the medical management group was 12 compared to the intervention group, which was 49. There was no significant difference between the two when it comes to presence of ischemic ECG changes and 2D-echo results (i.e., mean ejection fraction and presence of wall motion abnormality) (Table 4).

There was a trend towards inpatient mortality among patients who were managed medically compared to the intervention group, although this was not significantly different (32% versus 23%, $p > 0.05$). The 1-year all-cause mortality, however, was similar (52% versus 54%, $p > 0.05$) (Tables 5(a) and 5(b)).

4. Discussion

The main findings of this study show that age and troponin level appear to play a role in the current clinical decision making for patients with suspected poststroke ACS. Troponin level appears to significantly correlate with 1-year all-cause mortality. In the management of poststroke acute coronary syndrome, optimal medical therapy had similar inpatient and all-cause mortality compared to PCI and/or CABG. Although there was a trend towards inpatient mortality among patients who were managed medically compared to the intervention group, it was not found to be statistically significant ($p > 0.05$) (Tables 5(a) and 5(b)). The 1-year all-cause mortality rates were also found to be similar between the two groups, with 52% for the medical management groups and 54% for the intervention group.

Most patients who had acute coronary syndrome after an acute ischemic stroke did not have any symptoms that pertain to the ACS. Only around 30% had chest pain. This may be explained by language or cognitive impairments that occur in the setting of acute ischemic stroke. Alternatively, it is possible that many of the cases presented as a silent myocardial infarction. The patients' troponin levels, however, reflect a significant amount of cardiac injury, being remarkably elevated to a mean of 18. This emphasizes the importance of cardiac evaluation in acute ischemic stroke patients, even without obvious typical symptoms.

In a study by Chalela et al., troponin elevation was found to occur in 6% of patients with acute ischemic stroke. In another study, 53.4% of the patients admitted for acute ischemic stroke have elevated troponin, although only 6.6% met the criteria for acute coronary syndrome [10]. Interestingly, the study also showed that elevated troponin levels correlated with older age, history of coronary artery disease, congestive heart failure, diabetes mellitus, and renal disease [11]. An elevated troponin level was also associated with severity of stroke [10], poor outcomes, and death [12]. Troponin levels were associated with predicting a modified Rankin score, a measure to determine the degree of disability in doing activities of daily living, of 5 (bedridden) or 6 (death) [12]. Furthermore, a study by Scheitz et al. showed that an elevated troponin level was an independent predictor of poor outcome and in-hospital mortality [13]. In our study, the troponin levels revealed being significantly related to 1-year all-cause mortality, with 15 out of the 82 patients dying within 1 year of the ischemic stroke (Tables 5(a) and 5(b)). In contrast

TABLE 3: Patient characteristics of those who underwent medical management versus intervention (stent or CABG).

	Medical management	Stent or CABG	p value
N (%)	69 (84%)	13 (16%)	
Mean age (years)	73 ± 13	67 ± 7	$p = 0.02$
Gender			
Female	38 (88%)	5 (12%)	$p = 0.21$
Male	31 (80%)	8 (20%)	
Race			$p = 0.6$
Caucasian	20 (83%)	4 (17%)	
African American	42 (82%)	9 (18%)	
Hispanic	5 (100%)	0 (0%)	
Asian	2 (100%)	0 (0%)	
Mean length of stay (days)	12 ± 10	25 ± 21	$p = 0.005$
Comorbidities			
Coronary artery disease	29 (80%)	7 (20%)	$p = 0.3$
Body mass index > 30	17 (77%)	5 (23%)	$p = 0.44$
Hypertension	66 (83%)	13 (17%)	$p = 0.5$
Hyperlipidemia	32 (86%)	5 (14%)	$p = 0.41$
Diabetes mellitus	39 (85%)	7 (15%)	$p = 0.5$
Chronic kidney disease	20 (83%)	4 (17%)	$p = 0.5$
Congestive heart failure	30 (79%)	8 (21%)	$p = 0.18$
Coronary artery disease equivalents	12 (80%)	3 (20%)	$p = 0.8$
Smoker	15 (75%)	5 (25%)	$p = 0.17$

TABLE 4: Cardiac evaluation results of patients who underwent medical management versus intervention (stent or CABG).

	Medical management	Stent + CABG	Stat test	p value
Mean peak troponin	12 ± 17	49 ± 64	Kruskal-Wallis	0.005
Ischemic ECG changes				
With	62	10	Fisher exact	0.19
Without	7	3		
2D-echocardiogram				
Mean ejection	40 ± 18	38 ± 17	t-test	0.64
Wall motion abnormality				
Present	39	8	Chi-square	0.11
Absent	30	5		

to Scheitz's study, our data did not show that troponin level is associated with inpatient mortality. However, because results across multiple studies have been different, it remains to be determined if troponin level correlates only with the severity of stroke or whether it is an independent predictor of death [14].

A clinical review by Davis et al. showed that the most frequent ECG abnormalities in acute stroke patients were prolonged QT interval and ST-T changes [15]. In a study by Dogan et al., on the other hand, 65% of patients had ischemia-like ECG changes with the most common one being T-wave inversion [16]. In our study, presence of ischemic ECG changes was found in 88% of the patients and similarly to Dogan's study the most common abnormality was T-wave inversion (89%). Although Dogan's study showed that ST-segment changes were an independent predictor of mortality, a large scale study by Goldstein showed that ischemic

ECG changes were not associated with mortality in stroke patients [17]. Our study was consistent with Goldstein's results showing that ischemic ECG changes did not correlate with inpatient mortality or 1-year all-cause mortality (Tables 5(a) and 5(b)).

Our study revealed that patients who had acute coronary syndrome in the setting of acute ischemic stroke had low ejection fraction and wall motion abnormalities. The mean EF of our patients is 40, which is close to the results of a study by Bulsara et al., where the mean EF of the patients was 33%. In Bulsara's study, the findings in the ECGs did not match the wall motion abnormalities in the 2D-echocardiograms [18]. Our study, however, showed that wall motion abnormalities correlated with the ischemic changes found in the ECG (Table 2). In a study done with subarachnoid hemorrhage patients, wall hypokinesis was present in the first 2 days and there was partial or complete resolution of the wall motion

TABLE 5: (a) Inpatient mortality of cases who underwent medical management versus intervention (stent or CABG). (b) 1-year all-cause mortality of patients who underwent medical management versus intervention (stent or CABG).

(a)

	Inpatient mortality		Inpatient mortality		RR	95% CI	Stat test	p value
	Number	%	Yes	No				
Mean peak troponin								
High	8	32	8	13	1.36	0.69–2.67	Chi-square	0.37
Low	17	68	17	44				
Ischemic ECG changes								
Present	8	32	8	13	1.3669	0.69–2.69	Fisher exact	0.26
Absent	17	68	17	44				
Management								
Stent/CABG	3	12	8	13	1.36	0.69–2.67	Chi-square	0.37
Medical	22	88	17	44				

(b)

	1-year all-cause mortality		1-year all-cause mortality		RR	95% CI	Stat test	p value
	Number	%	Yes	No				
Mean peak troponin								
High	15	34.88	15	6	1.55	1.06–2.28	Chi-square	0.04
Low	28	65.12	28	33				
Ischemic ECG changes								
Present	38	88.37	38	34	1.05	0.54–2.03	Fisher exact	0.56
Absent	5	11.63	5	5				
Management								
Stent/CABG	7	16.28	7	6	1.03	0.59–1.7	Chi-square	0.57
Medical	36	83.72	36	33				

abnormalities during the hospitalization [19]. Due to the retrospective nature of our study, we were not able to follow the 2D-echocardiograms of our patients during their hospital stay.

In our study, 67% of patients with acute coronary syndrome and acute ischemic stroke did not undergo cardiac catheterization. There are several factors that may have influenced this management decision. One is the size of the stroke. Patients who are deemed at risk of hemorrhagic conversion do not undergo cardiac catheterization during the same admission. The procedure may then be scheduled 3–6 months after the stroke. It is also important to note that 29% of the patients in the study had chronic kidney disease. In elderly patients, it is not uncommon to encounter patients and family members refusing cardiac catheterization because of higher risk of requiring hemodialysis.

Our study also found that older age is associated with greater likelihood of conservative management (Table 3). This may be because the risks of cardiac catheterization sometimes outweigh the benefits in frail, elderly patients. The level of troponin also plays a role in deciding the management. The higher it is, the more likely the patient will undergo cardiac catheterization as this may imply larger cardiac damage (Table 4). Apart from the age and troponin level, the two groups (patients who were managed conservatively and those

who underwent cardiac catheterization) did not have any significant difference in terms of comorbidities (Table 3). Since the cooccurrence of acute coronary syndrome and acute ischemic stroke is not common, this study is limited by its sample size. There is a trend seen in medical management group and inpatient mortality; however, the limited sample size may account for why it is not statistically significant.

In conclusion, when clinical characteristics and cardiac work-up of the medical management group and the intervention group were compared, the only significant difference was that medical management group had older individuals (73 versus 67 years), lower mean peak troponin levels (12 versus 49), and lower mean length of stay (12 versus 25 days). Troponin levels revealed being significantly related to 1-year all-cause mortality, but not to inpatient mortality. Optimal medical therapy had similar inpatient and all-cause mortality compared to PCI and/or CABG.

5. Limitations of the Study

Given the retrospective nature of our study, variables like severity of stroke, MRI findings for the location of the stroke, patient frailty, and other related variables were missing in our patient records and were not included in the study. Sixty-seven percent of the patients in the study also did not undergo cardiac catheterization. Finally, it is possible that the elevated troponin levels seen in our patient group were secondary to catecholamine surge caused by the stroke.

Authors' Contributions

All authors contributed to the conceptual planning, data collection, analysis, and writing of the manuscript.

References

[1] K. C. Johnston, J. Y. Li, P. D. Lyden et al., "Medical and neurological complications of ischemic stroke: experience from the RANTTAS trial," *Stroke*, vol. 29, no. 2, pp. 447–453, 1998.

[2] P. L. Chin, J. Kaminski, and M. Rout, "Myocardial infarction coincident with cerebrovascular accidents in the elderly," *Age and Ageing*, vol. 6, no. 1, pp. 29–37, 1977.

[3] F. L. Silver, J. W. Norris, A. J. Lewis, and V. C. Hachinski, "Early mortality following stroke: a prospective review," *Stroke*, vol. 15, no. 3, pp. 492–496, 1984.

[4] E. Touzé, O. Varenne, G. Chatellier, S. Peyrard, P. M. Rothwell, and J.-L. Mas, "Risk of myocardial infarction and vascular death after transient ischemic attack and ischemic stroke: a systematic review and meta-analysis," *Stroke*, vol. 36, no. 12, pp. 2748–2755, 2005.

[5] T. Kono, H. Morita, T. Kuroiwa, H. Onaka, H. Takatsuka, and A. Fujiwara, "Left ventricular wall motion abnormalities in patients with subarachnoid hemorrhage: neurogenic stunned myocardium," *Journal of the American College of Cardiology*, vol. 24, no. 3, pp. 636–640, 1994.

[6] B. R. Chambers and J. W. Norris, "Outcome in patients with asymptomatic neck bruits," *New England Journal of Medicine*, vol. 315, no. 14, pp. 860–865, 1986.

[7] J. L. Wilterdink, K. L. Furie, and J. D. Easton, "Cardiac evaluation of stroke patients," *Neurology*, vol. 51, no. 3, pp. S23–S26, 1998.

[8] E. A. Amsterdam, N. K. Wenger, and R. G. Brindis, "2014 AHA/ACC guideline for the management of patients with non-ST-elevation acute coronary syndromes," *Circulation*, vol. 130, pp. e344–e426, 2014.

[9] H. Nguyen and J. G. Zaroff, "Neurogenic stunned myocardium," *Current Neurology and Neuroscience Reports*, vol. 9, no. 6, pp. 486–491, 2009.

[10] J. A. Chalela, M. A. Ezzeddine, L. Davis, and S. Warach, "Myocardial injury in acute stroke: a troponin I study," *Neurocritical Care*, vol. 1, no. 3, pp. 343–346, 2004.

[11] K. W. Faiz, B. Thommessen, G. Einvik, P. H. Brekke, T. Omland, and O. M. Rønning, "Determinants of high sensitivity cardiac troponin T elevation in acute ischemic stroke," *BMC Neurology*, vol. 14, article 96, 2014.

[12] J. Ghali, D. Allison, T. Kleinig et al., "Elevated serum concentrations of troponin T in acute stroke: what do they mean?" *Journal of Clinical Neuroscience*, vol. 17, no. 1, pp. 69–73, 2010.

[13] J. F. Scheitz, M. Endres, H.-C. Mochmann, H. J. Audebert, and C. H. Nolte, "Frequency, determinants and outcome of elevated troponin in acute ischemic stroke patients," *International Journal of Cardiology*, vol. 157, no. 2, pp. 239–242, 2012.

[14] G. Kerr, G. Ray, O. Wu, D. J. Stott, and P. Langhorne, "levated troponin after stroke: a systematic review," *Cerebrovascular Diseases*, vol. 28, no. 3, pp. 220–226, 2009.

[15] T. P. Davis, J. Alexander, and M. Lesch, "Electrocardiographic changes associated with acute cerebrovascular disease: a clinical review," *Progress in Cardiovascular Diseases*, vol. 36, no. 3, pp. 245–260, 1993.

[16] A. Dogan, E. Tunc, M. Ozturk, M. Kerman, and G. Akhan, "Electrocardiographic changes in patients with ischaemic stroke and their prognostic importance," *International Journal of Clinical Practice*, vol. 58, no. 5, pp. 436–440, 2004.

[17] D. S. Goldstein, "The electrocardiogram in stroke: relationship to pathophysiological type and comparison with prior tracings," *Stroke*, vol. 10, no. 3, pp. 253–259, 1979.

[18] K. R. Bulsara, M. J. McGirt, L. Liao et al., "Use of the peak troponin value to differentiate myocardial infarction from reversible neurogenic left ventricular dysfunction associated with aneurysmal subarachnoid hemorrhage," *Journal of Neurosurgery*, vol. 98, no. 3, pp. 524–528, 2003.

[19] N. Banki, A. Kopelnik, P. Tung et al., "Prospective analysis of prevalence, distribution, and rate of recovery of left ventricular systolic dysfunction in patients with subarachnoid hemorrhage," *Journal of Neurosurgery*, vol. 105, no. 1, pp. 15–20, 2006.

4

Kansas City Cardiomyopathy Questionnaire Utility in Prediction of 30-Day Readmission Rate in Patients with Chronic Heart Failure

Shengchuan Dai,[1,2] Manoucher Manoucheri,[1] Junhong Gui,[1]
Xiang Zhu,[3] Divyanshu Malhotra,[1] Shenjing Li,[4] Jason D'souza,[1] Fnu Virkram,[1]
Aditya Chada,[1] and Haibing Jiang[1]

[1]Internal Medicine Residency Program, Department of Medicine, Florida Hospital Orlando, Orlando, FL, USA
[2]Division of Cardiology, University of Illinois at Chicago, Chicago, IL, USA
[3]Center for Interventional Endoscopy, Florida Hospital Orlando, Orlando, FL, USA
[4]Division of Cardiology, University of South Dakota, Vermillion, SD, USA

Correspondence should be addressed to Shengchuan Dai; sdai240@gmail.com
and Manoucher Manoucheri; manoucher.manoucheri.md@flhosp.org

Academic Editor: Stephan von Haehling

Background. Heart failure (HF) is one of the most common diagnoses associated with hospital readmission. We designed this prospective study to evaluate whether Kansas City Cardiomyopathy Questionnaire (KCCQ) score is associated with 30-day readmission in patients hospitalized with decompensated HF. *Methods and Results*. We enrolled 240 patients who met the study criteria. Forty-eight (20%) patients were readmitted for decompensated HF within thirty days of hospital discharge, and 192 (80%) patients were not readmitted. Compared to readmitted patients, nonreadmitted patients had a higher average KCCQ score (40.8 versus 32.6, $P = 0.019$) before discharge. Multivariate analyses showed that a high KCCQ score was associated with low HF readmission rate (adjusted OR = 0.566, $P = 0.022$). The c-statistic for the base model (age + gender) was 0.617. The combination of home medication and lab tests on the base model resulted in an integrated discrimination improvement (IDI) increase of 3.9%. On that basis, the KCQQ further increased IDI of 2.7%. *Conclusions*. The KCCQ score determined before hospital discharge was significantly associated with 30-day readmission rate in patients with HF, which may provide a clinically useful measure and could significantly improve readmission prediction reliability when combined with other clinical components.

1. Introduction

It is estimated that heart failure (HF) affects over 5.7 million Americans with 870,000 new cases diagnosed each year. The predicted prevalence is estimated to increase 46% from 2012 to 2030, resulting in over 8 million individuals suffering with HF [1]. The cost of caring for HF patients was about $30.7 billion in 2012 and is estimated to increase by 127% to $69.7 billion by 2030 [1]. Despite advances in understanding and treatment, the mortality rate of HF remains extremely high with 50% of patients dying within 5 years of initial diagnosis [2].

Readmission of HF after hospitalization is common, and unfortunately many of these readmissions are predictable and possibly preventable [2, 3]. Although new data showed reduction in Medicare hospital readmission rates [4], HF is still one of the most common diagnoses associated with 30-day readmission; an analysis of 2007 to 2009 Medicare claims-based data showed that 24.8 percent of beneficiaries admitted with HF were readmitted within 30 days and 35.2 percent of those readmissions were for HF [5]. These concerning statistics paved the way for a stronger focus on tools to predict and prevent such readmissions.

The Kansas City Cardiomyopathy Questionnaire (KCCQ) was a tool initially designed to provide a better description of health-related quality of life in patients with HF [6]. This questionnaire identified the following clinically relevant domains: physical limitations (question 1), symptoms (frequency [questions 3, 5, 7, and 9], severity [questions 4, 6, and 8], and change over time [question 2]), self-efficacy and knowledge (questions 11, 12), social interference (question 16), and health-related quality of life (questions 13–15) [6]. Previous studies have shown that KCCQ score correlated with survival and hospitalization in patients with HF [7] and was an independent predictor of poor prognosis in this patient population [8]. In addition, KCCQ score measured 1 week after hospital discharge independently predicted one-year survival free of cardiovascular readmission [9]. More recently, KCCQ has also been studied during acute HF hospitalization and demonstrated sensitivity to acute changes, but score changes during hospitalization did not predict short-term readmission [10], although it was a relatively small study, with a sample size of only 52 patients, and it did not investigate the relationship between KCCQ score and HF readmission. Therefore, whether KCCQ score can be used to predict the short-term readmission has yet to be completely evaluated.

To address these gaps in knowledge and explore the feasibility of using the KCCQ score to predict the short-term HF readmission, we designed and conducted this prospective study.

2. Methods

The study was approved by the Florida Hospital Institutional Review Board and conducted in accordance with the Declaration of Helsinki. The study was conducted at Florida Hospital, Orlando Campus. Patients who were admitted to the HF unit were screened and enrolled for the study. The inclusion criteria were patients admitted with decompensated HF with ejection fraction (EF) less than or equal to 40% and age between 20 and 89 years. Exclusion criteria were noncardiac disease with a life expectancy of less than one year, HF due to uncorrected valvular heart disease, psychiatric illness interfering with an appropriate follow-up, inability to understand study procedure, and inability to provide informed consent. Primary endpoint was 30-day readmission rate and the KCCQ score. Admission comorbid conditions, demographics, laboratory, echocardiographic data, and medications on discharge were secondary endpoints.

For every patient who met the study criteria, a trained research assistant explained the study to the patient and administered the KCCQ after a written informed consent was obtained. The assessment was generally completed within 1–3 days before discharge. A follow-up conversation was performed over the telephone 30 days after discharge to determine if rehospitalization occurred or not. Postdischarge readmission information was gathered through follow-up interview with the patient.

To evaluate associations between KCCQ score and readmission within 30 days after discharge, we first compared the difference between the nonreadmission group and readmission group in terms of the KCCQ scores, demographic characteristics, comorbidity, medications, and laboratory data using univariate analysis. In the univariate analysis, t-test was used for continuous variable, and Fisher's exact test was used for count number analysis. We then performed multivariate

analysis to investigate how each clinical factor was associated with HF readmissions after controlling for the other factors. In the multivariate analysis, logistic regression models were used, and adjusted odds ratios (OR) were estimated for each factor hypothesized to predict HF readmission. We included HF readmission as a dependent variable and all potential factors as independent predictors in the logistic regression irrespective of whether they showed a significant difference between readmission and nonreadmission groups in the univariate analysis.

After the multivariate analysis, we further constructed five simplified prediction models and evaluated the importance of KCCQ score in the final model through comparing area under receiver operating characteristic curve (ROC) of each model. In this analysis, we also used integrated discrimination improvement (IDI), described by Pencina et al., to measure the average increase in model sensitivity penalized for average decrease in specificity with the addition of new variables [11]. In the prediction models, age was transformed to every 10-year increment, ejection fraction to every 10% decrease, KCCQ score to every 25-point increment, and sodium level to binary variable (<135 or ≥135).

Two hundred and twenty-eight (228, or 95%) patients had complete data for all variables. However, 12 (5%) patients had missing data in either age or race. As no nested missing pattern was detected, multiple imputation models were used for data imputation. As age was a continuous variable and race was a binary variable, normal linear regression was used for age while logistic regression was used for race imputation. All analyses were performed by Stata version 14 (StataCorp., 2015). All P values were two-tailed, and $\alpha < 0.05$ was set as the level of statistical significance for all tests.

3. Results

In total, 240 patients were enrolled in the study. Forty-eight (20%) patients were readmitted within 30 days after discharge for HF while 192 (80%) patients were not readmitted or readmitted for reasons other than HF (Table 1). There was no significant difference between the nonreadmitted and readmitted patients in terms of average age (63.0 versus 59.9 yrs, $P = 0.163$), initial length of hospital stay (11.2 versus 9.7 days, $P = 0.420$), or percentage of white patients (59.9% versus 56.3%, $P = 0.743$). However, a significant difference between these two groups was noted on comparing gender, with male patients being more prone to being readmitted than female (85.4% versus 68.8% for male and 14.6% versus 31.3% for female, $P = 0.020$). None of the comorbidities showed significant difference in the relative frequency between the readmission and nonreadmission group (Table 1).

The KCCQ score, lab test results on admission, and discharge medications were compared between the nonreadmitted and readmitted patients (Table 2). The average KCCQ score was significantly higher in the nonreadmitted patients than in readmitted patients (40.8 versus 32.6, $P = 0.019$). Compared to readmitted patients, nonreadmitted patients had a higher ejection fraction on admission (24.7% versus 21.8%, $P = 0.021$). However, no significant difference was detected on comparing discharge medications, blood sodium

TABLE 1: Summary of demographic characteristics and medical history between HF readmission and nonreadmission within 30 days after discharge.

Demographic characteristics	Readmission within 30 days after discharge		
	No (n = 192)	Yes (n = 48)	P value
Age, yrs, mean (SD)	63.0 (13.6)	59.9 (14.5)	0.163
LOS, days, mean (SD)	11.2 (11.6)	9.7 (7.6)	0.420
Race			0.743
White	115 (59.9)	27 (56.3)	
Other	77 (40.1)	21 (43.8)	
Gender			0.020
Female	60 (31.3)	7 (14.6)	
Male	132 (68.8)	41 (85.4)	
Comorbidity			
CAD	137 (71.4)	28 (58.3)	0.085
MI	75 (39.1)	20 (41.7)	0.744
DM	103 (53.7)	26 (54.2)	1.000
Hypertension	156 (81.3)	38 (79.2)	0.838
COPD	44 (22.9)	10 (20.8)	0.848
ICD	100 (52.1)	22 (45.8)	0.519
LVAD	8 (4.2)	2 (4.2)	1.000
History of prior stroke	19 (9.9)	1 (2.1)	0.139
Obesity	52 (27.1)	13 (27.1)	1.000
At least one comorbidity	186 (96.9)	46 (95.8)	0.662

Note. Numbers in the parenthesis are percentage except indicated.

TABLE 2: Summary of KCCQ score, lab tests, and discharge medication between HF readmission and nonreadmission within 30 days after discharge.

Demographic characteristics	Readmission within 30 days after discharge		
	No (n = 192)	Yes (n = 48)	P value
KCCQ score, mean (SD)	40.8 (22.2)	32.6 (18.5)	0.019
Lab on admission			
Sodium, mean (SD)	137.6 (4.7)	137.5 (5.6)	0.915
HGB, mean (SD)	12.1 (2.1)	11.9 (2.1)	0.622
Ejection fraction	24.7 (7.4)	21.8 (8.8)	0.021
Discharge medication			
Beta blocker	172 (89.6)	43 (89.6)	1.000
ACE/ARB	110 (57.3)	25 (52.1)	0.520
Diuretic	168 (87.5)	40 (83.3)	0.478
Lipid-lowering	126 (65.6)	29 (60.4)	0.504
Aldosterone antagonist	98 (51.0)	23 (47.9)	0.748
Digoxin	60 (31.3)	15 (31.3)	1.000
Hydralazine	30 (15.6)	5 (10.4)	0.494
Nitrates	39 (20.3)	6 (12.5)	0.301
Inotrope	46 (24.0)	13 (27.1)	0.708

Note. Numbers in the parenthesis are percentage except indicated.

level, or HGB between the two groups of patients in the univariate analysis (Table 2).

To further investigate the effect of each independent variable while controlling other covariates, multivariate analyses were performed (Table 3 and Figure 1). The results showed that the KCCQ score and EF were negatively associated with readmission rate (adjusted OR = 0.566 and 1.903 and P = 0.022 and 0.021, resp.) and that males were more likely to be readmitted than females (adjusted OR = 5.589, P = 0.001). Interestingly, patients with MI were more likely (adjusted OR = 2.849, P = 0.049) and patients with CAD were less likely to be readmitted (adjusted OR = 0.231, P = 0.012), compared to patients with other comorbidities. One possible interpretation could be that patients who have had a myocardial infarction are more likely to have wall motion abnormalities and fixed myocardial defects and thus a lower ejection fraction than those with nonobstructive coronary artery disease without an MI, leading to opposite contribution to HF readmission.

In order to evaluate how much contribution the KCCQ score made in predicting HF readmission, we developed a model by including seven factors besides KCCQ score (model 5) based on the multivariate regression results, published literature, and models. The c-statistic indicated

that model 5 which included KCCQ score and all other potential predictors had the highest c-statistic value (0.710) among other reduced models without KCCQ score (Figure 2). As seen in Table 4, the IDI analysis demonstrated that the discriminatory performance of model 5 improved by 6.6% from the base model (model 1) that only included age and gender and by 2.7% from the reduced model (model 4) including all factors but the KCCQ score (this is the absolute increment; when compared with model 4, the IDI of the full model with KCCQ, model 5, increased by 2.7/3.9 = 69%). On the other hand, as an established independent factor associated with HF readmission [12, 13], EF increased the IDI from 1.3% (model 3) to 3.9% (model 4). These results suggested that the KCCQ score, as a single independent variable, is one of the important factors that could potentially be used for predicting readmission rates of HF patients within 30 days after discharge, and a combination of all these important factors would offer the greatest incremental gain.

4. Discussion

In this prospective study, we found that the KCCQ score was significantly associated with short-term HF readmission rate. It contributed to improving the c-statistics of a model based on age, gender, medications, laboratory data, and LVEF available at discharge from 0.670 to 0.710 and raised the

Kansas City Cardiomyopathy Questionnaire Utility in Prediction of 30-Day Readmission Rate in Patients...

21

TABLE 3: Summary of multivariate analysis investigating the effects of demographic characteristics, medical history, discharge medication, lab test, and overall KCCQ score on readmission rate within 30 days after discharge ($n = 240$).

Factor	Adjusted OR	SE	95% CI	P value
Age	0.990	0.145	0.742–1.320	0.946
White	0.821	0.348	0.358–1.884	0.642
Male	5.589	2.962	1.979–15.79	0.001
CAD	0.231	0.135	0.074–0.724	0.012
MI	2.849	1.514	1.005–8.074	0.049
DM	0.877	0.369	0.384–2.001	0.754
Hypertension	0.815	0.405	0.308–2.157	0.681
COPD	1.084	0.514	0.429–2.744	0.864
ICD	0.648	0.271	0.286–1.471	0.299
LVAD	0.710	0.650	0.118–4.275	0.709
History of prior stroke	0.150	0.171	0.016–1.402	0.096
Obesity	1.377	0.658	0.540–3.511	0.503
Beta blocker	1.096	0.713	0.306–3.920	0.888
ACE/ARB	0.734	0.299	0.331–1.629	0.447
Diuretic	0.438	0.257	0.138–1.384	0.159
Lipid-lowering	1.186	0.511	0.509–2.761	0.693
Aldosterone antagonist	0.873	0.360	0.389–1.957	0.741
Digoxin	1.137	0.47	0.506–2.554	0.756
Hydralazine	0.639	0.402	0.186–2.193	0.476
Nitrates	0.443	0.271	0.134–1.467	0.182
Inotrope	0.799	0.378	0.316–2.022	0.636
Sodium	1.791	0.815	0.734–4.368	0.200
Hgb	0.810	0.087	0.655–1.000	0.050
Ejection fraction	1.903	0.532	1.100–3.292	0.021
KCCQ	0.566	0.141	0.347–0.922	0.022

TABLE 4: Prognostic value of readmission within 30 days after discharge of different models comparing to model 1 with only demographic predictors.

Model	c-statistics	IDI increase (%)	P value
Model 1: age + gender	0.617	—	—
Model 2: age + gender + beta_blocker + ace/arb	0.647	0.9	0.123
Model 3: age + gender + beta_blocker + ace/arb + sodium + hgb	0.656	1.3	0.081
Model 4: age + gender + beta_blocker + ace/arb + sodium + hgb + ef	0.670	3.9	0.005
Model 5: age + gender + beta_blocker + ace/arb + sodium + hgb + ef + KCCQ	0.710	6.6	<0.001

IDI by 2.7%, which suggested that it may be helpful in predicting 30-day readmission and thus significantly improve prediction reliability when combined with other critical components. These findings may provide some help to guide follow-up strategies towards delivering optimal care, such as encouraging patients with lower KCCQ to have an early follow-up [14].

Lots of efforts have been made to identify the predictable factors that are associated with high risk of being readmitted, which has been quite challenging until now. In this study, we found that HF patients who had lower KCCQ score at time of discharge and lower EF and of male gender seemed to be more prone for readmission within 30 days. These findings were similar to some studies but not others. As a matter of fact, no specific patient or hospital factors have been shown to

consistently predict 30-day readmission after hospitalization for HF. In a systematic review of 112 studies describing the association between traditional patient characteristics and readmission after hospitalization for HF, left ventricular EF, as well as other factors such as demographic characteristics, comorbid conditions, and New York Heart Association class, was associated with readmission in only a minority of cases [13]. In another meta-analysis of 69 studies and 144 factors for short-term readmission, noncardiovascular comorbidities, poor physical condition, history of admission, and failure to use evidence-based medication, rather than cardiovascular comorbidities, age, or gender, were more strongly associated with short-term readmission [15].

The KCCQ scores have been demonstrated to have much greater sensitivity to clinical changes in HF patients than

Factor	OR (95% CI)
Age	0.99 (0.74, 1.32)
White	0.82 (0.36, 1.88)
Male	5.59 (1.98, 15.79)
CAD	0.23 (0.07, 0.72)
MI	2.85 (1.00, 8.07)
DM	0.88 (0.38, 2.00)
Hypertension	0.82 (0.31, 2.16)
COPD	1.08 (0.43, 2.74)
ICD	0.65 (0.29, 1.47)
LVAD	0.71 (0.12, 4.28)
History of prior stroke	0.15 (0.02, 1.40)
Obesity	1.38 (0.54, 3.51)
Beta blocker	1.10 (0.31, 3.92)
ACE/ARB	0.73 (0.33, 1.63)
Diuretic	0.44 (0.14, 1.38)
Lipid-lowering	1.19 (0.51, 2.76)
Aldosterone antagonist	0.87 (0.39, 1.96)
Digoxin	1.14 (0.51, 2.55)
Hydralazine	0.64 (0.19, 2.19)
Nitrates	0.44 (0.13, 1.47)
Inotrope	0.80 (0.32, 2.02)
Sodium	1.79 (0.73, 4.37)
Hgb	0.81 (0.65, 1.00)
Ejection fraction	1.90 (1.10, 3.29)
KCCQ	0.57 (0.35, 0.92)

Adjusted OR

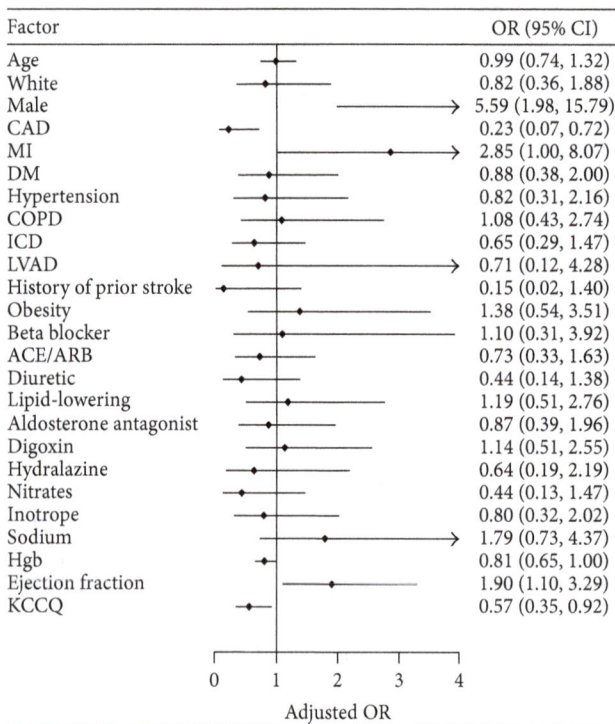

FIGURE 1: Adjusted odds ratios of readmission within 30 days after discharge derived from multivariate logistic regression analysis.

Model 1 ROC area: 0.6172 — Model 2 ROC area: 0.6465
Model 3 ROC area: 0.6559 — Model 4 ROC area: 0.6704
Model 5 ROC area: 0.7098 — Reference

FIGURE 2: Comparison of ROC area among different models. Model 1: logit (read30) = age + gender; model 2: logit (read30) = age + gender + beta_blocker + ace/arb; model 3: logit (read30) = age + gender + beta_blocker + ace/arb + sodium + hgb; model 4: logit (read30) = age + gender + beta_blocker + ace/arb + sodium + hgb + ef; and model 5: logit (read30) = age + gender + beta_blocker + ace/arb + sodium + hgb + ef + KCCQ. read30: readmission in 30 days.

the New York Heart Association (NYHA) functional classification, Minnesota Living with Heart Failure Questionnaire (LiHFe), and Short Form-36 (SF-36) [6]. The EVEREST trial suggested that the KCCQ is an important prognostic indicator of readmission within one year after discharge [9]. In their study, patients with KCCQ scores < 25 (worse health status) had more than threefold increased risk of the combined endpoint of rehospitalization and mortality than those in the best health status tier (KCCQ score > 75). More recently, KCCQ score was used to assess the feasibility of reflecting the changes of acute HF during hospitalization and predicting 30-day readmission. The authors found that it was feasible to use the KCCQ during acute HF hospitalizations and was sensitive to clinical improvement, but score changes during hospitalization did not predict 30-day readmission. However, this study was a relatively small study that included only 54 patients and was focused on KCCQ score differences during hospitalization between nonreadmission and admission groups [10]. In contrast, more than 240 patients were enrolled in our study and the KCCQ score was higher in nonreadmitted HF patients and was independently associated with lower 30-day readmission.

As mentioned above, there are multiple factors contributing to HF readmission; therefore, risk prediction models including and weighing all relevant factors were developed. In these models, discrimination, defined by the area under the receiver operating characteristic (ROC) curve, is used to tell how well a model can separate those who will have the outcome from those who will not have the outcome of interest. In this case, if the predicted risks

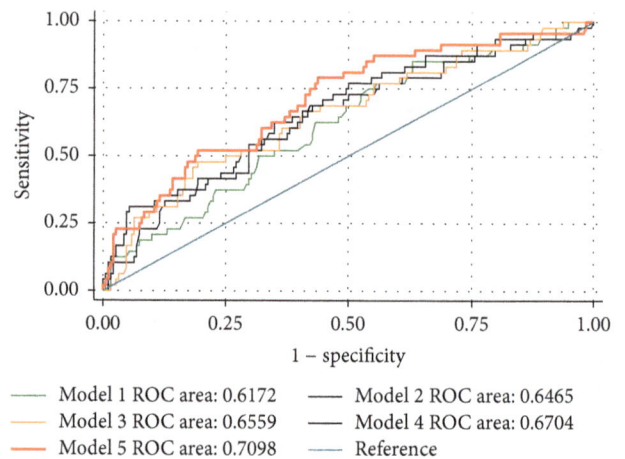

for readmitted patients are all higher than for patients who are not readmitted, the model discriminates perfectly with c-statistic of 1. Conversely, if risk prediction is no better than chance, the c-statistic is 0.5. Models are typically considered reasonable when the c-statistic is greater than 0.7 and strong when the c-statistic is greater than 0.8 [16]. For 30-day readmission after HF hospitalization, several models have been developed. Only two models have generated c-statistics greater than 0.6 after studying both derivation and validation cohorts. One of them is the automated model developed by Amarasingham et al. incorporating data from the electronic health record at the time of hospitalization [17]. The other model combined claims-based demographic and comorbidity data with clinical data including vital signs, laboratory values, and measured left ventricular ejection fraction [18]. However, neither of the two models included KCCQ scores. Given only 48 readmissions in our study population, we included only 7 parameters besides the KCCQ score in the full model (model 5). Low EF and gender (men) resulting in increased odds ratios for readmission in the multivariate analysis were included; we also included information about medications, beta-blocker and ACE inhibitor/ARB, which had demonstrated lowering HF mortality [19–21], and sodium and Hgb, which may affect HF rehospitalization and mortality [22, 23] and have been used in other models (http://www.readmissionscore.org/heart_failure.php), although they were not independently associated with readmission in the multivariate analysis. The full model (model 5), which included the KCCQ score, increased the c-statistics of 0.617 in base model 1 based on age and gender to 0.710, with an IDI increase of 6.6%. Given that many other possible risk factors have not been included in this model, such as GFR and BNP, this model may not be perfect, although its *c*-statistics was greater than 0.7, and may exaggerate the contribution of the KCCQ score. However, our results suggested that the contribution of KCCQ for predicting short-term HF readmission could potentially be as important as LVEF.

The present findings should be considered within the context of the study's limitations. This study was performed in a single-community medical center, and further studies in other centers or multiple centers need to be done to validate our findings. We only administered the KCCQ one time during the hospitalization, which would not reflect changes between admission, during hospitalization, and after hospitalization. We did not collect some relevant medical history, such as history of admission due to heart failure in the past; physical examination findings; some other labs such as GFR and BNP, or chest X-ray findings. These factors could also be important in the risk prediction model.

Abbreviations

KCCQ: Kansas City Cardiomyopathy Questionnaire
HF: Heart failure
HRQL: Health-related quality of life
EF: Ejection fraction
LVEF: Left ventricular ejection fraction
OR: Odds ratios
CAD: Coronary artery disease
MI: Myocardial infarction
DM: Diabetes mellitus
COPD: Chronic obstructive pulmonary disease
ICD: Implantable cardioverter-defibrillator
LVAD: Left ventricular assist device
ACE: Angiotensin converting enzyme
ARBs: Angiotensin receptor blockers
HGB: Hemoglobin
IDI: Integrated discrimination improvement
NYHA: New York Heart Association
ROC: Receiver operating characteristic
GFR: Glomerular filtration rate
BNP: Brain natriuretic peptide.

Additional Points

Competency in Medical Knowledge. Heart failure is one of the most common diagnoses associated with readmission. KCCQ score provided important prognostic information for predicting 30-day readmission and it can significantly improve prediction reliability along with other critical components. *Translational Outlook.* Additional clinical studies need to be done in multiple centers with a larger sample size to validate our finding. Future research should include relevant physical examination findings and chest X-ray findings, which could be important in the risk prediction model.

Competing Interests

The authors declare that they have no competing interests.

Authors' Contributions

Shengchuan Dai and Junhong Gui contributed equally to the manuscript.

Acknowledgments

The authors wish to acknowledge the following participating doctors from Florida Hospital Orlando who helped with data collection: Maria Amin (MD); Saroj Khadka (MD); Prabhava Bagla (MD); and Zoltan Varga (MD, Ph.D.).

References

[1] D. Mozaffarian, E. J. Benjamin, A. S. Go et al., "Heart disease and stroke statistics—2015 update: a report from the american heart association," *Circulation*, vol. 131, no. 4, pp. e29–e322, 2015.

[2] S. F. Jencks, M. V. Williams, and E. A. Coleman, "Rehospitalizations among patients in the medicare fee-for-service program," *The New England Journal of Medicine*, vol. 360, no. 14, pp. 1418–1428, 2009.

[3] H. M. Krumholz, J. Amatruda, G. L. Smith et al., "Randomized trial of an education and support intervention to prevent readmission of patients with heart failure," *Journal of the American College of Cardiology*, vol. 39, no. 1, pp. 83–89, 2002.

[4] G. Gerhardt, A. Yemane, P. Hickman, A. Oelschlaeger, E. Rollins, and N. Brennan, "Medicare readmission rates showed meaningful decline in 2012," *Medicare and Medicaid Research Review*, vol. 3, no. 2, 2013.

[5] K. Dharmarajan, A. F. Hsieh, Z. Lin et al., "Diagnoses and timing of 30-day readmissions after hospitalization for heart failure, acute myocardial infarction, or pneumonia," *The Journal of the American Medical Association*, vol. 309, no. 4, pp. 355–363, 2013.

[6] C. P. Green, C. B. Porter, D. R. Bresnahan, and J. A. Spertus, "Development and evaluation of the Kansas City Cardiomyopathy Questionnaire: a new health status measure for heart failure," *Journal of the American College of Cardiology*, vol. 35, no. 5, pp. 1245–1255, 2000.

[7] G. E. Soto, P. Jones, W. S. Weintraub, H. M. Krumholz, and J. A. Spertus, "Prognostic value of health status in patients with heart failure after acute myocardial infarction," *Circulation*, vol. 110, no. 5, pp. 546–551, 2004.

[8] P. A. Heidenreich, J. A. Spertus, P. G. Jones et al., "Health status identifies heart failure outpatients at risk for hospitalization or death," *Journal of the American College of Cardiology*, vol. 47, no. 4, pp. 752–756, 2006.

[9] S. M. Dunlay, M. Gheorghiade, K. J. Reid et al., "Critical elements of clinical follow-up after hospital discharge for heart failure: insights from the EVEREST trial," *European Journal of Heart Failure*, vol. 12, no. 4, pp. 367–374, 2010.

[10] K. Sauser, J. A. Spertus, L. Pierchala, E. Davis, and P. S. Pang, "Quality of life assessment for acute heart failure patients from emergency department presentation through 30 days after discharge: a pilot study with the kansas city cardiomyopathy questionnaire," *Journal of Cardiac Failure*, vol. 20, no. 1, pp. 18–22, 2014.

[11] M. J. Pencina, R. B. D'Agostino, and R. B. D'Agostino Jr., "Evaluating the added predictive ability of a new marker: from area under the roc curve to reclassification and beyond," *Statistics in Medicine*, vol. 27, no. 2, pp. 157–172, 2008.

[12] K. J. Harjai, E. Nunez, T. Turgut et al., "The independent effects of left ventricular ejection fraction on short-term outcomes and resource utilization following hospitalization for heart failure," *Clinical Cardiology*, vol. 22, no. 3, pp. 184–190, 1999.

[13] J. S. Ross, G. K. Mulvey, B. Stauffer et al., "Statistical models and patient predictors of readmission for heart failure: a systematic review," *Archives of Internal Medicine*, vol. 168, no. 13, pp. 1371–1386, 2008.

[14] K. K. Lee, J. Yang, A. F. Hernandez, A. E. Steimle, and A. S. Go, "Post-discharge follow-up characteristics associated with 30-day readmission after heart failure hospitalization," *Medical Care*, vol. 54, no. 4, pp. 365–372, 2016.

[15] M. Saito, K. Negishi, and T. H. Marwick, "Meta-analysis of risks for short-term readmission in patients with heart failure," *The American Journal of Cardiology*, vol. 117, no. 4, pp. 626–632, 2016.

[16] D. W. Hosmer Jr., S. Lemeshow, and R. X. Sturdivant, Eds., *Applied Logistic Regression*, John Wiley & Sons, New York, NY, USA, 2nd edition, 2000.

[17] R. Amarasingham, B. J. Moore, Y. P. Tabak et al., "An automated model to identify heart failure patients at risk for 30-day readmission or death using electronic medical record data," *Medical Care*, vol. 48, no. 11, pp. 981–988, 2010.

[18] B. G. Hammill, L. H. Curtis, G. C. Fonarow et al., "Incremental value of clinical data beyond claims data in predicting 30-day outcomes after heart failure hospitalization," *Circulation: Cardiovascular Quality and Outcomes*, vol. 4, no. 1, pp. 60–67, 2011.

[19] J. M. Foody, M. H. Farrell, and H. M. Krumholz, "β-Blocker therapy in heart failure: scientific review," *The Journal of the American Medical Association*, vol. 287, no. 7, pp. 883–889, 2002.

[20] M. D. Flather, S. Yusuf, L. Kober et al., "Long-term ace-inhibitor therapy in patients with heart failure or left-ventricular dysfunction: a systematic overview of data from individual patients. Ace-inhibitor myocardial infarction collaborative group," *The Lancet*, vol. 355, no. 9215, pp. 1575–1581, 2000.

[21] M. A. Pfeffer, J. J. V. McMurray, E. J. Velazquez et al., "Valsartan, captopril, or both in myocardial infarction complicated by heart failure, left ventricular dysfunction, or both," *The New England Journal of Medicine*, vol. 349, no. 20, pp. 1893–1906, 2003.

[22] A. Romanovsky, S. Bagshaw, and M. H. Rosner, "Hyponatremia and congestive heart failure: a marker of increased mortality and a target for therapy," *International Journal of Nephrology*, vol. 2011, Article ID 732746, 7 pages, 2011.

[23] Y.-D. Tang and S. D. Katz, "Anemia in chronic heart failure: prevalence, etiology, clinical correlates, and treatment options," *Circulation*, vol. 113, no. 20, pp. 2454–2461, 2006.

5

Divorce and Severity of Coronary Artery Disease: A Multicenter Study

Amin Daoulah,[1] Mushabab Al-Murayeh,[2] Salem Al-kaabi,[3] Amir Lotfi,[4] Osama E. Elkhateeb,[5] Salem M. Al-Faifi,[6] Saleh Alqahtani,[7] James Stewart,[8] Jon Heavey,[9] William T. Hurley,[9] Mohamed N. Alama,[10] Mazen Faden,[11] Mohamed Al-Shehri,[2] Ali Youssef,[12] and Alawi A. Alsheikh-Ali[13,14]

[1] Section of Adult Cardiology, Cardiovascular Department, King Faisal Specialist Hospital & Research Center, Jeddah, Saudi Arabia

[2] Cardiovascular Department, Armed Forces Hospital Southern Region, Khamis Mushayt, Saudi Arabia

[3] Cardiology Department, Zayed Military Hospital, Abu Dhabi, UAE

[4] Division of Cardiology, Baystate Medical Center, Tufts University School of Medicine, Springfield, MA, USA

[5] Cardiac Center, King Abdullah Medical City, Holy Capital, Makkah, Saudi Arabia

[6] Section of Pulmonology, Internal Medicine Department, King Faisal Specialist Hospital & Research Center, Jeddah, Saudi Arabia

[7] Division of Gastroenterology and Hepatology, The Johns Hopkins Hospital, 1830 East Monument Street, Suite 428, Baltimore, MD 21287, USA

[8] Anesthesiology Department, King Faisal Specialist Hospital & Research Center, Riyadh, Saudi Arabia

[9] Emergency Medicine Department, Cleveland Clinic Foundation, Cleveland, OH, USA

[10] Cardiology Unit, King Abdul Aziz University Hospital, Jeddah, Saudi Arabia

[11] Anesthesiology Department, King Abdul Aziz University Hospital, Jeddah, Saudi Arabia

[12] Suez Canal University, Ismailia, Egypt

[13] College of Medicine, Mohammed Bin Rashid University of Medicine and Health Sciences, Dubai, UAE

[14] Institute of Cardiac Sciences, Sheikh Khalifa Medical City, Abu Dhabi, UAE

Correspondence should be addressed to Amin Daoulah; amindaoulah@yahoo.com

Academic Editor: Stephan von Haehling

The association between marital status and coronary artery disease (CAD) is supported by numerous epidemiological studies. While divorce may have an adverse effect on cardiac outcomes, the relationship between divorce and severe CAD is unclear. We conducted a multicenter, observational study of consecutive patients undergoing coronary angiography during the period between April 1, 2013, and March 30, 2014. Of 1,068 patients, 124 (12%) were divorced. Divorce was more frequent among women (27%) compared to men (6%). Most divorced patients had been divorced only once (49%), but a subset had been divorced 2 (38%) or ≥3 (12%) times. After adjusting for baseline differences, there was no significant association between divorce and severe CAD in men. In women, there was a significant adjusted association between divorce and severe MVD (OR 2.31 [1.16, 4.59]) or LMD (OR 5.91 [2.19, 15.99]). The modification of the association between divorce and severe CAD by gender was statistically significant for severe LMD ($P_{interaction}$ 0.0008) and marginally significant for CAD ($P_{interaction}$ 0.05). Among women, there was a significant adjusted association between number of divorces and severe CAD (OR 2.4 [95% CI 1.2, 4.5]), MVD (OR 2.0 [95% CI 1.4, 3.0]), and LMD (OR 3.4 [95% CI 1.9, 5.9]). In conclusion, divorce, particularly multiple divorces, is associated with severe CAD, MVD, and LMD in women but not in men.

1. Introduction

Coronary artery disease (CAD) is a major cause of death globally [1, 2]. Modifiable risk factors such as abnormal lipids, smoking, hypertension, diabetes, abdominal obesity, psychosocial factors, lack of daily consumption of fruits and vegetables, and lack of regular physical activity account for the majority of the increased risk for cardiovascular events worldwide in both sexes [3]. Previous cross-sectional studies have examined the association between marital status and health outcomes [4–6]. A number of studies have shown divorce to have a negative impact on cardiovascular health [7–9]. Studies additionally reveal that women suffer more economic and emotional distress as a result of a divorce compared to men [10–13]. A recent study demonstrated that cumulative exposure to divorce increases the risks of myocardial infarction, and women with multiple divorces are at an even higher risk. However, this analysis of myocardial infarction was based on self-reported data [14]. We therefore conducted a study examining the association between divorce and severity of CAD among men and women undergoing coronary angiography for clinical indications.

2. Methods

2.1. Study Design. The details regarding the design, methods, and endpoints of this multicenter, cross-sectional observational study came from the Polygamy and Risk of Coronary Artery Disease in Men Undergoing Angiography [15]. This study was undertaken to assess the relationship between divorce and severe CAD. It was approved by King Faisal Specialist Hospital & Research Center Institutional Review Board and reviewed for waiver by the institutional review board of each of the participating hospitals. An invitation letter was given to all participants who affirmed verbal consent prior to their enrollment.

2.2. Selection Criteria. All patients undergoing coronary angiography for clinical indications were recruited from five hospitals in two Gulf countries (The Kingdom of Saudi Arabia and The United Arab Emirates), during the period between April 1, 2013, and March 30, 2014. These hospitals are tertiary cardiac centers with large patient volumes and advanced cardiac care capabilities. There were no exclusion criteria.

2.3. Data Collection. All data were collected prospectively. Two separate data forms, general and angiographic, were filled out by the assigned physician. Both forms were completed prior to the patients discharge from the hospital. All data forms were reviewed by the respective cardiologists and then sent to the principle investigator, who also checked the forms prior to submission for analysis.

Measures and Variables. Contents of personal data form (collected through interview) are as follows:

(i) Demographic data: age, ethnic background

(ii) Physiologic status: hypertension, diabetes, dyslipidemia, and BMI

(iii) Life style: smoking history

(iv) Past medical history: coronary artery disease, percutaneous coronary intervention, coronary artery bypass surgery, cerebral vascular disease, peripheral arterial disease, congestive heart failure, atrial fibrillation, and chronic kidney disease

(v) Socioeconomic data: occupation (unemployed, private sector, government sector, and self-employed), living in rural or urban area, highest level of education completed (illiterate, secondary school, and higher education), and monthly income (<1300, 1300 to 2600, 2600 to 5300, >5300 USA Dollars)

(vi) Current marital status: divorced (single or multiple times) or not divorced which includes single, married, and widowed status

Contents of angiographic data form (collected from chart review of patient files) are as follows:

(i) Reason for coronary angiography (elective versus urgent/emergent)

(ii) CAD: number of vessels involved and severity of stenosis

(iii) Treatment (medical versus revascularization)

2.4. Definitions. Severe CAD was defined as ≥70% luminal stenosis in a major epicardial vessel or ≥50% stenosis in the left main coronary artery (LMD). Multivessel disease (MVD) was defined as having more than one coronary artery with stenosis ≥70%.

2.5. Statistical Analysis. Standard summary statistics were used to describe the cohort. Continuous variables are presented as mean ± standard deviation and were compared across multiple groups using the analysis of variance test. Categorical variables are presented as percentages and compared using the Chi-square test. The associations between divorce and severe CAD, MVD, and LMD were assessed using logistic regression models and quantified with odds ratios. Adjusted regression models included the following explanatory variables: age, gender, community setting (urban versus rural), employment, income level, education level, indication for angiography, and other variables that differed by divorce status in univariate comparisons ($P < 0.1$). All statistical tests were two-sided and significance was set at the conventional P value of less than 0.05. No adjustments for multiple comparisons were made.

3. Results

3.1. Characteristics of Patients and Coronary Angiogram Findings. Overall characteristics of patients and coronary angiogram findings are shown in Table 1. A detailed description can be found in [15].

3.2. Patient Characteristics Stratified by Divorce Status. Of the 1,068 patients enrolled, 124 (12%) were divorced. Among the 297 women, 81 were divorced (27%). Among the 771 men, only 43 were divorced (6%), $P < 0.0001$ (Table 1). Most

TABLE 1: Baseline characteristics of the overall cohort stratified by divorce status and gender.

	All patients				Men (n = 771)			Women (n = 297)		
	All (n = 1,068)	No divorce (n = 944)	Divorce (n = 124)	P value	No divorce (n = 728)	Divorce (n = 43)	P value	No divorce (n = 216)	Divorce (n = 81)	P value
Age (yr)	59 ± 13	59 ± 13	58 ± 12	0.1895	59 ± 13	57 ± 15	0.2753	60 ± 13	58 ± 10	0.1178
BMI (kg/m^2)	28 ± 6	28 ± 6	29 ± 6	0.1415	28 ± 6	28 ± 5	0.6331	29 ± 8	29 ± 7	0.6193
Rural (%)	26	26	23	0.3775	27	35	0.2552	24	16	0.1363
Diabetes mellitus (%)	56	57	48	0.0398	57	44	0.1421	63	49	0.0339
Hypertension (%)	60	59	66	0.0910	57	63	0.4367	67	69	0.6861
Smoking (%)	43	45	34	0.0258	54	70	0.0399	14	15	0.8421
Dyslipidemia (%)	64	65	60	0.2818	66	56	0.1693	60	62	0.7530
Past history (%)										
Coronary artery Disease	43	43	44	0.9011	45	36	0.2439	38	48	0.1116
PCI	23	23	21	0.6652	23	26	0.7092	21	19	0.5977
CABG	6	6	9	0.2455	6	5	0.6836	6	11	0.1356
Atrial fibrillation	6	5	11	0.0075	4	14	0.004	8	10	0.6752
CHF	14	13	17	0.2756	13	14	0.8854	14	19	0.3217
CVA	5	4	7	0.2632	4	7	0.3389	5	6	0.7134
CKD	16	15	19	0.2127	14	23	0.1008	18	17	0.8771
Depression	9	10	7	0.3920	8	0	0.0521	15	11	0.4099
PAD	4	3	6	0.1158	2	5	0.3015	6	6	0.8384
Ethnicity (%)				0.5333			0.2300			0.9455
Arabic Gulf	89	88	91		87	91		92	91	
Arabic non-Gulf	5	6	3		6	0		4	5	
Non-Arabic	6	6	6		7	9		4	4	
Monthly income (%)				0.0902			0.3803			0.6616
<$1300	58	57	69		51	44		78	83	
$1300–2600	24	26	17		29	26		15	12	
$2600–5300	11	11	12		13	26		4	5	
>$5300	7	6	2		7	4		3	0	
Job category (%)				<0.0001			0.1572			0.0722
Jobless	39	35	68		21	28		82	89	
Private sector	13	14	2		18	5		2	1	
Government sector	35	37	21		43	49		15	6	
Self-employed	13	14	9		18	18		1	4	
Education levels (%)				0.2948			0.5954			0.3363
Illiterate	49	48	57		42	49		68	62	
Secondary school	34	34	31		38	32		21	29	
Higher education	17	18	12		20	19		11	9	
Indication for CAG (%)				0.0047			0.3064			0.0017
Elective	48	49	41		46	40		57	42	
NSTEACS	46	45	58		48	58		38	58	

TABLE 1: Continued.

	All patients				Men (n = 771)			Women (n = 297)		
	All (n = 1,068)	No divorce (n = 944)	Divorce (n = 124)	P value	No divorce (n = 728)	Divorce (n = 43)	P value	No divorce (n = 216)	Divorce (n = 81)	P value
STEMI	6	6	1		6	2		6	0	
Findings on CAG (%)										
Any CAD	68	68	66	0.6272	73	67	0.4232	52	65	0.0426
Single vessel disease	20	22	11		23	12		19	11	
Double vessel disease	25	25	23		26	37		22	16	
Triple vessel disease	23	22	32		24	19		12	38	
Multivessel disease	48	47	55	0.0824	50	56	0.4857	34	54	0.0013
Left main disease	12	11	12	0.7194	13	2	0.0354	3	17	<0.0001
Intervention (%)				0.2298			0.2279			<0.0001
Medical therapy	37	37	34		34	30		50	36	
PCI	45	45	42		46	58		40	33	
CABG	18	18	24		20	12		10	31	

DM, diabetes mellitus; CAD, BMI, body mass index; CAD, coronary artery disease; PCI, percutaneous coronary intervention; CABG, coronary artery bypass grafting; AF, atrial fibrillation; CHF, congestive heart failure; CVA, cerebrovascular accident; CKD, chronic kidney disease; PAD, peripheral arterial disease; $, USA Dollars; Ph.D., a doctor of philosophy; STEMI, ST segment elevation myocardial infarction; NSTEACS, non-ST-segment elevation acute coronary syndromes; CAG, coronary angiography.

TABLE 2: Adjusted association of divorce with severe CAD in the overall cohort and separately in men and women.[*]

| | All patients | | Men | | Women | | P |
	Crude odds ratio	Adjusted odds ratio	Crude odds ratio	Adjusted odds ratio	Crude odds ratio	Adjusted odds ratio	interaction
Any CAD	0.90 [0.60, 1.33]	0.85 [0.42, 1.73]	0.77 [0.40, 1.49]	0.39 [0.14, 1.09]	1.68 [0.98, 2.85]	1.30 [0.51, 3.34]	0.0533
MVD	1.41 [0.97, 2.06]	1.76 [1.09, 2.83]	1.24 [0.67, 2.31]	1.16 [0.57, 2.35]	2.34 [1.39, 3.96]	2.31 [1.16, 4.59]	0.1640
LMD	1.11 [0.63, 1.98]	1.46 [0.77, 2.76]	0.15 [0.02, 1.13]	0.14 [0.02, 1.02]	6.24 [2.42, 16.12]	5.91 [2.19, 15.99]	0.0008

[*] The adjusted regression models included the following explanatory variables: age, gender, community setting (urban versus rural), employment, income level, education level, indication for angiography, and all other variables that differed by divorce status in univariate comparisons with a $P < 0.1$.

divorced patients had been divorced only once (49%), but some had a history of 2 (38%) or 3 (12%) divorces. One patient had been divorced 4 times. Divorced patients were less likely to have a history of diabetes mellitus or smoking. They were more likely to be unemployed and have a history of atrial fibrillation. Indication for coronary angiogram differed significantly by divorce status with divorced patients more often undergoing coronary angiogram for NSTEACS and less often for STEMI or elective indications. Presence of severe CAD, MVD, or LMD and the subsequent management did not significantly differ by divorce status (Table 1). Additionally, after adjusting for baseline differences and indication for angiogram, a history of divorce was still not significantly associated with severe CAD (OR 0.85 [0.42, 1.73]), MVD (OR 1.76 [1.09, 2.83]), or LMD (OR 1.46 [0.77, 2.76]) (Table 2).

3.3. Patient Characteristics Stratified by Divorce Status and Gender. Compared to nondivorced men, divorced men were more likely to be smokers and to have a history of atrial fibrillation and less likely to have LMD on coronary angiogram. Compared to nondivorced women, divorced women were less likely to have diabetes and more likely to have undergone coronary angiogram for NSEACS (Table 1). In univariate analyses, divorced women were more likely to have severe CAD (65% versus. 52%, P 0.042), MVD (54% versus 34%, P 0.001), or LMD (17% versus. 3%, $P < 0.0001$) compared to nondivorced women. Consequently, divorced women were more likely to require surgical revascularization (31% versus 10%, $P < 0.0001$) (Table 1). After adjusting for baseline characteristics and indications for coronary angiogram, there was no significant association between divorce and severe CAD in men. In women, there was an association between divorce and severe MVD (OR 2.31 [1.16, 4.59]) or LMD (OR 5.91 [2.19, 15.99]). The modification of the association between divorce and severe CAD by gender was statistically significant for severe LMD ($P_{interaction}$ 0.0008) and marginally significant for severe CAD ($P_{interaction}$ 0.05) (Table 2). Notably, the modification by gender of the association between divorce and severe CAD or LMD was qualitative such that divorce appeared to have an adverse effect in women and trended toward a decrease in severe CAD in men.

3.4. Number of Divorces and Coronary Artery Disease in Women. To further assess the relationship between divorce and severe CAD in women, we examined the association between number of divorces and severe CAD in women. In univariate analyses, there was a significant association

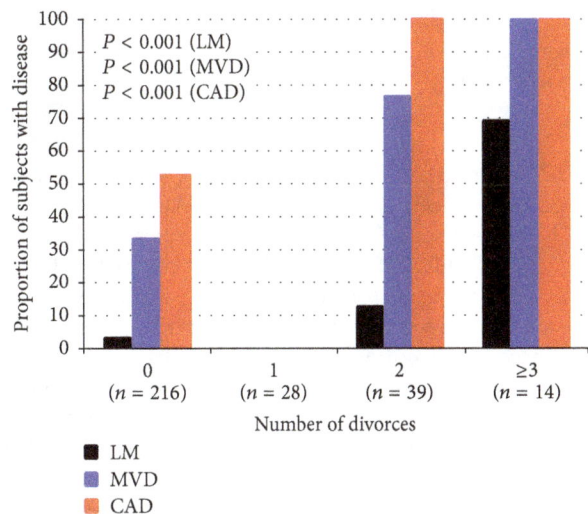

FIGURE 1: Relationship between number of divorces and severe CAD, MVD, and LMD in women.

between the number of divorces and severe CAD, MVD, and LMD in women (Figure 1). The adverse association between divorce and severe CAD appeared to be confined to women with multiple divorces, particularly those with 3 or more divorces, in whom the frequency of severe MVD and LMD was significantly higher than women with 1 or 2 divorces (Figure 1). After adjusting for baseline differences, there remained a significant association between number of divorces and severe CAD (OR 2.4 [95% CI 1.2, 4.5]), MVD (OR 2.0 [95% CI 1.4, 3.0]), and LMD (OR 3.4 [95% CI 1.9, 5.9]). In addition, the number of diseased coronary arteries differed significantly between divorced versus nondivorced women, with the former having a significantly higher rate of severe MVD (38% versus. 12%, $P < 0.001$) (Figure 2).

4. Discussion

Our study is the first to look at the association between divorce, including multiple divorces, and severe CAD using coronary angiography in men and women for clinical indications. After adjusting for baseline characteristics and indications for coronary angiogram, a number of observations were made. For women, there was a significant association between divorce, particularly multiple divorces, and severe

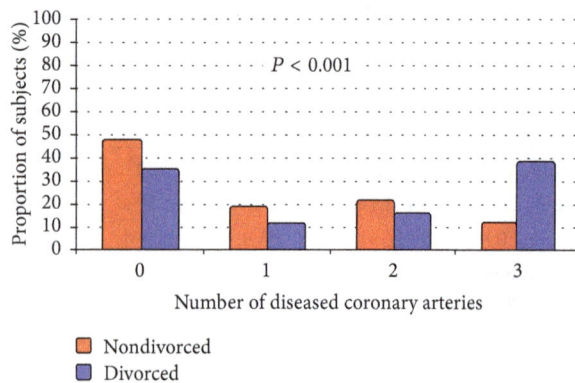

FIGURE 2: Number of diseased coronary arteries stratified by divorce status in women.

CAD, MVD, and LMD, while in men, there was no significant association between divorce and severe CAD.

The current statistics from the Ministry of Justice in the Kingdom of Saudi Arabia revealed that approximately 30% of married couples get divorced [16]. Rates of divorce and marriage are difficult to compare globally; many variables lead to differences between these rates, and cohabitation should be considered when comparing global rates. Data from an international report from the Social Trends Institute, the sustainable demographic dividend, demonstrated that the marriage rate in Saudi Arabia is 5.1 per 1000 adult population and in the UK is 4.4 and in the USA is 7.3. The divorce rate is 1.1 per 1000 adult population in Saudi Arabia, 2.4 in the UK, and 3.6 in the USA This may indicate global cultural differences, making it difficult to apply the results of this study globally [17].

Previous cross-sectional studies have examined the association between marital status and health outcomes [4–6]. Molloy et al. studied the extent to which known cardiovascular risk factors contribute to the association between marital status and cardiovascular mortality. They found that health behavior, psychological distress, and metabolic dysregulation contributed to cardiovascular risk in varying degrees [6]. A number of studies have shown divorce to have a negative impact on cardiovascular health [7–9, 14]. Venters et al. found that separated or divorced persons had the highest rates of hospitalization for heart attack and stroke [7]. In another study by Koskenvuo et al., effects of divorce as well as associations with social class were analyzed. They saw higher rates of ischemic heart disease among divorced persons and those in lower social classes [8]. The negative impact of divorce appears to be of limited duration. Adjustment to divorce seems to occur over several years. In women undergoing multiple divorces, the negative impact may have a longer relative duration, having been experienced multiple times over a limited period. Dupre et al. used prospective data to examine the associations between several marital trajectories, mortality, and potential factors contributing to the associations. They found complex associations between marital trajectories and mortality, including significantly higher hazard ratios for men and women currently divorced, women with multiple divorces, and men and women who were recently divorced (within 1–4 years). They found a

significantly lower risk of mortality among women divorced for 10 or more years, speculating that the stresses of divorce decline over time due to the ability to adjust to changes in socioeconomic resources, health behaviors, and health status challenges of divorce [9]. Multiple divorces provide the potential for increased financial, emotional, and social stress in needing to maintain multiple households. A recent study demonstrated that cumulative exposure to divorce increased the risks of myocardial infarction and women with multiple divorces were at an even higher risk [14]. However, this analysis of myocardial infarction was based on self-reported data, which may be less accurate than medical evaluation [18–21]. In traditional Middle Eastern societies, divorce produces significant emotional stress for women, more so than men. Such societies are primarily male-dominated with much greater challenges to social status, employment, and housing for divorced women. Community and family support are often minimal or absent for women going through divorce. This is in distinction from western societies, where women have lower levels of emotional stress after divorce than men. Recent societal developments, such as increased education and employment of women, may lessen such stressors, but they remain [22–24]. Diabetes, a traditional risk factor of coronary artery disease, was lower in divorced compared to nondivorced women. Other known traditional risk factors such as smoking, dyslipidemia, and hypertension were not significantly different. On the other hand, unemployment and low income levels, socioeconomic factors associated with coronary artery disease, were higher in divorced women. Multiple interrelated socioeconomic factors, such as unemployment, low income, and divorce status may produce a risk of severe coronary artery disease that meets or exceeds that of traditional risk factors such as diabetes [25].

Several explanations may contribute to the association between divorce, particularly multiple divorces and the severe CAD, MVD, and LMD in women. It is possible that following divorce, women delay seeking care for CAD related symptoms until it has progressed into more severe disease. This may be due to a less robust support system available to divorced women [26–28]. Divorce may additionally have a negative impact on a woman's economic and emotional well-being, which reduces her ability to prevent, detect, and treat cardiovascular-related illness [10–13]. The acute and chronic stress associated with divorce may also play a role [29, 30]. It is likely that biological mechanisms related to the stress of divorce can increase cortisol levels and hemoglobin A1C, may have a role in blood pressure reactivity, reduce sleep time, impair efforts to be physically active, and lead to poor dietary habits [6, 31–36]. Variability in plaque characteristics has recently been shown to correlate with the presentation of CAD. This variability may provide clues to the mechanisms of differential development and presentations of CAD in men and women. For example, culprit plaque rupture and thin-cap fibroatheroma (TCFA) are more prevalent in STEMI patients compared to patients with stable angina, for example. There are multiple factors that affect and increase the risk of plaque rupture. In one meta-analysis, TCFA and smoking were found to be the only predictors for plaque rupture. It would be interesting to compare the plaque burden and plaque rupture between divorced and nondivorced populations. An optical coherence tomography (OCT) study of such a cohort could potentially identify differences in plaque characteristics [37]. In addition, the emotional and economic turmoil a woman faces following a divorce may have negative consequences on adherence to instructions for disease management, including adherence to prescribed medications. This may lead to worsened vascular pathology [38–40]. Although divorce in men appeared to have a trend toward a decrease in severe LMD ($P_{\text{interaction}}$ 0.0008) and CAD ($P_{\text{interaction}}$ 0.05), the clinical significance remains unclear. Further studies are required to confirm our findings and to investigate the mechanism underlying these findings to help us identify possible interventions to reduce these risks.

Study strengths are that it is the first to look at the association between divorce, especially multiple divorces, and severe CAD using coronary angiography from Gulf Regions.

Study Limitations. Our study had an adequate sample size (1068), but the number of divorced subjects was small (124). The time intervals from divorce to the cardiac catheterization were not recorded; this interval may have influenced the findings. Failing to take into account this time interval and including a significant number of patients with a prior history of CAD (43%) may potentially lead to a reverse causality to the study results. Our study population was selected to undergo coronary angiography if clinically indicated, and, as such, cannot be generalized to all divorced subjects in a healthy population. Unmeasured confounding variables such as dietary habit, physical activity, level of intimacy, inflammatory or stress markers, or other unconsidered variables may have influenced the association.

5. Conclusion

Divorce, particularly multiple divorces, is associated with severe CAD, MVD, and LMD in women but not in men. However, future research studies need to measure the time from divorce to clinical presentation and to investigate the mechanism underlying these findings in men and women. Our recommendation from a clinical/public health standpoint is that perhaps programs should be considered to provide greater support to individuals when they become divorced and greater clinical monitoring is indicated.

Authors' Contributions

Amin Daoulah participated in study design; acquisition of the data; review of clinical records; analysis and interpretation of the data; drafting of the manuscript; and revision of the manuscript for important content. Alawi A. Alsheikh-Ali participated in data analysis and interpretation of the data and critical revision of the manuscript. All other authors participated equally in data collection and data reviewing.

Acknowledgments

The authors would like to sincerely thank all patients who agreed to participate in this study. The manuscript was presented at the Asia Pacific Society of Cardiology Congress in Abu Dhabi, United Arab Emirates (April 29–May 2 2015) and published in Global Heart Volume 10, Issue 2, Supplement, Pages e26 (APSC2015-1163).

References

[1] M. Heron, "Deaths, leading causes for, 2012," *National Vital Statistics Reports*, vol. 64, pp. 1–93, 2015.

[2] A. H. Mokdad, S. Jaber, M. I. Abdel Aziz et al., "The state of health in the Arab world, 1990-2010: An analysis of the burden of diseases, injuries, and risk factors," *The Lancet*, vol. 383, no. 9914, pp. 309–320, 2014.

[3] S. Yusuf, S. Hawken, S. Ounpuu et al., "INTERHEART Study Investigators. Effect of potentially modifiable risk factors associated with myocardial infarction in 52 countries (the INTERHEART study): case-control study," *Lancet*, vol. 364, no. 9438, pp. 937–952, 2004.

[4] M. Blom, A. Georgiades, K. D. László, H. Alinaghizadeh, I. Janszky, and S. Ahnve, "Work and marital status in relation to depressive symptoms and social support among women with coronary artery disease," *Journal of Women's Health*, vol. 16, no. 9, pp. 1305–1316, 2007.

[5] B. Lindegard and M. J. S. Langman, "Marital state, alcohol consumption, and liability to myocardial infarction, stroke, diabetes mellitus, or hypertension in men from Gothenburg," *British Medical Journal (Clinical Research Edition)*, vol. 291, no. 6508, pp. 1529–1533, 1985.

[6] G. J. Molloy, E. Stamatakis, G. Randall, and M. Hamer, "Marital status, gender and cardiovascular mortality: behavioural, psychological distress and metabolic explanations," *Social Science and Medicine*, vol. 69, no. 2, pp. 223–228, 2009.

[7] M. Venters, D. R. Jacobs Jr., P. Pirie, R. V. Luepker, A. R. Folsom, and R. F. Gillum, "Marital status and cardiovascular risk: the Minnesota heart survey and the Minnesota heart health program," *Preventive Medicine*, vol. 15, no. 6, pp. 591–605, 1986.

[8] M. Koskenvuo, J. Kaprio, M. Romo, and H. Langinvainio, "Incidence and prognosis of ischaemic heart disease with respect to marital status and social class. A national record linkage study," *Journal of Epidemiology and Community Health*, vol. 35, no. 3, pp. 192–196, 1981.

[9] M. E. Dupre, A. N. Beck, and S. O. Meadows, "Marital trajectories and mortality among US adults," *The American Journal of Epidemiology*, vol. 170, no. 5, pp. 546–555, 2009.

[10] M. E. Hughes and L. J. Waite, "Marital biography and health at mid-life," *Journal of Health and Social Behavior*, vol. 50, no. 3, pp. 344–358, 2009.

[11] A. E. Barrett, "Marital trajectories and mental health," *Journal of Health and Social Behavior*, vol. 41, no. 4, pp. 451–464, 2000.

[12] T. A. LaPierre, "The enduring effects of marital status on subsequent depressive symptoms among women: Investigating the roles of psychological, social and financial resources," *Journal of Epidemiology and Community Health*, vol. 66, no. 11, pp. 1056–1062, 2012.

[13] P. J. Smock, W. D. Manning, and S. Gupta, "The effect of marriage and divorce on women's economic well-being," *American Sociological Review*, vol. 64, no. 6, pp. 794–812, 1999.

[14] M. E. Dupre, L. K. George, G. Liu, and E. D. Peterson, "Association between divorce and risks for acute myocardial infarction," *Circulation: Cardiovascular Quality and Outcomes*, vol. 8, no. 3, pp. 244–251, 2015.

[15] A. Daoulah, A. Lotfi, M. Al-Murayeh et al., "Polygamy and risk of coronary artery disease in men undergoing angiography: an observational study," *International Journal of Vascular Medicine*, vol. 2017, Article ID 1925176, 6 pages, 2017.

[16] Saudi National Portal, "Saudi Reports and Statistics," 2007, https://www.saudi.gov.sa/wps/portal/saudi/aboutKingdom/reportsAndStatistics.

[17] W. Bradford, *The Sustainable Demographic Dividend: What Do Marriage and ertility Have to Do with the Economy*, Social Trends Institute, New York, NY, USA, 2011.

[18] Y. Okura, L. H. Urban, D. W. Mahoney, S. J. Jacobsen, and R. J. Rodeheffer, "Agreement between self-report questionnaires and medical record data was substantial for diabetes, hypertension, myocardial infarction, and stroke but not for heart failure," *Journal of Clinical Epidemiology*, vol. 57, no. 10, pp. 1096–1103, 2004.

[19] S. Tretli, P. G. Lund-Larsen, and O. P. Foss, "Reliability of questionnaire information on cardiovascular disease and diabetes: cardiovascular disease study in Finnmark county," *Journal of Epidemiology and Community Health*, vol. 36, no. 4, pp. 269–273, 1982.

[20] M. Machón, L. Arriola, N. Larrañaga et al., "Validity of self-reported prevalent cases of stroke and acute myocardial infarction in the Spanish cohort of the EPIC study," *Journal of Epidemiology and Community Health*, vol. 67, no. 1, pp. 71–75, 2013.

[21] S. D. Harlow and M. S. Linet, "Agreement between questionnaire data and medical records. The evidence for accuracy of recall," *American Journal of Epidemiology*, vol. 129, no. 2, pp. 233–248, 1989.

[22] M. M. Haj-Yahia, "Wife abuse and battering in the sociocultural context of Arab society," *Family Process*, vol. 39, no. 2, pp. 237–255, 2000.

[23] O. Cohen and R. Savaya, "Adjustment to divorce: A preliminary study among Muslim Arab citizens of Israel," *Family Process*, vol. 42, no. 2, pp. 269–290, 2003.

[24] O. Cohen and R. Savaya, ""Broken Glass": The Divorced Woman in Moslem Arab Society in Israel," *Family Process*, vol. 36, no. 3, pp. 225–245, 1997.

[25] A. Daoulah, O. E. Elkhateeb, S. A. Nasseri et al., "Socioeconomic factors and severity of coronary artery disease in patients undergoing coronary angiography: a multicentre study of arabian gulf states," *The Open Cardiovascular Medicine Journal*, vol. 11, no. 1, pp. 47–57, 2017.

[26] F. Rivero, T. Bastante, J. Cuesta et al., "Factors associated with delays in seeking medical attention in patients with ST-segment elevation acute coronary syndrome," *Revista Española de Cardiología (English Edition)*, vol. 69, no. 3, pp. 279–285, 2016.

[27] H. Alshahrani, R. McConkey, J. Wilson, M. Youssef, and D. Fitzsimons, "Female gender doubles pre-hospital delay times for patients experiencing ST segment elevation myocardial infarction in Saudi Arabia," *European Journal of Cardiovascular Nursing*, vol. 13, no. 5, pp. 399–407, 2014.

[28] M. Ferraz-Torres, T. Belzunegui-Otano, B. Marín-Fernandez, Ó. Martinez-Garcia, and B. Ibañez-Beroiz, "Differences in the treatment and evolution of acute coronary syndromes according to gender: What are the causes?" *Journal of Clinical Nursing*, vol. 24, no. 17-18, pp. 2468–2477, 2015.

[29] A. Steptoe and M. Kivimäki, "Stress and cardiovascular disease," *Nature Reviews Cardiology*, vol. 9, no. 6, pp. 360–370, 2012.

[30] K. Orth-Gomér, S. P. Wamala, M. Horsten, K. Schenck-Gustafsson, N. Schneiderman, and M. A. Mittleman, "Marital stress worsens prognosis in women with coronary heart disease: the Stockholm Female Coronary Risk Study," *The Journal of the American Medical Association*, vol. 284, no. 23, pp. 3008–3014, 2000.

[31] D. A. Sbarra, R. W. Law, L. A. Lee, and A. E. Mason, "Marital dissolution and blood pressure reactivity: evidence for the specificity of emotional intrusion-hyperarousal and task-rated emotional difficulty," *Psychosomatic Medicine*, vol. 71, no. 5, pp. 532–540, 2009.

[32] S. W. Tobe, A. Kiss, S. Sainsbury, M. Jesin, R. Geerts, and B. Baker, "The impact of job strain and marital cohesion on ambulatory blood pressure during 1 year: the double exposure study," *American Journal of Hypertension*, vol. 20, no. 2, pp. 148–153, 2007.

[33] M. S. Tryon, R. DeCant, and K. D. Laugero, "Having your cake and eating it too: a habit of comfort food may link chronic social stress exposure and acute stress-induced cortisol hyporesponsiveness," *Physiology and Behavior*, vol. 114-115, pp. 32–37, 2013.

[34] C. J. Roberts, I. C. Campbell, and N. Troop, "Increases in weight during chronic stress are partially associated with a switch in food choice towards increased carbohydrate and saturated fat intake," *European Eating Disorders Review*, vol. 22, no. 1, pp. 77–82, 2014.

[35] M. A. Stults-Kolehmainen and R. Sinha, "The effects of stress on physical activity and exercise," *Sports Medicine*, vol. 44, no. 1, pp. 81–121, 2014.

[36] T. L. Crain, L. B. Hammer, T. Bodner et al., "Work-family conflict, family-supportive supervisor behaviors (FSSB), and sleep outcomes," *Journal of Occupational Health Psychology*, vol. 19, no. 2, pp. 155–167, 2014.

[37] M. Iannaccone, G. Quadri, S. Taha et al., "Prevalence and predictors of culprit plaque rupture at OCT in patients with coronary artery disease: A meta-Analysis," *European Heart Journal Cardiovascular Imaging*, vol. 17, no. 10, pp. 1128–1137, 2016.

[38] J. R. Wu, T. A. Lennie, and M. L. Chung, "Medication adherence mediates the relationship between marital status and event-free survival in patients with heart failure," *Circulation*, vol. 120, article S516, 2009.

[39] G. J. Molloy, M. Hamer, G. Randall, and Y. Chida, "Marital status and cardiac rehabilitation attendance: a meta-analysis," *European Journal of Cardiovascular Prevention and Rehabilitation*, vol. 15, no. 5, pp. 557–561, 2008.

[40] R. Reviere and I. W. Eberstein, "Work, marital status, and heart disease," *Health Care for Women International*, vol. 13, no. 4, pp. 393–399, 1992.

6

Postinfarct Left Ventricular Remodelling: A Prevailing Cause of Heart Failure

Alessio Galli and Federico Lombardi

Cardiovascular Diseases Unit, Fondazione IRCCS Ca' Granda Ospedale Maggiore Policlinico, Department of Clinical and Community Sciences, University of Milan, Via F. Sforza 35, 20122 Milan, Italy

Correspondence should be addressed to Alessio Galli; aleg170389@gmail.com

Academic Editor: Stephan von Haehling

Heart failure is a chronic disease with high morbidity and mortality, which represents a growing challenge in medicine. A major risk factor for heart failure with reduced ejection fraction is a history of myocardial infarction. The expansion of a large infarct scar and subsequent regional ventricular dilatation can cause postinfarct remodelling, leading to significant enlargement of the left ventricular chamber. It has a negative prognostic value, because it precedes the clinical manifestations of heart failure. The characteristics of the infarcted myocardium predicting postinfarct remodelling can be studied with cardiac magnetic resonance and experimental imaging modalities such as diffusion tensor imaging can identify the changes in the architecture of myocardial fibers. This review discusses all the aspects related to postinfarct left ventricular remodelling: definition, pathogenesis, diagnosis, consequences, and available therapies, together with experimental interventions that show promising results against postinfarct remodelling and heart failure.

1. Introduction

The number of persons surviving an acute coronary syndrome has increased in the last decade [1], as a consequence of several improvements in the care of patients: more effective therapies, the development of a network of emergency intervention, door-to-balloon time of 90 minutes or less in the growing number of hospitals equipped to perform a primary percutaneous coronary intervention (PPCI) and better understanding of alarm symptoms of coronary heart disease among people [2–5]. All these elements contribute to reduce the loss of viable myocardial tissue in patients with myocardial infarction. However, in spite of a significant reduction in short-term mortality in patients with myocardial infarction, it has been observed an increase in long-term morbidity due to chronic heart disease, as shown by the statistics of hospital discharges for heart failure in the United States in the last 30 years (from about 440.000 in 1980 to 1.023.000 in 2010) [1].

In the United States, it is estimated that about 860.000 persons survive a first or recurrent heart attack every year

[1], leading to an equal increase in the number of patients at risk of developing heart failure, the disease with the highest social and economic cost in western countries (57.757 deaths with $31 billion per year in the United States) [1]. Heart failure is a chronic and progressive disease characterized by a symptomatic impairment in cardiac function [6]. 5.1 million adult Americans live with it, and it is estimated that by 2030 more than 8 million adults living in the United States will have heart failure. Mortality is high, reaching 50% at 5 years from diagnosis of heart failure [1]. Heart failure is divided into two categories: heart failure with reduced ejection fraction (HFrEF), accounting for 50 to 70% of cases, and heart failure with preserved ejection fraction (HFpEF). A left ventricular ejection fraction (LVEF) $\geq$ 50% discriminates HFpEF from HFrEF, indicating a diastolic dysfunction more than systolic dysfunction [7].

The American Heart Association and the American College of Cardiology jointly released a classification of chronic heart failure based on four stages, with disease severity increasing from the first to the fourth stage [8]. Stage A is the presence of risk factors for heart failure without structural heart disease, stage B is the presence of a structural heart disease without symptoms, stage C is symptomatic heart failure, and stage D is symptomatic heart failure that is refractory to medical therapy. Structural heart diseases include ventricular hypertrophy in hypertensive patients, valvular diseases, cardiomyopathies, and scars due to previous myocardial infarctions [8]. Notwithstanding a reduction of about 50% of infarct size with modern revascularization strategies as compared with no reperfusion [9], heart failure develops within 5 years of a first myocardial infarction in 8% of men and 18% of women between 45 and 64 years of age [1]. As the incidence of heart failure increases with age, it is likely that the higher incidence in women is due to an older age at the time of first myocardial infarction [1]. Animal models of myocardial infarction and cardiac imaging on patients with ischemic cardiomyopathy revealed that heart failure is preceded by an increase in ventricular volumes [10, 11]. This process has been termed postinfarct ventricular remodelling, and it implies an enlargement of left ventricular chamber, which passes from an elliptical to a more spherical shape [10]. This change is described by an increase in sphericity index [12], that is, the ratio between the actual left ventricular volume and the volume of a sphere whose diameter is equal to the major axis of the left ventricle. Normal values for sphericity index are 0.29 ± 0.7 at end diastole and 0.15 ± 0.8 at end systole [13].

It is known that chronic β adrenergic stimulation and renin-angiotensin system activation promote postinfarct remodelling, and long-term use of drugs that inhibit these two pathways is nowadays the best strategy to prevent heart failure in patients with a history of myocardial infarction [6, 8].

The knowledge of mechanical and molecular factors leading to ventricular remodelling could guide the development of new targeted therapies against heart failure.

2. Definition and Pathogenesis

2.1. Definition and Diagnosis of Postinfarct Ventricular Remodelling. Postinfarct ventricular remodelling develops in about 30% patients with a history of myocardial infarction [14]. As remodelling depends on infarct size [15, 16], it is likely that its prevalence is higher in the subgroup of patients without any or successful reperfusion. In a recent survey on patients admitted to 80% of the intensive coronary care units of Italian hospitals, only 60% of patients with ST-elevation acute coronary syndromes could be treated with reperfusion [17].

Ventricular remodelling is a predictor of heart failure, and for this reason it assumes a negative prognostic value [10].

An arbitrary definition of ventricular remodelling, but widely adopted in follow-up studies [18, 19], is an increase of at least 20% of left ventricular end-diastolic ventricular volume (LVEDV) from the first postinfarction imaging. However, as the first imaging study with cardiac magnetic resonance is usually performed a few days after myocardial infarction, early ventricular remodelling, which is the phase of remodelling that occurs in the first hours after myocardial infarction, could not be recognized, leading to an underestimation of the final ventricular dilatation [14].

Left ventricular remodelling is characterized by a progressive increase in both end-diastolic (LVEDV) and end-systolic volumes (LVESV). The increase in LVESV can precede the increase in LVEDV, as a consequence of an impaired systolic function that causes a reduction in stroke volume [14, 20].

The imaging modalities used to noninvasively assess ventricular volumes and function are echocardiography, radionuclide ventriculography, and cardiac magnetic resonance (CMR) [21]. In particular, cine CMR is the preferred method because it allows for a more accurate estimate of cardiac volumes, but it is not yet available in all hospitals [22, 23].

Ventricular volumes are best expressed as volume indices, which are obtained by dividing the volumes by the body surface area. Normal values for LVEDVI and LVESVI are $75 \pm 20\,\mathrm{mL/m^2}$ and $25 \pm 7\,\mathrm{mL/m^2}$, respectively, [24]. Volume indices allow for a reduction in interindividual variance that also depends on wider ventricular chambers in men than women [24, 25].

A reduction in left ventricular ejection fraction (LVEF) is often observed during postinfarct remodelling, predicting heart failure and increased mortality. Normal values of LVEF are $67 \pm 8\%$ [21] and depend on a preserved global systolic function [10, 26]. However, initial ventricular remodelling is not always associated with a reduction in LVEF, as this measure of systolic function can remain unchanged or even increase in the months following an acute myocardial infarction, even in the presence of an enlargement of ventricular chambers [27].

2.2. Pathogenesis. Ventricular remodelling accompanies different heart diseases, such as dilatative nonischemic cardiomyopathy and cardiac hypertrophy in chronic hypertension and implies a change in myocardial anatomical structure [28]. Postinfarct remodelling is a specific type of left ventricular remodelling that is a consequence of an increase in both preload and afterload causing an enlargement of ventricular chamber and a hypertrophy of normal myocardium [28]. The increase in preload is sustained by the phenomenon of infarct expansion, which is an enlargement of infarct scar [29]. This causes a regional increase in the ventricular volume subtended by the expanded infarcted myocardial wall.

In infarcted myocardium, ventricular contraction is not symmetrical, because the necrotic segments have lost their contractility [30]. As a result, the force generated by the normal remote myocardium during contraction is not counterbalanced by an equal and opposite force, and the infarcted ventricular wall is thus stretched by an increased wall tension that is not homogeneously distributed in the left ventricle [31] (Figure 1). This phenomenon might explain why the infarcted wall usually has longer contraction times than the healthy remote myocardium. In effect, the infarcted wall has to counteract a greater resultant force, and its prolonged time to peak systolic velocity can be detected as an asynchrony of ventricular wall motion [32]. This wall motion defect has been recognized as a risk factor for the development of remodelling, and it can be assessed with echocardiography or cine CMR [33, 34].

It is likely that some segments might recover a normal or near normal contractility in the months after myocardial

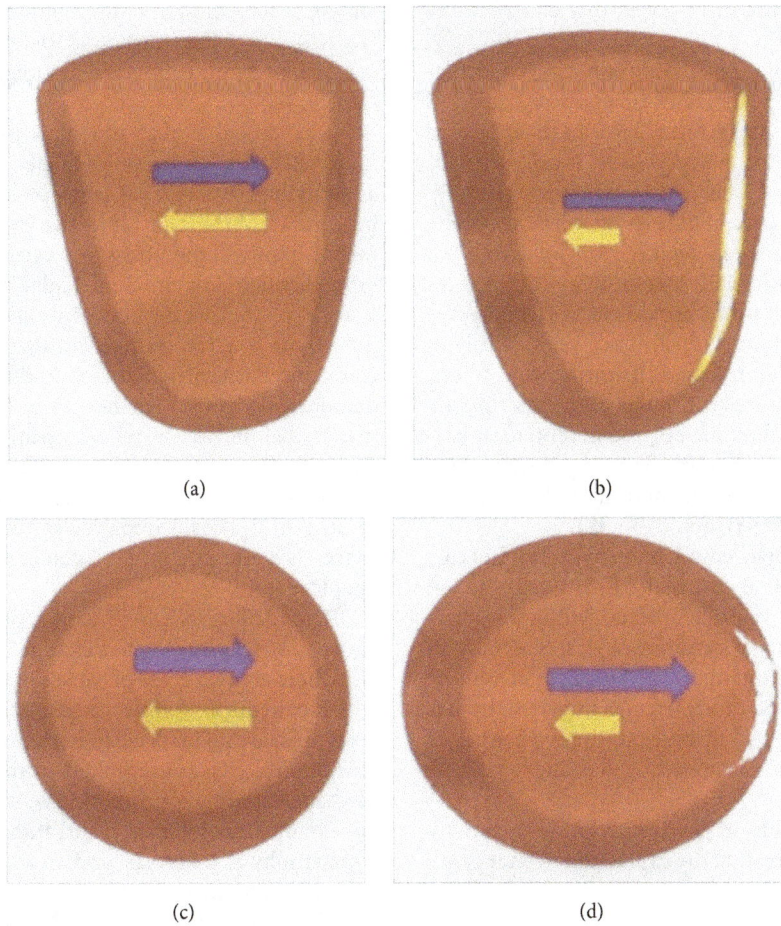

FIGURE 1: In a normal ventricle, the force generated by myocardial contraction is balanced (a and c). When there is an infarct scar (white), the infarcted segment is stretched by the force generated by the remote normal myocardium (b and d). As a result, the infarct scar expands and the infarcted wall becomes thinner, while the remote myocardium becomes hypertrophic to maintain a normal global cardiac function (d). Arrows indicate the vectors of forces generated by opposite left ventricular segments during systole.

infarction [30], because of the end of myocardial stunning [9, 35]. This is a reversible form of ischemia-reperfusion injury consisting in a dysfunction of myocardial tissue in the salvaged area at risk. As it is reversible, it is improbable that myocardial stunning contributes to ventricular remodelling. However, in transmural infarcts, some segments can remain hypokinetic, akinetic, or dyskinetic in areas where irreversible injury took place, causing a permanent regional ventricular dysfunction [30].

To maintain a normal stoke volume with a reduced number of normally working myocardial segments, the healthy myocardium has to produce a greater pressure [28]. The increase in workload (afterload) on healthy myocardium causes a hypertrophy of cardiomyocytes [28]. This phenomenon has been observed both in animal models of myocardial infarction [36] and more recently in men, using diffusion CMR tractography [37, 38]. Tractography with cardiac magnetic resonance has been recently introduced as a novel experimental imaging that allows for an in vivo study of the structure of the myocardial fibers that compose the ventricular wall [21, 39].

Diffusion CMR is capable of detecting the direction of H_2O molecules diffusing in solution. Direction of myocardial fibers can thus be identified, because water mainly diffuses along the major axis of cardiomyocytes [21, 39].

The ventricular wall is composed of three layers of fibers with different orientation that rotate from the subepicardial to the subendocardial layer by almost 180° [21, 39].

The external layer is composed of left-handed helical fibers that constitute the anterior basal and the posterior apical portions of the left ventricle and encircle the ventricular chamber with an orientation between −90° and −30°, having its long axis as 0° [21, 39]. Subendocardial fibers have an opposite orientation, with a course from the posterior basal segments of the left ventricle to the anterior apical wall. Subendocardial fibers are right-handed helical fibers and make with the long axis of the ventricle an axis between +30° and +90° [21, 39]. Fibers in the midmyocardial wall, between the subepicardial and the subendocardial layers, are circumferential and are parallel to the short axis of the left ventricle [21, 39]. In noninfarcted heart, the thickness of fibers is similar between the three layers that compose the ventricular wall [21, 37–39].

After a myocardial infarction, diffusion CMR tractography evidences the disappearance of subendocardial fibers and a hypertrophy of the subepicardial layer in the infarcted segments [37–39]. However, the hypertrophy is not sufficient to prevent the thinning of infarcted ventricular wall [12]. The areas with no fibers correspond to infarct scar, where dead cardiomyocytes have been replaced by collagen [39]. Traditional CMR can identify with precision this area of irreversible myocardial injury, which appears as delayed hyperenhancement with gadolinium. Postinfarct remodelling is characterized by a structural change in myocardial fibers, which is present not only in ventricular segments directly damaged by myocardial infarction, but also in remote, apparently healthy, myocardial regions. In effect, in patients with a previous myocardial infarction, subendocardial fibers in the remote myocardium are hypertrophic [37, 38].

In postinfarct ventricular remodelling, hypertrophic cardiomyocytes are longer than normal cardiac cells. In an animal model, postinfarct ventricular remodelling was characterized by a lengthening of cardiomyocytes especially in the area surrounding the infarct scar, but also in remote myocardium [36]. This type of ventricular hypertrophy has been termed eccentric and contributes to the worsening of ventricular dilatation during remodelling. It is due to volume overload [28].

Cardiomyocytes modify their transcriptional activity during remodelling, reactivating the expression of fetal genes that are normally silenced during adult life [40]. These include genes encoding for structural heart proteins, which allow for the lengthening of cardiomyocytes through the addition of new sarcomeres in series [41]. Myofibrils undergo a qualitative alteration, because cardiomyocytes reduce the synthesis of isoform α of myosin heavy chain (α-MHC) to increase the production of isoform β (β-MHC) [40, 42]. This change is associated not only with a reduced energetic requirement to cardiac muscle, but also with a reduced contractility of sarcomeres [43]. The force generated by each contractile unit is further decreased by the reduction in the mean number of myofibrils per sarcomere [44].

HDAC inhibitors (HDACi) are a class of anticancer drugs designed to modulate gene expression in cancer cells [45]. In animal models, HDACi were also effective against pathologic cardiac hypertrophy [45, 46]. Treatment with HDACi blocked the fetal cardiac gene program that is activated in heart failure and increased the ratio of α-MHC to β-MHC [46]. The knowledge of the transcriptional changes associated with ventricular remodelling and heart failure might prompt the discovery of new drugs capable of modulating the expression of specific genes involved in the disease, possibly with limited untoward effects.

As heart has poor, if not absent, regenerative capacity, cardiac hypertrophy that occurs during postinfarct remodelling is accompanied by an increase in extracellular matrix, which is mainly constituted by collagen [47, 48]. This phenomenon is due to an increased activity of cardiac fibroblasts in response to different soluble fibrogenic mediators, such as transforming growth factor-β (TGF-β) and systemic and local activation of renin-angiotensin-aldosterone system (RAAS) [28]. The mediators of the RAAS that promote ventricular remodelling are angiotensin II and aldosterone [28].

It is probable that the increase in wall stress in the infarcted heart that becomes dilated during remodelling [31], as described by Laplace's law, accelerates collagen synthesis by cardiac fibroblasts [28]. The expansion of extracellular matrix reduces the stress on cardiomyocytes, but on the other hand it impairs ventricular function [28]. In effect, a negative correlation between extracellular matrix volume in remote myocardium quantified by contrast-enhanced CMR and left ventricular ejection fraction (LVEF) has been demonstrated [48]. Furthermore, the extent of interstitial myocardial fibrosis correlates positively with mortality [49]. An excess of extracellular matrix becomes maladaptive when diffusion of oxygen, fatty acids, and glucose from capillaries to cardiomyocytes is impaired by an increased extravascular space. Chronic deficit of oxygen can lead cardiomyocytes to apoptosis [50].

Remodelling is a pathologic process that involves the entire ventricle, leading to a change in its global structure [10, 28]. There are two types of causes of remodelling: mechanical and biochemical. While mechanical causes, as previously described, are an increase in both preload and afterload [28], biochemical causes are linked to the production of soluble mediators capable of promoting ventricular remodelling [28]. For example, angiotensin II and aldosterone stimulate cardiac hypertrophy and fibrosis, and an increase in catecholamines helps to maintain a normal cardiac output in front of the contractile dysfunction of infarcted segments [28, 44, 51]. Many other soluble factors are produced by cardiac cells in response to various types of potential damage, for example, ischemia-reperfusion injury [52, 53] or mechanical strain [54]. This explains the link between mechanical and biochemical causes of postinfarct remodelling.

Chronic volume overload and increased adrenergic tone promote metalloproteinases activity [55]. These proteolytic enzymes break down collagen cross-links, thus weakening myocardial wall and worsening ventricular chamber dilatation [28]. MMP-9 probably is the most important metalloproteinase involved in ventricular remodelling [56]. It has been suggested that collagen degradation during postinfarct remodelling is due to an imbalance between the activity of matrix metalloproteinases and tissue inhibitors of matrix metalloproteinases, in particular of TIMP-1 and TIMP-2 [57]. Increased plasma levels of MMPs, TIMPs, and collagen-derived peptides have been detected in patients with postinfarct ventricular remodelling, indicating an increased collagen turnover [56–58].

Cardiomyocytes become hypertrophic in response to integrin-mediated mechanotransduction [54] and soluble factors produced during myocardial stress [28]. Some of these ligands are growth factors with a protective role, promoting cell survival upon activation of tyrosine kinase receptors (Table 1) [28, 59]. Other ligands have a dual activity, with either adaptive or maladaptive roles, depending on concentration and duration of stress (Table 1) [28]. For example, angiotensin II can promote cell survival through the

TABLE 1: Molecular pathways of ventricular remodelling. Many mediators have either an adaptive role (in bold) at low doses or a maladaptive role, with chronic/intense stimulation.

	Molecular pathways activated by interaction with receptor	Effects on cardiomyocytes
Soluble mediator		
Angiotensin II [28]	JNK **ERK**	Apoptosis Cell survival and growth
ROS [28, 60]	Cell damage **JAK/STAT**	Apoptosis Cell survival and growth
TNF-α [28, 61, 62]	NF-κB **NF-κB**	Apoptosis Cell survival and growth
Growth factors (IGF-1, PDGF, GDF-15, HGF, and NRG-1) [28, 59, 63, 64]	**PI3K/AKT** **RAS/RAF/MEK/ERK**	Cell survival and growth
Cardiotrophin-1 [28, 65]	**JAK/STAT**	Cell survival and growth
Cytosolic calcium [59, 66, 67]	Calpains (calcium-activated proteases) **Calcineurin/NFAT**	Apoptosis Cell survival and growth
Catecholamines [68, 69] (β-adrenergic signalling)	PKA **ERK**	Apoptosis Cell survival and growth
Mechanical sensing of myocardial stretch		
Integrins [54]	**FAK**	Cell survival and growth

JNK: Jun N-terminal kinase; ERK: extracellular-regulated kinase; JAK/STAT: Janus kinase/signal transducers and activators of transcription; ROS: reactive oxygen species; TNF-α: tumor necrosis factor-α; TRADD: TNF receptor-associated death domain; NF-κB: nuclear factor-κB; IGF-1: insulin-like growth factor-1; PDGF: platelet-derived growth factor; GDF-15: growth differentiation factor-15; HGF: hepatocyte growth factor; NRG-1: neuregulin-1; PI3K/AKT: phosphatidylinositol 3-kinase/AKT; NFAT: nuclear factor of activated T cells; PKA: protein kinase A; FAK: focal adhesion kinase.

pathway of the extracellular-regulated kinase (ERK), but an excess of the angiotensin receptor activity during ventricular remodelling leads to the activation of the Jun N-terminal kinase (JNK) pathway and consequently to cardiomyocyte apoptosis [28]. Like angiotensin II, other mediators with dual activity have growth-promoting effects on cardiomyocytes at low doses, but they cause apoptosis at high concentrations or with chronic exposure [28].

3. Predictors of Remodelling

3.1. Predictors of Postinfarct Ventricular Remodelling. Ventricular remodelling usually develops in patients with a history of ST segment elevation myocardial infarction (STEMI), which produces an infarct scar with a transmural extent [15]. There are many predictors of ventricular remodelling that can be assessed with different cardiac imaging modalities. Patients who develop postinfarct left ventricular remodelling usually have a greater LVESV and a lower LVEF as postinfarct baseline characteristics [16]. The best independent predictor of left ventricular remodelling is infarct size, which can be quantified as the percentage of left ventricular mass with late gadolinium enhancement on CMR images [15, 83]. Anterior infarcts are usually larger, because the anterior interventricular branch of the left coronary artery is the most important arteriosus vessel to the heart.

During an acute myocardial infarction, plasma levels of cardiac troponins and creatine kinase-MB positively correlate with infarct size determined by CMR, and very high levels predict an increase in ventricular volumes and a reduction in

LVEF [20, 84]. A 10% increase in cardiac mortality for every 10% increment in infarct size has been estimated [85].

It is believed that heart failure develops when at least 25% of the left ventricular myocardial mass is lost [5]. The greatest number of cardiomyocytes dies during an acute myocardial infarction or during reperfusion, as a consequence of ischemia-reperfusion lethal injury [9, 35], but cardiomyocytes can also undergo apoptosis because of the chronic myocardial stress of postinfarct remodelling [86].

Other predictors of ventricular remodelling are the irreversible forms of ischemia-reperfusion injury of the cardiac microvasculature, which are microvascular obstruction (MVO) and intramyocardial hemorrhage (IMH) [87–90].

MVO is identified as a hypointense area within the infarcted myocardium on CMR images of early and late gadolinium enhancement (Figure 2) [91–94]. This phenomenon, that is, the no-reflow of myocardial tissue, can be observed in up to 50% of patients with STEMI [94]. In many studies, it has been diagnosed as a low angiographic myocardial blush/perfusion grade, or a ST segment resolution <70% after primary percutaneous coronary intervention [92–94].

IMH is associated with a large infarct size and a large area of MVO [95]. Its presence and extension can be assessed with CMR using T2* mapping, because of the superparamagnetic properties of iron-containing hemoglobin degradation products that reduce myocardial signal in the hemorrhagic area [87, 95, 96]. The association between IMH and postinfarct remodelling might be explained by chronic inflammation and impaired healing of infarcted tissue [97], owing to the presence of a chronic iron deposit within the necrotic

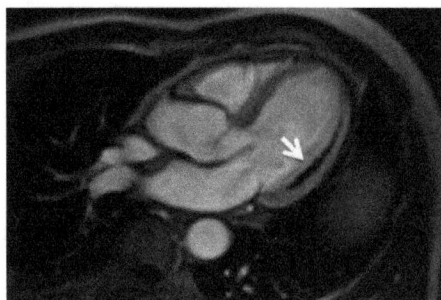

FIGURE 2: Microvascular obstruction (arrow) as shown by early gadolinium enhancement in a patient with acute myocardial infarction (CMR study).

myocardium [98]. Free iron catalyzes the production of free radicals, which cause oxidative stress [99]. Furthermore, the intramyocardial hemorrhage seems to worsen the systolic dysfunction of infarcted segments, promoting infarct expansion and ventricular dilatation [100].

MVO and IMH are also independent predictors of major adverse cardiac events (MACE), including cardiac death, stroke, myocardial infarction, and hospitalization for heart failure: hazard ratio (HR) for MVO is 2.79 (95% CI: 1.25–6.25, $p = 0.012$) [101], and HR for IMH is 1.17 (95% CI: 1.03–1.33, $p = 0.01$) [89].

After a myocardial infarction, the most frequent of the posterior basal segments, a dysfunction of a papillary muscle can occur, leading to a mitral regurgitation [14, 28]. The blood volume of the regurgitation increases the ventricular preload, contributing to remodelling. For this reason, a clinically significant mitral regurgitation is a risk factor for postinfarct ventricular remodelling [28, 102]. The progressive enlargement of the ventricular chamber worsens further the function of the mitral valve, through the dilatation of the mitral annulus [14, 28].

The presence of an aortic stenosis or hypertension may worsen postinfarct left ventricular remodelling [103, 104]. These conditions are associated with an increase in afterload, which contributes to hypertrophic remodelling of myocardial wall. It has been shown that replacement of a severely stenotic aortic valve and therapy to lower blood pressure in hypertensive patients could ameliorate concentric left ventricular hypertrophy [105, 106], but there are no data on postinfarct remodelling.

3.2. Biomarkers of Ventricular Remodelling. Cardiac magnetic resonance, which is the preferred imaging modality for the assessment of ventricular volumes and function, has been used to validate several putative biomarkers of ventricular remodelling. However, the clinical role of these biomarkers in predicting postinfarct remodelling needs further investigation.

A positive correlation has been found between ventricular remodelling and plasma levels of some enzymes that contribute to extracellular matrix remodelling, such as matrix metalloproteinases (MMP-2 and MMP-9) and tissue inhibitors of metalloproteinases (TIMPs) [58, 107].

Other plasma proteins whose levels positively correlate with ventricular remodelling are tissue plasminogen activator (t-PA) [58], a fibrinolytic enzyme that might play a causative role in postreperfusion intramyocardial hemorrhage [108] and that might contribute to extracellular matrix remodelling [109], terminal peptides derived from procollagen [58], some markers of systemic inflammation such as interleukin-1β and C-reactive protein (CRP) [58, 110], and some growth factors, such as hepatocyte growth factor (HGF), and growth differentiation factor-15 (GDF-15) [58].

The atrial natriuretic peptide (ANP), the brain natriuretic peptide (BNP), and the N-terminal fragment of its precursor (NT-proBNP) are produced by cardiomyocytes, and their blood levels increase with increasing myocardial wall stretch. In addition to their well known prognostic value in patients with heart failure, high levels of natriuretic peptides or NT-proBNP after myocardial infarction predict an increase in ventricular volumes, which is postinfarct remodelling [58, 108].

4. Consequences of Postinfarct Remodelling

Parameters that define left ventricular remodelling are consolidated surrogate end points [10]. In a meta-analysis, therapies that reduce end-systolic and end-diastolic volume, or that increase left ventricular ejection fraction, improve survival of patients. The use of surrogate end points in clinical trials is often advantageous, because it may render necessary fewer patients to demonstrate a statistically significant efficacy of one treatment. However, conclusions in clinical trials should never be based only on surrogate end points, but also on clinical events such as death or hospitalization for heart failure.

When a patient develops postinfarct left ventricular remodelling, he is at increased risk of heart failure or sudden death due to a lethal arrhythmia [11]. The qualitative alteration of left ventricular geometry and myocardial structure, together with increased fibrosis, predispose to anomalies in potential conduction that can result in reentrant arrhythmias [111]. Furthermore, the cellular changes that supervene during remodelling might increase the electrical automatism of ventricular myocytes [112]. Calcium overload in the cytosol is a trigger for arrhythmias sustained by afterdepolarizations, which are anomalous depolarizations that follow the normal action potential of cardiomyocytes [113]. They are often referred to as triggered activity [113].

Eccentric hypertrophy, as that observed during postinfarct ventricular remodelling, is associated with a threefold increase in the risk of major adverse cardiac events, including death from cardiovascular causes, reinfarction, heart failure, stroke, and cardiac arrest (HR: 3.1; 95% CI: 1.9–4.8, $p < 0.01$) [11]. Ventricular end-diastolic and end-systolic volumes directly correlate with mortality and rate of hospitalization for heart failure: Solomon and coworkers reported a hazard ratio of 1.06 (95% CI: 1.02–1.11, $p = 0.009$) per 10 mL increase in end-diastolic volume and of 1.11 (95% CI: 1.04–1.19, $p = 0.001$) per 10 mL increase in end-systolic volume [70]. Heart failure that develops following postinfarct remodelling is characterized by a reduced ejection fraction, because the

TABLE 2: Therapies capable of inducing reverse remodelling.

	Mechanism of action	Notes
Class of drugs		
ACE inhibitors/ARBs [70, 71]	RAAS antagonism	
Antialdosterone diuretics [72]	RAAS antagonism	
β-blockers [73]	Reduce cardiotoxic effects of chronic β-adrenergic stimulation and improve heart responsiveness to physiological adrenergic stimulation	
NO donors plus hydralazine [74]	Increase cGMP and reduce preload	
MMPs inhibitors [75]	Inhibit ECM remodelling	Experimental. No evidences in humans
rNRG-1 [76, 77]	Promotes cardiomyocyte survival pathways	Experimental
Type of mechanical intervention		
CRT [44, 78]	Increases GSK-3β activity and improves LV contractility	Eligibility: patients with symptomatic HF and LBBB
LVAD [44, 79]	Reduces LV workload	Eligibility: patients with severe HF as bridge to recovery or bridge to heart transplant
Mitral valve surgery [80]	Reduces LV workload	Eligibility: patients with severe mitral regurgitation
Diastolic cardiac restraint devices [81, 82]	Reduce myocardial wall tension	Experimental

ACE: angiotensin-converting enzyme; ARBs: angiotensin receptor blockers; RAAS: renin-angiotensin-aldosterone system; NO nitric oxide; cGMP: cyclic guanosine monophosphate; MMPs: matrix metalloproteinases; ECM: extracellular matrix; rNRG-1: recombinant human neuregulin-1; CRT: cardiac resynchronization therapy; GSK-3β: glycogen synthase kinase-3β; LV: left ventricle; HF: heart failure; LBBB: left bundle branch block; LVAD: left ventricular assist device.

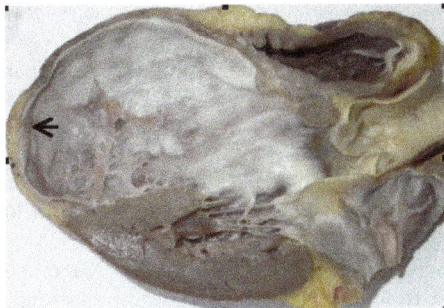

FIGURE 3: The expansion of a wide anterior and transmural infarct scar often leads to the formation of an apical left ventricular aneurysm that predisposes to left ventricular thrombosis. In this case, postinfarct remodelling is characterized by a great apical dilatation of the left ventricular chamber, together with a thinning of the infarcted segments (arrow).

infarcted myocardium has a suboptimal systolic function. A 5-unit decrease in LVEF is associated with about 30% increase in the risk of death or hospitalization for heart failure (HR: 1.29; 95% CI: 1.14–1.49, $p < 0.001$) [70].

Infarct scar expansion during postinfarct remodelling sometimes causes a great regional dilatation of ventricular chamber, which is a ventricular aneurysm (Figure 3). This process is usually observed with wide myocardial infarctions in the territory of the anterior interventricular artery. The myocardial wall of the ventricular aneurysm is constituted by the transmural infarct scar, with infarcted segments that are akinetic or dyskinetic [114].

The slow blood flow in the cavity of the ventricular aneurysm can lead to the formation of an intracardiac thrombus. Among 100 patients with an anterior ST segment elevation myocardial infarction and LVEF <40%, 27 patients had a left ventricular thrombus, as assessed by contrast-enhanced CMR [115]. A left ventricular thrombus is asymptomatic in the majority of cases, but it is associated with a low but significant risk of systemic thromboembolism (10–15% of cases), including strokes and transient ischemic attacks [114]. For this reason, patients with an intracardiac thrombus should be treated with anticoagulants [114].

5. Therapies against Postinfarct Remodelling

There are clinical evidences that postinfarct remodelling can be prevented or, in some cases, reversed [44]. This process has been termed reverse remodelling, and it could be accomplished with either pharmacologic or mechanical interventions, or with a combined approach. While mechanical approaches require surgery and are reserved to patients with symptomatic heart failure who meet strict eligibility criteria, drugs are the preferred strategy for treating patients with mild heart failure or for preventing postinfarct ventricular remodelling. Table 2 summarizes the current therapies that are capable of inducing reverse remodelling, together with some of the experimental interventions that have been effective in pilot trials.

Angiotensin-converting enzyme inhibitors (ACEi) and angiotensin receptor blockers (ARBs) have consolidated efficacy as antiremodelling drugs [70, 71], because of their action as antagonists of the renin-angiotensin-aldosterone system (RAAS) that plays a major causative role in ventricular fibrosis. A combined therapy with an ACEi or an ARB and an antialdosterone diuretic is more effective than a monotherapy in reversing remodelling [71].

The recent PARADIGM-HF multicenter randomized controlled trial [116] tested a drug that is a combination of the ARB valsartan and the neprilysin inhibitor sacubitril on 8399 patients with heart failure and a reduced LVEF, reporting a reduction of 20% in death from cardiovascular causes or hospitalization for heart failure as compared with the ACE inhibitor enalapril alone at maximum dosage ($p < 0.001$). Neprilysin is and endopeptidase that degrades several vasoactive peptides, such as natriuretic peptides, bradykinin, and adrenomedullin [116]. It is likely that increasing all these substances in blood through neprilysin inhibition protects the heart from remodelling, in particular when it is associated with the inhibition of the RAAS. It is desirable that a meta-analysis of large clinical trials confirms the efficacy and safety of this new combined approach, before it enters clinical practice in the management of heart failure.

Together with ACEi, ARBs and antialdosterone diuretics, β-blockers are the current mainstay of pharmacologic therapy against postinfarct remodelling [73].

Adrenergic stimulation allows for the maintenance of an adequate global cardiac function after acute myocardial infarction, by increasing the contractility of viable myocardium. However, chronic β-adrenergic overstimulation has cardiotoxic effects, leading to left ventricular dilatation and systolic dysfunction [68, 69]. β-blockers might improve autonomic control of failing heart by increasing the number of β-receptors on cardiomyocytes and by modulating their activity [44, 117]. Apart from its beneficial effects on remodelling, a long-term therapy with β-blockers reduces mortality after an acute myocardial infarction, by reducing the risk of a lethal arrhythmia [118].

Nitric oxide (NO) donors such as nitrates have well known beneficial effects in patients with heart failure [44, 74] and might induce reverse remodelling by reducing the preload, as well as increasing cyclic guanosine monophosphate (cGMP) in cardiomyocytes [44, 119]. cGMP protects cardiac cells from apoptosis [44, 119, 120].

As the major risk factor for postinfarct remodelling is infarct size [20], therapies against ischemia-reperfusion injury during acute coronary syndromes should be expected to prevent postinfarct remodelling. As a proof of concept, experimental therapies that improve myocardial salvage during PPCI, such as cyclosporine and ischemic postconditioning, have been associated with maintenance of left ventricular volumes, but larger confirmatory trials are required [121].

Other promising approaches are stem cells and gene therapy, which have shown interesting results in pilot trials on adjunctive therapy of myocardial infarction and heart failure, and that might reverse postinfarct remodelling [5, 122].

6. Conclusions

Therapies with proven efficacy against postinfarct remodelling exist, and research is bringing new discoveries in the pathogenesis of postinfarct remodelling into the field of clinical practice and therapy. Heart failure is one of the most important causes of morbidity and mortality worldwide, and patients with postinfarct remodelling show the highest risk of symptomatic heart failure. For this reason, the battle of medicine against heart failure is against postinfarct remodelling, which means that the prevention is better than the cure.

Acknowledgments

The authors thank Dr. Edgardo Bonacina, Director of the Anatomic Pathology Unit of Niguarda Ca' Granda Hospital, for permission on Figure 3. This study is partially supported by an unconditioned grant of Fondazione Polizzotto.

References

[1] A. S. Go, D. Mozaffarian, V. L. Roger et al., "Heart disease and stroke statistics—2014 update: a report from the American heart association," *Circulation*, vol. 129, no. 3, pp. e28–e292, 2014.

[2] P. T. O'Gara, F. G. Kushner, D. D. Ascheim et al., "2013 ACCF/AHA Guideline for the management of ST-elevation myocardial infarction: a report of the American College of Cardiology Foundation/American Heart Association Task Force on Practice Guidelines," *Journal of the American College of Cardiology*, vol. 61, no. 4, pp. e78–e140, 2013.

[3] E. C. Keeley and L. D. Hillis, "Primary PCI for myocardial infarction with ST-segment elevation," *The New England Journal of Medicine*, vol. 356, no. 1, pp. 47–54, 2007.

[4] D. S. Menees, E. D. Peterson, Y. Wang et al., "Door-to-balloon time and mortality among patients undergoing primary PCI," *The New England Journal of Medicine*, vol. 369, no. 10, pp. 901–909, 2013.

[5] S. Windecker, J. J. Bax, A. Myat, G. W. Stone, and M. S. Marber, "Future treatment strategies in ST-segment elevation myocardial infarction," *The Lancet*, vol. 382, no. 9892, pp. 644–657, 2013.

[6] J. J. V. McMurray, S. Adamopoulos, S. D. Anker et al., "ESC Guidelines for the diagnosis and treatment of acute and chronic heart failure 2012: the Task Force for the Diagnosis and Treatment of Acute and Chronic Heart Failure 2012 of the European Society of Cardiology. Developed in collaboration with the Heart Failure Association (HFA) of the ESC," *European Heart Journal*, vol. 33, no. 14, pp. 1787–1847, 2012.

[7] A. Dhingra, A. Garg, S. Kaur et al., "Epidemiology of heart failure with preserved ejection fraction," *Current Heart Failure Reports*, vol. 11, no. 4, pp. 354–365, 2014.

[8] S. A. Hunt, D. W. Baker, M. H. Chin et al., "ACC/AHA guidelines for the evaluation and management of chronic heart failure in the adult: executive summary: a report of the American College of Cardiology/American Heart Association task force on practice guidelines (committee to revise the 1995 guidelines for the evaluation and management of heart failure) developed in collaboration with the International Society for Heart and Lung Transplantation Endorsed by the Heart Failure Society of America," *Journal of the American College of Cardiology*, vol. 38, no. 7, pp. 2101–2113, 2001.

[9] G. M. Fröhlich, P. Meier, S. K. White, D. M. Yellon, and D. J. Hausenloy, "Myocardial reperfusion injury: looking beyond primary PCI," *European Heart Journal*, vol. 34, no. 23, pp. 1714–1724, 2013.

[10] M. A. Konstam, D. G. Kramer, A. R. Patel, M. S. Maron, and J. E. Udelson, "Left ventricular remodeling in heart failure: current concepts in clinical significance and assessment," *JACC: Cardiovascular Imaging*, vol. 4, no. 1, pp. 98–108, 2011.

[11] A. Verma, A. Meris, H. Skali et al., "Prognostic implications of left ventricular mass and geometry following myocardial infarction: the VALIANT (Valsartan in Acute Myocardial Infarction) Echocardiographic Study," *JACC: Cardiovascular Imaging*, vol. 1, no. 5, pp. 582–591, 2008.

[12] J. Ganame, G. Messalli, P. G. Masci et al., "Time course of infarct healing and left ventricular remodelling in patients with reperfused ST segment elevation myocardial infarction using comprehensive magnetic resonance imaging," *European Radiology*, vol. 21, no. 4, pp. 693–701, 2011.

[13] J. J. Gomez-Doblas, J. Schor, P. Vignola et al., "Left ventricular geometry and operative mortality in patients undergoing mitral valve replacement," *Clinical Cardiology*, vol. 24, no. 11, pp. 717–722, 2001.

[14] F. A. Flachskampf, M. Schmid, C. Rost, S. Achenbach, A. N. Demaria, and W. G. Daniel, "Cardiac imaging after myocardial infarction," *European Heart Journal*, vol. 32, no. 3, pp. 272–283, 2011.

[15] P. G. Masci, J. Ganame, M. Francone et al., "Relationship between location and size of myocardial infarction and their reciprocal influences on post-infarction left ventricular remodelling," *European Heart Journal*, vol. 32, no. 13, pp. 1640–1648, 2011.

[16] T. Springeling, S. W. Kirschbaum, A. Rossi et al., "Late cardiac remodeling after primary percutaneous coronary intervention—five-year cardiac magnetic resonance imaging follow-up," *Circulation Journal*, vol. 77, no. 1, pp. 81–88, 2013.

[17] G. Casella, M. Cassin, F. Chiarella et al., "Epidemiology and patterns of care of patients admitted to Italian Intensive Cardiac Care units: the BLITZ-3 registry," *Journal of Cardiovascular Medicine*, vol. 11, no. 6, pp. 450–461, 2010.

[18] L. Bolognese, A. N. Neskovic, G. Parodi et al., "Left ventricular remodeling after primary coronary angioplasty: patterns of left ventricular dilation and long-term prognostic implications," *Circulation*, vol. 106, no. 18, pp. 2351–2357, 2002.

[19] C. Savoye, O. Equine, O. Tricot et al., "Left ventricular remodeling after anterior wall acute myocardial infarction in modern clinical practice (from the REmodelage VEntriculaire [REVE] Study Group)," *The American Journal of Cardiology*, vol. 98, no. 9, pp. 1144–1149, 2006.

[20] G. K. Lund, A. Stork, K. Muellerleile et al., "Prediction of left ventricular remodeling and analysis of infarct resorption in patients with reperfused myocardial infarcts by using contrast-enhanced MR imaging," *Radiology*, vol. 245, no. 1, pp. 95–102, 2007.

[21] C. M. Kramer, A. J. Sinusas, D. E. Sosnovik, B. A. French, and F. M. Bengel, "Multimodality imaging of myocardial injury and remodeling," *Journal of Nuclear Medicine*, vol. 51, no. 1, pp. 107S–121S, 2010.

[22] K. H. Darasz, S. R. Underwood, J. Bayliss et al., "Measurement of left ventricular volume after anterior myocardial infarction: comparison of magnetic resonance imaging, echocardiography, and radionuclide ventriculography," *International Journal of Cardiovascular Imaging*, vol. 18, no. 2, pp. 135–142, 2002.

[23] S. Prasad and D. Pennell, "Measurement of left ventricular volume after anterior myocardial infarction: comparison of magnetic resonance imaging, echo and radionuclide ventriculography," *The International Journal of Cardiovascular Imaging*, vol. 18, no. 5, pp. 387–390, 2002.

[24] A. S. Fauci, E. Braunwald, D. L. Kasper et al., *Harrison's Principles of Internal Medicine*, McGraw-Hill, 17th edition, 2008.

[25] S.-A. Chang, Y. H. Choe, S. Y. Jang, S. M. Kim, S.-C. Lee, and J. K. Oh, "Assessment of left and right ventricular parameters in healthy Korean volunteers using cardiac magnetic resonance imaging: change in ventricular volume and function based on age, gender and body surface area," *International Journal of Cardiovascular Imaging*, vol. 28, no. 2, pp. 141–147, 2012.

[26] J. P. Curtis, S. I. Sokol, Y. Wang et al., "The association of left ventricular ejection fraction, mortality, and cause of death in stable outpatients with heart failure," *Journal of the American College of Cardiology*, vol. 42, no. 4, pp. 736–742, 2003.

[27] C. M. Kramer, W. J. Rogers, T. M. Theobald, T. P. Power, G. Geskin, and N. Reichek, "Dissociation between changes in intramyocardial function and left ventricular volumes in the eight weeks after first anterior myocardial infarction," *Journal of the American College of Cardiology*, vol. 30, no. 7, pp. 1625–1632, 1997.

[28] L. H. Opie, P. J. Commerford, B. J. Gersh, and M. A. Pfeffer, "Controversies in ventricular remodelling," *The Lancet*, vol. 367, no. 9507, pp. 356–367, 2006.

[29] H. B. Hillenbrand, J. Sandstede, S. Störk et al., "Remodeling of the infarct territory in the time course of infarct healing in humans," *Magnetic Resonance Materials in Physics, Biology and Medicine*, vol. 24, no. 5, pp. 277–284, 2011.

[30] J. J. W. Sandstede, C. Lipke, W. Kenn, M. Beer, T. Pabst, and D. Hahn, "Cine MR imaging after myocardial infarction—assessment and follow-up of regional and global left ventricular function," *International Journal of Cardiac Imaging*, vol. 15, no. 6, pp. 435–440, 1999.

[31] L. Zhong, Y. Su, S.-Y. Yeo, R.-S. Tan, D. N. Ghista, and G. Kassab, "Left ventricular regional wall curvedness and wall stress in patients with ischemic dilated cardiomyopathy," *The American Journal of Physiology—Heart and Circulatory Physiology*, vol. 296, no. 3, pp. H573–H584, 2009.

[32] Y. Zhang, A. K. Y. Chan, C.-M. Yu et al., "Left ventricular systolic asynchrony after acute myocardial infarction in patients with narrow QRS complexes," *American Heart Journal*, vol. 149, no. 3, pp. 497–503, 2005.

[33] S.-A. Chang, H.-J. Chang, S. I. Choi et al., "Usefulness of left ventricular dyssynchrony after acute myocardial infarction, assessed by a tagging magnetic resonance image derived metric, as a determinant of ventricular remodeling," *The American Journal of Cardiology*, vol. 104, no. 1, pp. 19–23, 2009.

[34] Y. Zhang, G. W. Yip, A. K. Y. Chan et al., "Left ventricular systolic dyssynchrony is a predictor of cardiac remodeling after myocardial infarction," *American Heart Journal*, vol. 156, no. 6, pp. 1124–1132, 2008.

[35] D. M. Yellon and D. J. Hausenloy, "Myocardial reperfusion injury," *The New England Journal of Medicine*, vol. 357, no. 11, pp. 1074–1135, 2007.

[36] C. M. Kramer, W. J. Rogers, C. S. Park et al., "Regional myocyte hypertrophy parallels regional myocardial dysfunction during post-infarct remodeling," *Journal of Molecular and Cellular Cardiology*, vol. 30, no. 9, pp. 1773–1778, 1998.

[37] M.-T. Wu, W.-Y. I. Tseng, M.-Y. M. Su et al., "Diffusion tensor magnetic resonance imaging mapping the fiber architecture

remoding in human myocardium after infarction: correlation with viability and wall motion," *Circulation*, vol. 114, no. 10, pp. 1036–1045, 2006.

[38] M.-T. Wu, M.-Y. Su, Y.-L. Huang et al., "Sequential changes of myocardial microstructure in patients postmyocardial infarction by diffusion-tensor cardiac MR: correlation with left ventricular structure and function," *Circulation: Cardiovascular Imaging*, vol. 2, no. 1, pp. 32–40, 2009.

[39] C. Mekkaoui, S. Huang, H. H. Chen et al., "Fiber architecture in remodeled myocardium revealed with a quantitative diffusion CMR tractography framework and histological validation," *Journal of Cardiovascular Magnetic Resonance*, vol. 14, no. 1, article 70, 2012.

[40] J. Machackova, J. Barta, and N. S. Dhalla, "Myofibrillar remodelling in cardiac hypertrophy, heart failure and cardiomyopathies," *Canadian Journal of Cardiology*, vol. 22, no. 11, pp. 953–968, 2006.

[41] W. Grossman and W. J. Paulus, "Myocardial stress and hypertrophy: a complex interface between biophysics and cardiac remodeling," *Journal of Clinical Investigation*, vol. 123, no. 9, pp. 3701–3703, 2013.

[42] S. Miyata, W. Minobe, M. R. Bristow, and L. A. Leinwand, "Myosin heavy chain isoform expression in the failing and nonfailing human heart," *Circulation Research*, vol. 86, no. 4, pp. 386–390, 2000.

[43] M. Krenz and J. Robbins, "Impact of beta-myosin heavy chain expression on cardiac function during stress," *Journal of the American College of Cardiology*, vol. 44, no. 12, pp. 2390–2397, 2004.

[44] N. Koitabashi and D. A. Kass, "Reverse remodeling in heart failure-mechanisms and therapeutic opportunities," *Nature Reviews Cardiology*, vol. 9, no. 3, pp. 147–157, 2012.

[45] L. H. Lehmann, B. C. Worst, D. A. Stanmore, and J. Backs, "Histone deacetylase signaling in cardioprotection," *Cellular and Molecular Life Sciences*, vol. 71, no. 9, pp. 1673–1690, 2014.

[46] C. L. Antos, T. A. McKinsey, M. Dreitz et al., "Dose-dependent blockade to cardiomyocyte hypertrophy by histone deacetylase inhibitors," *The Journal of Biological Chemistry*, vol. 278, no. 31, pp. 28930–28937, 2003.

[47] W. Chan, S. J. Duffy, D. A. White et al., "Acute left ventricular remodeling following myocardial infarction: coupling of regional healing with remote extracellular matrix expansion," *JACC: Cardiovascular Imaging*, vol. 5, no. 9, pp. 884–893, 2012.

[48] M. Ugander, A. J. Oki, L.-Y. Hsu et al., "Extracellular volume imaging by magnetic resonance imaging provides insights into overt and sub-clinical myocardial pathology," *European Heart Journal*, vol. 33, no. 10, pp. 1268–1278, 2012.

[49] T. C. Wong, K. Piehler, C. G. Meier et al., "Association between extracellular matrix expansion quantified by cardiovascular magnetic resonance and short-term mortality," *Circulation*, vol. 126, no. 10, pp. 1206–1216, 2012.

[50] W. Xin, X. Li, X. Lu, K. Niu, and J. Cai, "Involvement of endoplasmic reticulum stress-associated apoptosis in a heart failure model induced by chronic myocardial ischemia," *International Journal of Molecular Medicine*, vol. 27, no. 4, pp. 503–509, 2011.

[51] J. J. Gajarsa and R. A. Kloner, "Left ventricular remodeling in the post-infarction heart: a review of cellular, molecular mechanisms, and therapeutic modalities," *Heart Failure Reviews*, vol. 16, no. 1, pp. 13–21, 2011.

[52] D. J. Hausenloy and D. M. Yellon, "Reperfusion injury salvage kinase signalling: taking a RISK for cardioprotection," *Heart Failure Reviews*, vol. 12, no. 3-4, pp. 217–234, 2007.

[53] T. Kempf, M. Eden, J. Strelau et al., "The transforming growth factor-β superfamily member growth-differentiation factor-15 protects the heart from ischemia/reperfusion injury," *Circulation Research*, vol. 98, no. 3, pp. 351–360, 2006.

[54] R. K. Harston and D. Kuppuswamy, "Integrins are the necessary links to hypertrophic growth in cardiomyocytes," *Journal of Signal Transduction*, vol. 2011, Article ID 521742, 8 pages, 2011.

[55] C. Banfi, V. Cavalca, F. Veglia et al., "Neurohormonal activation is associated with increased levels of plasma matrix metalloproteinase-2 in human heart failure," *European Heart Journal*, vol. 26, no. 5, pp. 481–488, 2005.

[56] J. Sundström, J. C. Evans, E. J. Benjamin et al., "Relations of plasma matrix metalloproteinase-9 to clinical cardiovascular risk factors and echocardiographic left ventricular measures: the Framingham heart study," *Circulation*, vol. 109, no. 23, pp. 2850–2856, 2004.

[57] S. Heymans, B. Schroen, P. Vermeersch et al., "Increased cardiac expression of tissue inhibitor of metalloproteinase-1 and tissue inhibitor of metalloproteinase-2 is related to cardiac fibrosis and dysfunction in the chronic pressure-overloaded human heart," *Circulation*, vol. 112, no. 8, pp. 1136–1144, 2005.

[58] M. Fertin, E. Dubois, A. Belliard, P. Amouyel, F. Pinet, and C. Bauters, "Usefulness of circulating biomarkers for the prediction of left ventricular remodeling after myocardial infarction," *American Journal of Cardiology*, vol. 110, no. 2, pp. 277–283, 2012.

[59] T. Force and K. L. Kolaja, "Cardiotoxicity of kinase inhibitors: the prediction and translation of preclinical models to clinical outcomes," *Nature Reviews Drug Discovery*, vol. 10, no. 2, pp. 111–126, 2011.

[60] N. R. Madamanchi, S. Li, C. Patterson, and M. S. Runge, "Reactive oxygen species regulate heat-shock protein 70 via the JAK/STAT pathway," *Arteriosclerosis, Thrombosis, and Vascular Biology*, vol. 21, no. 3, pp. 321–326, 2001.

[61] M. Hori and O. Yamaguchi, "Is tumor necrosis factor-α friend or foe for chronic heart failure?" *Circulation Research*, vol. 113, no. 5, pp. 492–494, 2013.

[62] J. W. Gordon, J. A. Shaw, and L. A. Kirshenbaum, "Multiple facets of NF-κB in the heart: to be or not to NF-κB," *Circulation Research*, vol. 108, no. 9, pp. 1122–1132, 2011.

[63] G. M. Ellison, D. Torella, S. Dellegrottaglie et al., "Endogenous cardiac stem cell activation by insulin-like growth factor-1/hepatocyte growth factor intracoronary injection fosters survival and regeneration of the infarcted pig heart," *Journal of the American College of Cardiology*, vol. 58, no. 9, pp. 977–986, 2011.

[64] G. M. Cote, D. B. Sawyer, and B. A. Chabner, "ERBB2 inhibition and heart failure," *The New England Journal of Medicine*, vol. 367, no. 22, pp. 2150–2153, 2012.

[65] M. Jougasaki, "Cardiotrophin-1 in cardiovascular regulation," *Advances in Clinical Chemistry*, vol. 52, pp. 41–76, 2010.

[66] E. Letavernier, L. Zafrani, J. Perez, B. Letavernier, J.-P. Haymann, and L. Baud, "The role of calpains in myocardial remodelling and heart failure," *Cardiovascular Research*, vol. 96, no. 1, pp. 38–45, 2012.

[67] W. T. Pu, Q. Ma, and S. Izumo, "NFAT transcription factors are critical survival factors that inhibit cardiomyocyte apoptosis during phenylephrine stimulation in vitro," *Circulation Research*, vol. 92, no. 7, pp. 725–731, 2003.

[68] X. Zhang, C. Szeto, E. Gao et al., "Cardiotoxic and cardioprotective features of chronic β-Adrenergic signaling," *Circulation Research*, vol. 112, no. 3, pp. 498–509, 2013.

[69] R. S. Whelan, K. Konstantinidis, R.-P. Xiao, and R. N. Kitsis, "Cardiomyocyte life-death decisions in response to chronic β-adrenergic signaling," *Circulation Research*, vol. 112, no. 3, pp. 408–410, 2013.

[70] S. D. Solomon, H. Skali, N. S. Anavekar et al., "Changes in ventricular size and function in patients treated with valsartan, captopril, or both after myocardial infarction," *Circulation*, vol. 111, no. 25, pp. 3411–3419, 2005.

[71] R. E. Foster, D. B. Johnson, F. Barilla et al., "Changes in left ventricular mass and volumes in patients receiving angiotensin-converting enzyme inhibitor therapy for left ventricular dysfunction after Q-wave myocardial infarction," *American Heart Journal*, vol. 136, no. 2, pp. 269–275, 1998.

[72] M. Hayashi, T. Tsutamoto, A. Wada et al., "Immediate administration of mineralocorticoid receptor antagonist spironolactone prevents post-infarct left ventricular remodeling associated with suppression of a marker of myocardial collagen synthesis in patients with first anterior acute myocardial infarction," *Circulation*, vol. 107, no. 20, pp. 2559–2565, 2003.

[73] J. N. Cohn, R. Ferrari, and N. Sharpe, "Cardiac remodelling—concepts and clinical implications: a consensus paper from an international forum on cardiac remodeling. Behalf of an International Forum on Cardiac Remodeling," *Journal of the American College of Cardiology*, vol. 35, pp. 569–582, 2000.

[74] A. L. Taylor, S. Ziesche, C. Yancy et al., "Combination of isosorbide dinitrate and hydralazine in blacks with heart failure," *The New England Journal of Medicine*, vol. 351, no. 20, pp. 2049–2057, 2004.

[75] F. G. Spinale and F. Villarreal, "Targeting matrix metalloproteinases in heart disease: lessons from endogenous inhibitors," *Biochemical Pharmacology*, vol. 90, no. 1, pp. 7–15, 2014.

[76] A. Jabbour, C. S. Hayward, A. M. Keogh et al., "Parenteral administration of recombinant human neuregulin-1 to patients with stable chronic heart failure produces favourable acute and chronic haemodynamic responses," *European Journal of Heart Failure*, vol. 13, no. 1, pp. 83–92, 2011.

[77] R. Gao, J. Zhang, L. Cheng et al., "A phase II, randomized, double-blind, multicenter, based on standard therapy, placebo-controlled study of the efficacy and safety of recombinant human neuregulin-1 in patients with chronic heart failure," *Journal of the American College of Cardiology*, vol. 55, no. 18, pp. 1907–1914, 2010.

[78] S. Neubauer and C. Redwood, "New mechanisms and concepts for cardiac-resynchronization therapy," *The New England Journal of Medicine*, vol. 370, no. 12, pp. 1164–1166, 2014.

[79] S. Klotz, A. H. Jan Danser, and D. Burkhoff, "Impact of left ventricular assist device (LVAD) support on the cardiac reverse remodeling process," *Progress in Biophysics and Molecular Biology*, vol. 97, no. 2-3, pp. 479–496, 2008.

[80] K. Takeda, T. Sakaguchi, S. Miyagawa et al., "The extent of early left ventricular reverse remodelling is related to midterm outcomes after restrictive mitral annuloplasty in patients with non-ischaemic dilated cardiomyopathy and functional mitral regurgitation," *European Journal of Cardiothoracic Surgery*, vol. 41, no. 3, pp. 506–511, 2012.

[81] M. R. Costanzo, R. J. Ivanhoe, A. Kao et al., "Prospective evaluation of elastic restraint to lessen the effects of heart failure (PEERLESS-HF) trial," *Journal of Cardiac Failure*, vol. 18, no. 6, pp. 446–458, 2012.

[82] C. T. Klodell Jr., J. M. Aranda Jr., D. C. McGiffin et al., "Worldwide surgical experience with the Paracor HeartNet cardiac restraint device," *Journal of Thoracic and Cardiovascular Surgery*, vol. 135, no. 1, pp. 188–195, 2008.

[83] S. Ørn, C. Manhenke, I. S. Anand et al., "Effect of left ventricular scar size, location, and transmurality on left ventricular remodeling with healed myocardial infarction," *American Journal of Cardiology*, vol. 99, no. 8, pp. 1109–1114, 2007.

[84] J. Hallén, J. K. Jensen, M. W. Fagerland, A. S. Jaffe, and D. Atar, "Cardiac troponin I for the prediction of functional recovery and left ventricular remodelling following primary percutaneous coronary intervention for ST-elevation myocardial infarction," *Heart*, vol. 96, no. 23, pp. 1892–1897, 2010.

[85] R. Y. Kwong, A. K. Chan, K. A. Brown et al., "Impact of unrecognized myocardial scar detected by cardiac magnetic resonance imaging on event-free survival in patients presenting with signs or symptoms of coronary artery disease," *Circulation*, vol. 113, no. 23, pp. 2733–2743, 2006.

[86] E. Braunwald, "Heart failure," *JACC: Heart Failure*, vol. 1, no. 1, pp. 1–20, 2013.

[87] K. C. Wu, "CMR of microvascular obstruction and hemorrhage in myocardial infarction," *Journal of Cardiovascular Magnetic Resonance*, vol. 14, article 68, 2012.

[88] R. A. P. Weir, C. A. Murphy, C. J. Petrie et al., "Microvascular obstruction remains a portent of adverse remodeling in optimally treated patients with left ventricular systolic dysfunction after acute myocardial infarction," *Circulation: Cardiovascular Imaging*, vol. 3, no. 4, pp. 360–367, 2010.

[89] O. Husser, J. V. Monmeneu, J. Sanchis et al., "Cardiovascular magnetic resonance-derived intramyocardial hemorrhage after STEMI: influence on long-term prognosis, adverse left ventricular remodeling and relationship with microvascular obstruction," *International Journal of Cardiology*, vol. 167, no. 5, pp. 2047–2054, 2013.

[90] A. N. Mather, T. A. Fairbairn, S. G. Ball, J. P. Greenwood, and S. Plein, "Reperfusion haemorrhage as determined by cardiovascular MRI is a predictor of adverse left ventricular remodelling and markers of late arrhythmic risk," *Heart*, vol. 97, no. 6, pp. 453–459, 2011.

[91] J. C. Weaver and J. A. McCrohon, "Contrast-enhanced cardiac MRI in myocardial infarction," *Heart Lung and Circulation*, vol. 17, no. 4, pp. 290–298, 2008.

[92] B. G. Schwartz and R. A. Kloner, "Coronary no reflow," *Journal of Molecular and Cellular Cardiology*, vol. 52, no. 4, pp. 873–882, 2012.

[93] S. C. A. M. Bekkers, S. K. Yazdani, R. Virmani, and J. Waltenberger, "Microvascular obstruction: underlying pathophysiology and clinical diagnosis," *Journal of the American College of Cardiology*, vol. 55, no. 16, pp. 1649–1660, 2010.

[94] D. T. L. Wong, R. Puri, J. D. Richardson, M. I. Worthley, and S. G. Worthley, "Myocardial 'no-reflow'—diagnosis, pathophysiology and treatment," *International Journal of Cardiology*, vol. 167, no. 5, pp. 1798–1806, 2013.

[95] D. P. O'Regan, R. Ahmed, N. Karunanithy et al., "Reperfusion hemorrhage following acute myocardial infarction: assessment with T2* mapping and effect on measuring the area at risk," *Radiology*, vol. 250, no. 3, pp. 916–922, 2009.

[96] M. I. Zia, N. R. Ghugre, K. A. Connelly et al., "Characterizing myocardial edema and hemorrhage using quantitative T2 and T2* mapping at multiple time intervals post ST-segment elevation myocardial infarction," *Circulation: Cardiovascular Imaging*, vol. 5, no. 5, pp. 566–572, 2012.

[97] S. Frantz, J. Bauersachs, and G. Ertl, "Post-infarct remodelling: contribution of wound healing and inflammation," *Cardiovascular Research*, vol. 81, no. 3, pp. 474–481, 2009.

[98] A. Kali, A. Kumar, I. Cokic et al., "Chronic manifestation of postreperfusion intramyocardial hemorrhage as regional iron deposition: a cardiovascular magnetic resonance study with ex vivo validation," *Circulation: Cardiovascular Imaging*, vol. 6, no. 2, pp. 218–228, 2013.

[99] R. S. Britton, K. L. Leicester, and B. R. Bacon, "Iron toxicity and chelation therapy," *International Journal of Hematology*, vol. 76, no. 3, pp. 219–228, 2002.

[100] A. Kidambi, A. N. Mather, M. Motwani et al., "The effect of microvascular obstruction and intramyocardial hemorrhage on contractile recovery in reperfused myocardial infarction: insights from cardiovascular magnetic resonance," *Journal of Cardiovascular Magnetic Resonance*, vol. 15, article 58, 2013.

[101] G. Klug, A. Mayr, S. Schenk et al., "Prognostic value at 5 years of microvascular obstruction after acute myocardial infarction assessed by cardiovascular magnetic resonance," *Journal of Cardiovascular Magnetic Resonance*, vol. 14, no. 1, article 46, 2012.

[102] M. Soleimani, M. Khazalpour, G. Cheng et al., "Moderate mitral regurgitation accelerates left ventricular remodeling after posterolateral myocardial infarction," *Annals of Thoracic Surgery*, vol. 92, no. 5, pp. 1614–1620, 2011.

[103] A. N. Rassi, P. Pibarot, and S. Elmariah, "Left ventricular remodelling in aortic stenosis," *Canadian Journal of Cardiology*, vol. 30, no. 9, pp. 1004–1011, 2014.

[104] A. Ganau, R. B. Devereux, M. J. Roman et al., "Patterns of left ventricular hypertrophy and geometric remodeling in essential hypertension," *Journal of the American College of Cardiology*, vol. 19, no. 7, pp. 1550–1558, 1992.

[105] H. P. Krayenbuehl, O. M. Hess, E. S. Monrad, J. Schneider, G. Mall, and M. Turina, "Left ventricular myocardial structure in aortic valve disease before, intermediate, and late after aortic valve replacement," *Circulation*, vol. 79, no. 4, pp. 744–755, 1989.

[106] A. J. McLellan, M. P. Schlaich, A. J. Taylor et al., "Reverse cardiac remodeling after renal denervation: atrial electrophysiologic and structural changes associated with blood pressure lowering," *Heart Rhythm*, vol. 12, no. 5, pp. 982–990, 2015.

[107] L. Nilsson, J. Hallén, D. Atar, L. Jonasson, and E. Swahn, "Early measurements of plasma matrix metalloproteinase-2 predict infarct size and ventricular dysfunction in ST-elevation myocardial infarction," *Heart*, vol. 98, no. 1, pp. 31–36, 2012.

[108] C. J. French, A. K. M. T. Zaman, R. J. Kelm Jr., J. L. Spees, and B. E. Sobel, "Vascular rhexis: loss of integrity of coronary vasculature in mice subjected to myocardial infarction," *Experimental Biology and Medicine*, vol. 235, no. 8, pp. 966–973, 2010.

[109] P. Carmeliet, L. Moons, R. Lijnen et al., "Urokinase-generated plasmin activates matrix metalloproteinases during aneurysm formation," *Nature Genetics*, vol. 17, no. 4, pp. 439–444, 1997.

[110] S. Ørn, T. Ueland, C. Manhenke et al., "Increased interleukin-1β levels are associated with left ventricular hypertrophy and remodelling following acute ST segment elevation myocardial infarction treated by primary percutaneous coronary intervention," *Journal of Internal Medicine*, vol. 272, no. 3, pp. 267–276, 2012.

[111] J. G. Akar and F. G. Akar, "Mapping arrhythmias in the failing heart: from Langendorff to patient," *Journal of Electrocardiology*, vol. 39, no. 4, pp. S19–S23, 2006.

[112] M. Fernández-Velasco, N. Goren, G. Benito, J. Blanco-Rivero, L. Boscá, and C. Delgado, "Regional distribution of hyperpolarization-activated current (If) and hyperpolarization-activated cyclic nucleotide-gated channel mRNA expression in ventricular cells from control and hypertrophied rat hearts," *Journal of Physiology*, vol. 553, no. 2, pp. 395–405, 2003.

[113] H. A. Fozzard, "Afterdepolarizations and triggered activity," *Basic Research in Cardiology*, vol. 87, no. 2, pp. 105–113, 1992.

[114] U. O. Egolum, D. G. Stover, R. Anthony, A. M. Wasserman, D. Lenihan, and J. B. Damp, "Intracardiac thrombus: diagnosis, complications and management," *The American Journal of the Medical Sciences*, vol. 345, no. 5, pp. 391–395, 2013.

[115] R. A. P. Weir, T. N. Martin, C. J. Petrie et al., "Cardiac and extracardiac abnormalities detected by cardiac magnetic resonance in a post-myocardial infarction cohort," *Cardiology*, vol. 113, no. 1, pp. 1–8, 2009.

[116] J. J. V. McMurray, M. Packer, A. S. Desai et al., "Angiotensin-neprilysin inhibition versus enalapril in heart failure," *The New England Journal of Medicine*, vol. 371, no. 11, pp. 993–1004, 2014.

[117] K. Leineweber, P. Rohe, A. Beilfuß et al., "G-protein-coupled receptor kinase activity in human heart failure: effects of β-adrenoceptor blockade," *Cardiovascular Research*, vol. 66, no. 3, pp. 512–519, 2005.

[118] Å. Hjalmarson, "Effects of beta blockade on sudden cardiac death during acute myocardial infarction and the postinfarction period," *The American Journal of Cardiology*, vol. 80, no. 9, pp. 35J–39J, 1997.

[119] S. P. Jones and R. Bolli, "The ubiquitous role of nitric oxide in cardioprotection," *Journal of Molecular and Cellular Cardiology*, vol. 40, no. 1, pp. 16–23, 2006.

[120] J. Inserte and D. Garcia-Dorado, "The cGMP/PKG pathway as a common mediator of cardioprotection: translatability and mechanism," *British Journal of Pharmacology*, vol. 172, no. 8, pp. 1996–2009, 2015.

[121] R. A. Kloner, "Current state of clinical translation of cardioprotective agents for acute myocardial infarction," *Circulation Research*, vol. 113, no. 4, pp. 451–463, 2013.

[122] M. Jessup, B. Greenberg, D. Mancini et al., "Calcium upregulation by percutaneous administration of gene therapy in cardiac disease (CUPID): A phase 2 trial of intracoronary gene therapy of sarcoplasmic reticulum Ca^{2+}-ATPase in patients with advanced heart failure," *Circulation*, vol. 124, no. 3, pp. 304–313, 2011.

7

Association between Stable Coronary Artery Disease and In Vivo Thrombin Generation

Benjamin Valente-Acosta,[1,2] Manuel Alfonso Baños-González,[1,3]
Marco Antonio Peña-Duque,[1] Marco Antonio Martínez-Ríos,[1] Leslie Quintanar-Trejo,[1]
Gad Aptilon-Duque,[1] Mirthala Flores-García,[1] David Cruz-Robles,[1]
Guillermo Cardoso-Saldaña,[1] and Aurora de la Peña-Díaz[1,2]

[1]Instituto Nacional de Cardiología Ignacio Chávez, Grupo Genética Intervencionista, Departamentos de Biología Molecular,
 Hemodinámica, Endocrinología, 14080 México City, Mexico
[2]Departamento de Farmacología, Facultad de Medicina, Universidad Nacional Autónoma de México, 04510 México City, Mexico
[3]División Académica de Ciencias de la Salud, Universidad Juárez Autónoma de Tabasco, Hospital Regional de Alta Especialidad
 "Dr. Juan Graham Casasús", 86126 Villahermosa, TAB, Mexico

Correspondence should be addressed to Aurora de la Peña-Díaz; aurorade2002@yahoo.com

Academic Editor: Chim Choy Lang

Background. Thrombin has been implicated as a key molecule in atherosclerotic progression. Clinical evidence shows that thrombin generation is enhanced in atherosclerosis, but its role as a risk factor for coronary atherosclerotic burden has not been proven in coronary artery disease (CAD) stable patients. *Objectives*. To evaluate the association between TAT levels and homocysteine levels and the presence of coronary artery disease diagnosed by coronary angiography in patients with stable CAD. *Methods and Results*. We included 95 stable patients admitted to the Haemodynamics Department, including 63 patients with significant CAD and 32 patients without. We measured the thrombin-antithrombin complex (TAT) and homocysteine concentrations in all the patients. The CAD patients exhibited higher concentrations of TAT (40.76 μg/L versus 20.81 μg/L, $p = 0.002$) and homocysteine (11.36 μmol/L versus 8.81 μmol/L, $p < 0.01$) compared to the patients without significant CAD. Specifically, in patients with CAD+ the level of TAT level was associated with the severity of CAD being 36.17 ± 24.48 μg/L in the patients with bivascular obstruction and 42.77 ± 31.81 μg/L in trivascular coronary obstruction, $p = 0.002$. *Conclusions*. The level of in vivo thrombin generation, quantified as TAT complexes, is associated with the presence and severity of CAD assessed by coronary angiography in stable CAD patients.

1. Introduction

Coronary artery disease (CAD) has been recognized as a chronic inflammatory disease. Proinflammatory cytokines and adhesion molecules play an important role in its initiation and progression [1, 2] by initiating a crosstalk between inflammation and the haemostatic system [3].

A key molecule in the haemostatic system is thrombin, a serine protease that primarily converts soluble fibrinogen into fibrin [4]. Thrombin is neutralized by its physiological inhibitor antithrombin; thus, the thrombin-antithrombin (TAT) complex is believed to be a reliable marker of in vivo thrombin generation [5].

Thrombin is a pleiotropic enzyme, performing various actions to activate protease-activated receptors expressed on the endothelial cells, leukocytes, vascular smooth-muscle cells, fibroblasts, and platelets. These actions result in multiple proatherogenic cellular responses including the enhancement of endothelial dysfunction and permeability, oxidative stress, apoptosis, and the overexpression of inflammatory cytokines that promote atherosclerotic plaque formation [6–8].

The importance of thrombin as a key promoter of atherosclerosis has only been shown in animal models [9, 10]. Bea et al. cleverly showed that a direct thrombin inhibitor could reduce the progression of atherosclerosis in apolipoprotein

E-deficient mice through the inhibition of the transcription of multiple proinflammatory factors [9].

On the other hand, homocysteine (Hcy), an amino acid metabolized from methionine [11], enhances thrombin generation [12, 13]. High concentrations of homocysteine have been associated with an increased risk of atherosclerosis and arterial thrombosis [14].

In the clinical field, the evidence is inconsistent; some cross-sectional studies have shown a positive association between thrombin generation and aortic, carotid, and peripheral arterial atherosclerosis [15–17], whereas others have not [18–20].

In the present study, we aim to show the association between TAT levels as a marker for thrombin generation in vivo, homocysteine levels, and the presence and severity of coronary artery disease diagnosed by coronary angiography.

2. Material and Methods

2.1. Subjects. The study was performed in patients who were admitted to the Haemodynamics Department for a diagnostic coronary angiography because of stable chest pain, suspected for CAD. The study was carried out in the National Institute of Cardiology Ignacio Chavez.

The population included in our study consisted of 95 patients who underwent a coronary angiography, which was performed using femoral access in all patients. Patients were classified according to their coronary angiography as CAD+ when they had stenosis greater than 50% in at least one major coronary artery and as CAD− when they had no angiographic evidence of coronary occlusion.

The severity of coronary atherosclerosis was classified as one-, two-, or three-vessel disease according to the number of major coronary arteries that were stenotic.

We excluded patients who had undergone coronary bypass surgery or previous coronary intervention, those with infectious, neoplastic, or thyroid disease, kidney or liver failure, or a recent myocardial infarction, those who had been diagnosed with unstable angina within the last month, and those taking any type of anticoagulant.

For all the patients anthropometric measures and traditional risk factors were recorded. Individuals were considered to have diabetes mellitus type 2 if they had been previously diagnosed or were receiving hypoglycemic treatment and/or insulin. Individuals were considered to have hypertension if they had been previously diagnosed or were receiving an antihypertensive therapy. Dyslipidemia was defined as total cholesterol (TC) $\geq$ 200 mg/dL and/or low-density lipoprotein cholesterol (LDL-C) $\geq$ 130 mg/dL and/or triglycerides (TG) $\geq$ 150 mg/dL and/or high-density lipoprotein cholesterol (HDL-C) $\leq$ 40 mg/dL or by a previous diagnosis. Body mass index was calculated using a standard formula (weight (kg)/height (m)^2).

2.2. Laboratory Measurements. From each patient, we obtained a blood sample after a fast of at least 8 hours and always before the angiography. Venous blood (10 mL) was drawn and placed in a tube with EDTA as an anticoagulant. The sample was then centrifuged at 5000 rpm for 15 minutes. The plasma was immediately distributed into aliquots and stored at −70°C for less than 6 months. The samples were analyzed in blocks to reduce interassay variability.

The TC and TG were measured by enzymatic methods (Roche-Syntex/Boehringer Mannheim, Germany). High-density cholesterol (HDL-C) was quantified after precipitating lipoproteins containing apolipoprotein B with phospho-tungstate/Mg^{2+}. Low-density cholesterol (LDL-C) was estimated using the modified Friedewald formula. Accuracy and precision of lipid measurements were under periodic surveillance by the Centers for Disease Control and Prevention service (Atlanta, GA).

The plasma concentrations of total Hcy (tHcy) were determined with a commercially available immunonephelometric assay (Dade Behring), and the values were expressed in μmol/L. The TAT was quantified using an ELISA kit (Dade Behring), and the values were expressed in μg/L.

The institutional ethics committee approved the protocol and informed consent was obtained from each participant.

2.3. Statistical Analysis. We used descriptive statistics expressed as numbers (percentages) in categorical variables whereas continuous variables were expressed as mean ± standard deviation (SD) and the median with interquartile range values in accordance with their distribution. Student's *t*-test or the Mann-Whitney test was performed to compare the differences between continuous variables according to their distribution. The Kolmogorov-Smirnov test was used as evidence of normality. Significant differences between the categorical variables were evaluated using the Chi square test. The Pearson coefficient was used to evaluate the correlation of plasma tHcy and TAT concentrations.

We performed multivariate analyses using logistic regression to calculate independent association of the presence and severity of CAD with levels of TAT, Hcy, and traditional risk factors. Also, we performed a receiver operating characteristics curve (ROC) to establish the sensitivity and specificity of TAT for CAD diagnosis. Statistical calculations were performed using SPSS, version 15.

3. Results

Significant CAD was detected in 63 patients who were classified as CAD+ of which 31 were subclassified as bivascular and 32 as trivascular, whereas 32 patients did not have significant stenotic lesions; hence they were classified as CAD−.

The clinical and biochemical characteristics of the patients are shown in Tables 1 and 2, respectively. Hypertension, smoking, dyslipidemia, and diabetes mellitus type 2 are more prevalent in the patients with CAD+ than in CAD− patients. There was no statistically significant difference in the body mass index (BMI) between patients. Moreover, there were no differences in triglyceride or HDL-C levels. However, the TC and LDL-C levels were higher in CAD− patients.

The thrombin-antithrombin complex concentration was higher depending on the severity of the coronary artery

TABLE 1: Clinical characteristics of the CAD+ and CAD− groups.

Variables	CAD+ n = 63	CAD− n = 32	p
Age (SD)	60.97 ± 9.97	47.91 ± 6.23	<0.01
Sex (M/F)	59/4	22/10	<0.01
BMI (kg/m^2)	27.16 ± 3.61	28.2 ± 3.87	NS
DM2, n (%)	27 (42.9)	2 (6.3)	<0.01
Hypertension, n (%)	38 (60.3)	10 (31.3)	<0.01
Smokers, n (%)	11 (17.5)	5 (15.6)	NS
Dyslipidemia, n (%)	36 (57.1)	10 (31.3)	<0.05

The variables are expressed as the mean ± standard deviation (SD). A t-test was performed to compare the quantitative variables that exhibited a normal distribution; otherwise, a Mann-Whitney (nonparametric) test was performed. A Chi square distribution was calculated for the categorical variables. BMI = body mass index. DM2 = diabetes mellitus type 2.

TABLE 2: Biochemical characteristics of the CAD+ and CAD− groups.

Variables	CAD+ n = 63	CAD− n = 32	p
Total cholesterol	151 (121–188)	170.21 (144.47–209.61)	<0.05
LDL-C	90.12 (61.04–115.08)	113.85 (88.7–152.58)	<0.01
HDL-C	33 (29–40)	33.32 (28.76–38.45)	NS
Triglycerides	151 (116–206)	135.34 (92.55–187.15)	NS
TAT	28.55 (15.53–60.12)	19.15 (9.23–29.48)	<0.01
tHcy	11.2 (8.52–13.3)	7.56 (6.73–9.87)	<0.01

The variables are expressed as the median and the interquartile range 25th–75th (IQR). A t-test was performed to compare the quantitative variables that exhibited a normal distribution; otherwise, a Mann-Whitney (nonparametric) test was performed.

TABLE 3: TAT concentrations on the risk of CAD after adjusting for traditional CAD factors using conditional logistic regression model.

Risk factor	B coefficient	Odds ratio (95% CI)	p value
Age	0.133	1.142 (1.05–1.24)	<0.01
Male sex	2.806	16.54 (0.928–294.81)	NS
Diabetes mellitus	3.700	40.43 (3.193–512.05)	<0.01
Hypertension	1.234	3.43 (0.757–15.58)	NS
Dyslipidemia	1.125	3.08 (0.718–13.20)	NS
Homocysteine	0.116	1.123 (0.933–1.35)	NS
TAT	*0.47*	*1.048 (1.005–1.09)*	*0.02*

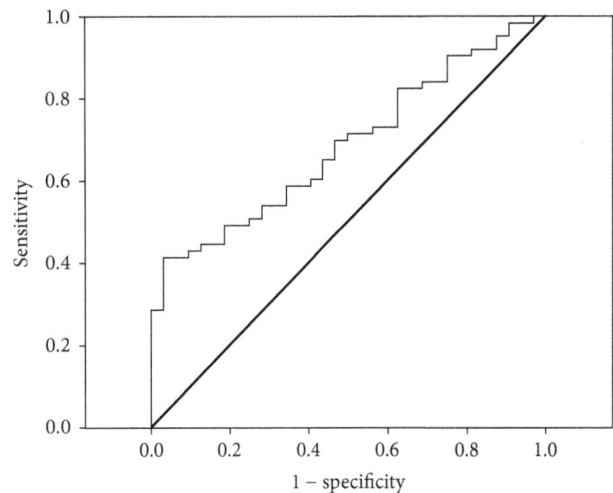

FIGURE 1: TAT sensitivity and specificity for CAD.

4. Discussion

disease. In the CAD− group, the average concentration was 20.81 ± 13.59 μg/L whereas it was 40.76 ± 29.47 in the CAD+ group (36.17 ± 24.48 μg/L in the patients with bivascular coronary artery disease and 42.77 ± 31.81 μg/L in the patients with a trivascular coronary obstruction, $p = 0.002$).

The concentration of total homocysteine was higher in the CAD+ group, at 11.36 ± 4.38, compared with 8.81 ± 3.72 in the CAD− group ($p < 0.01$). We found a positive correlation between the plasma concentrations of TAT and tHcy ($r = 0.234$, $p = 0.022$).

We analyzed the effect of high TAT concentrations on the risk of CAD in a multivariate logistic regression model which include adjustment for age, sex, diabetes mellitus type 2, hypertension, and dyslipidemia; a high TAT concentration increased the risk for CAD (OR 1.048 CI = 1.005–1.093, $p = 0.027$) as shown in Table 3. Conversely, tHcy was not related to a significant increase in risk (OR 1.123, CI = 0.933–1.352, $p = 0.219$).

We used ROC curves to determine the sensitivity and specificity of serum TAT in patients with CAD. The value for TAT level to detect CAD patients with a sensitivity of 50% and specificity of 75% was 28.49 μg/L. The area under the curve was 0.685 as shown in Figure 1.

In our study, we investigated the relationship between thrombin generation and coronary artery disease diagnosed by coronary angiography. In our population of 95 Mexican patients with clinically suspected CAD, we were able to diagnose 63 patients with significant atherosclerotic lesions and 32 without significant CAD. We found that the concentration of TAT complexes, as a marker of in vivo thrombin formation, is related to the presence of CAD. Furthermore, TAT level was associated with the severity of the atherosclerotic burden in patients with stable but significant CAD. These findings are consistent with a previous study carried on by Borissoff et al. which provided evidence of a positive association between thrombin generation and the presence of CAD assessed by computed tomography [21].

The relationship between atherosclerosis and thrombin begins with a process mediated by PARs that triggers a multitude of phenotypic drifts leading to an endothelial dysfunction [7]. Additionally, thrombin has been shown to augment levels of mRNA that encode monocyte chemoattractant protein 1 (MCP-1) [22], a well-characterized chemokine abundant in human atherosclerotic plaques [23].

Furthermore, the transcription of IL-6, IL-8, and other inflammatory molecules is modified by thrombin, facilitating the recruitment of monocytes from the circulation into the arterial vessel wall [24]. Moreover, atherosclerosis positively correlates with an enhanced synthesis of reactive oxygen species (ROS), which tends to initiate multiple proatherogenic effects by facilitating lipid peroxidation and apoptotic processes [7]. This leads to the formation of an advanced plaque that has a low thrombomodulin concentration, allowing thrombin to augment the inflammatory stimuli [25].

We were also able to find a positive correlation between the TAT and homocysteine concentrations that agrees with previous reports showing a relationship between the degrees of coagulation activation, especially the generation of thrombin and the homocysteine concentration, in patients with acute coronary syndrome [18, 23]. This relationship could be explained by the inhibition of protein C activation and the downregulation of thrombomodulin by high concentrations of homocysteine [26].

It has been proposed that the treatment of hyperhomocysteinemia with an 8-week course of vitamins B_{12} and B_6 could reduce the generation of thrombin [27]. This is important in our population because high concentrations of homocysteine can be caused by the thermolabile variant of the methylenetetrahydrofolate reductase whose frequency in the Mexican population is the highest worldwide [28].

New antithrombin agents, such as vorapaxar, have shown efficacy in reducing the risk of new cardiovascular events in secondary prevention strategy but also showed an increased hemorrhagic risk [29]; this raises new questions about whether patients with high baseline TAT benefited more of such therapy and compensate the hemorrhagic risk and the possible regression or attenuation of the atherosclerosis process [9, 30, 31].

Our study has some limitations, such as a small sample size enrolled in a single-center and a lack of patients with one-vessel disease, mostly due to the small sample size and the clinical characteristics of our population.

5. Conclusion

The level of thrombin generation, quantified as TAT complexes, is associated with the presence and severity of CAD assessed by coronary angiography in stable CAD patients.

Competing Interests

The authors state that they have no competing interests.

Acknowledgments

This work was supported by CONACYT 59896, DGAPA IN220308, Instituto Científico Pfizer, and by annual financial statement assigned to Aurora de la Peña Díaz at UNAM.

References

[1] R. Ross and B. Dodet, "Atherosclerosis is an inflammatory disease," *American Heart Journal*, vol. 138, no. 5, supplement, pp. S419–S420, 1999.

[2] P. Libby, Y. Okamoto, V. Z. Rocha, and E. Folco, "Inflammation in atherosclerosis: transition from theory to practice," *Circulation Journal*, vol. 74, no. 2, pp. 213–220, 2010.

[3] M. Levi, T. van der Poll, and H. R. Büller, "Bidirectional relation between inflammation and coagulation," *Circulation*, vol. 109, no. 22, pp. 2698–2704, 2004.

[4] J. T. B. Crawley, S. Zanardelli, C. K. N. K. Chion, and D. A. Lane, "The central role of thrombin in hemostasis," *Journal of Thrombosis and Haemostasis*, vol. 5, no. 1, pp. 95–101, 2007.

[5] E. Brodin, T. Børvik, P. M. Sandset, K. H. Bønaa, A. Nordøy, and J.-B. Hansen, "Coagulation activation in young survivors of myocardial infarction (MI)—a population-based case-control study," *Thrombosis and Haemostasis*, vol. 92, no. 1, pp. 178–184, 2004.

[6] J. I. Borissoff, H. M. H. Spronk, S. Heeneman, and H. Ten Cate, "Is thrombin a key player in the 'coagulation-atherogenesis' maze?" *Cardiovascular Research*, vol. 82, no. 3, pp. 392–403, 2009.

[7] L. Martorell, J. Martínez-González, C. Rodríguez, M. Gentile, O. Calvayrac, and L. Badimon, "Thrombin and protease-activated receptors (PARs) in atherothrombosis," *Thrombosis and Haemostasis*, vol. 99, no. 2, pp. 305–315, 2008.

[8] J. I. Borissoff, H. M. H. Spronk, and H. ten Cate, "The hemostatic system as a modulator of atherosclerosis," *The New England Journal of Medicine*, vol. 364, no. 18, pp. 1746–1760, 2011.

[9] F. Bea, J. Kreuzer, M. Preusch et al., "Melagatran reduces advanced atherosclerotic lesion size and may promote plaque stability in apolipoprotein E-deficient mice," *Arteriosclerosis, Thrombosis, and Vascular Biology*, vol. 26, no. 12, pp. 2787–2792, 2006.

[10] J. Khallou-Laschet, G. Caligiuri, E. Tupin et al., "Role of the intrinsic coagulation pathway in atherogenesis assessed in hemophilic apolipoprotein E knockout mice," *Arteriosclerosis, Thrombosis, and Vascular Biology*, vol. 25, no. 8, pp. e123–e126, 2005.

[11] B. A. Maron and J. Loscalzo, "Homocysteine," *Clinics in Laboratory Medicine*, vol. 26, no. 3, pp. 591–609, 2006.

[12] M. K. Al-Obaidi, H. Philippou, P. J. Stubbs et al., "Relationships between homocysteine, factor VIIa, and thrombin generation in acute coronary syndromes," *Circulation*, vol. 101, no. 4, pp. 372–377, 2000.

[13] G. Freyburger, S. Labrouche, G. Sassoust, F. Rouanet, S. Javorschi, and F. Parrot, "Mild hyperhomocysteinemia and hemostatic factors in patients with arterial vascular diseases," *Thrombosis and Haemostasis*, vol. 77, no. 3, pp. 466–471, 1997.

[14] J. Zhou and R. C. Austin, "Contributions of hyperhomocysteinemia to atherosclerosis: causal relationship and potential mechanisms," *BioFactors*, vol. 35, no. 2, pp. 120–129, 2009.

[15] M. Nylænde, A. Kroese, E. Stranden et al., "Prothrombotic activity is associated with the anatomical as well as the functional severity of peripheral arterial occlusive disease," *Thrombosis and Haemostasis*, vol. 95, no. 4, pp. 702–707, 2006.

[16] M. R. Di Tullio, S. Homma, Z. Jin, and R. L. Sacco, "Aortic atherosclerosis, hypercoagulability, and stroke. The APRIS (Aortic Plaque and Risk of Ischemic Stroke) study," *Journal of the American College of Cardiology*, vol. 52, no. 10, pp. 855–861, 2008.

[17] J. A. Páramo, J. Orbe, O. Beloqui et al., "Prothrombin fragment 1 + 2 is associated with carotid intima-media thickness in subjects free of clinical cardiovascular disease," *Stroke*, vol. 35, no. 5, pp. 1085–1089, 2004.

[18] J. Kienast, S. G. Thompson, C. Raskino et al., "Prothrombin activation fragment 1 + 2 and thrombin antithrombin III complexes in patients with angina pectoris: relation to the presence and severity of coronary atherosclerosis," *Thrombosis and Haemostasis*, vol. 70, no. 4, pp. 550–553, 1993.

[19] J. G. van der Bom, M. L. Bots, F. Haverkate et al., "Activation products of the haemostatic system in coronary, cerebrovascular and peripheral arterial disease," *Thrombosis and Haemostasis*, vol. 85, no. 2, pp. 234–239, 2001.

[20] P. Görög, C. D. Ridler, G. M. Rees, and I. B. Kovacs, "Evidence against hypercoagulability in coronary artery disease," *Thrombosis Research*, vol. 79, no. 4, pp. 377–385, 1995.

[21] J. I. Borissoff, I. A. Joosen, M. O. Versteylen, H. M. Spronk, H. Ten Cate, and L. Hofstra, "Accelerated in vivo thrombin formation independently predicts the presence and severity of CT angiographic coronary atherosclerosis," *JACC: Cardiovascular Imaging*, vol. 5, no. 12, pp. 1201–1210, 2012.

[22] F. Colotta, F. L. Sciacca, M. Sironi, W. Luini, M. J. Rabiet, and A. Mantovani, "Expression of monocyte chemotactic protein-1 by monocytes and endothelial cells exposed to thrombin," *American Journal of Pathology*, vol. 144, no. 5, pp. 975–985, 1994.

[23] N. A. Neiken, S. R. Coughlin, D. Gordon, and J. N. Wilcox, "Monocyte chemoattractant protein-1 in human atheromatous plaques," *The Journal of Clinical Investigation*, vol. 88, no. 4, pp. 1121–1127, 1991.

[24] S. Seehaus, K. Shahzad, M. Kashif et al., "Hypercoagulability inhibits monocyte transendothelial migration through protease-activated receptor-1-, Phospholipase-cβ-, phosphoinositide 3-kinase-, and nitric oxide-dependent signaling in monocytes and promotes plaque stability," *Circulation*, vol. 120, no. 9, pp. 774–784, 2009.

[25] J. I. Borissoff, S. Heeneman, E. Kilinç et al., "Early atherosclerosis exhibits an enhanced procoagulant state," *Circulation*, vol. 122, no. 8, pp. 821–830, 2010.

[26] T. Hayashi, G. Honda, and K. Suzuki, "An atherogenic stimulus homocysteine inhibits cofactor activity of thrombomodulin and enhances thrombomodulin expression in human umbilical vein endothelial cells," *Blood*, vol. 79, no. 11, pp. 2930–2936, 1992.

[27] A. Undas, T. B. Domagala, M. Jankowski, and A. Szczeklik, "Treatment of hyperhomocysteinemia with folic acid and vitamins B12 and B6 attenuates thrombin generation," *Thrombosis Research*, vol. 95, no. 6, pp. 281–288, 1999.

[28] B. Wilcken, F. Bamforth, Z. Li et al., "Geographical and ethnic variation of the 677C>T allele of 5, 10 methylenetetrahydrofolate reductase (MTHFR): findings from over 7000 newborns from 16 areas world wide," *Journal of Medical Genetics*, vol. 40, no. 8, pp. 619–625, 2003.

[29] D. A. Morrow, E. Braunwald, M. P. Bonaca et al., "Vorapaxar in the secondary prevention of atherothrombotic events," *The New England Journal of Medicine*, vol. 366, no. 15, pp. 1404–1413, 2012.

[30] R. C. Becker, J. H. Alexander, C. Dyke et al., "Effect of the novel direct factor Xa inhibitor DX-9065a on thrombin generation and inhibition among patients with stable atherosclerotic coronary artery disease," *Thrombosis Research*, vol. 117, no. 4, pp. 439–446, 2006.

[31] H.-J. Wei, Y.-H. Li, G.-Y. Shi et al., "Thrombomodulin domains attenuate atherosclerosis by inhibiting thrombin-induced endothelial cell activation," *Cardiovascular Research*, vol. 92, no. 2, pp. 317–327, 2011.

8

Factors Affecting Health Related Quality of Life in Hospitalized Patients with Heart Failure

Georgia Audi,[1] Aggeliki Korologou,[1] Ioannis Koutelekos,[1] Georgios Vasilopoulos,[1] Kostas Karakostas,[2] Kleanthi Makrygianaki,[3] and Maria Polikandrioti[1]

[1]Faculty of Health and Caring Professions, Department of Nursing, Technological Educational Institute of Athens, Athens, Greece
[2]Thriasio General Hospital, Elefsina, Athens, Greece
[3]Alexandra General Hospital, Athens, Greece

Correspondence should be addressed to Maria Polikandrioti; mpolik2006@yahoo.com

Academic Editor: Giuseppe Biondi-Zoccai

This study identified factors affecting health related quality of life (HRQOL) in 300 hospitalized patients with heart failure (HF). Data were collected by the completion of a questionnaire which included patients' characteristics and the Minnesota Living with Heart Failure Questionnaire (MLHFQ). Analysis of data showed that the median of the total score of MLHFQ was 46 and the median of the physical and mental state was 22 and 6, respectively. Also, participants who were householders or had "other" professions had lower score of 17 points and therefore better quality of life compared to patients who were civil/private employees ($p < 0.001$ and $p < 0.001$, resp.). Patients not receiving anxiolytics and antidepressants had lower quality of life scores of 6 and 15.5 points, respectively, compared to patients who received ($p = 0.003$ and $p < 0.001$, resp.). Patients with no prior hospitalization had lower score of 7 points compared to those with prior hospitalization ($p = 0.002$), whereas patients not retired due to the disease had higher score of 7 points ($p = 0.034$). Similar results were observed for the physical and mental state. Improvement of HF patients' quality of life should come to the forefront of clinical practice.

1. Introduction

Heart failure (HF) is a global public and clinical health problem that is expanding at an alarming rate due to the ageing of population and the improvement in diagnosis and treatment of cardiovascular disease [1–3].

More than 5.8 million in the United States and more than 23 million worldwide suffer from the disease [2, 3]. Each year, 550,000 new cases are diagnosed [2–4], while this number is predicted to reach 1.5 million annually by 2040 [4].

Disease prevalence is increasing with age; in more detail, it affects approximately 2–5% of adults aged 65–75 and >10% of adults aged 80 and older [5, 6]. HF is more frequent in men than in women [6].

This life-threatening disease is also associated with high morbidity, mortality, and rehospitalizations [2, 3]. After diagnosis of HF, survival estimates are 50% and 10% at 5 and 10 years, respectively [2]. In regard to severe HF, more than 50% of patients die within one year after diagnosis [2, 5].

Moreover, HF is responsible for 1 million hospitalizations, in the United States and Europe annually [7, 8]. After discharge, rates of rehospitalization approach 30% within 60 to 90 days [7]. Exacerbation of symptoms accounts for 50% of readmissions within six months [4].

Although HF may be caused by several medical states, the prevalent etiology is ischemic heart disease mainly in the western world. In more detail, approximately 36% of patients with myocardial infarction will develop heart failure after 7-8 years [9, 10].

HF imposes a tremendous burden on patients, care givers, society, and health care system of each country. Indeed, HF patients experience various physical and psychosocial problems that affect their health related quality of life (HRQOL) [1, 11]. HF patients' HRQOL is a valuable measure for the outcome of the disease [11].

To the best of our knowledge, little is known about determinants of HRQOL in the hospitalized HF population in Greece.

The aim of this study was to identify factors affecting health related quality of life (HRQOL) in hospitalized HF patients.

2. Methods

2.1. Study Population and Design. The sample of the study consisted of 300 hospitalized HF patients (167 men and 133 women) in cardiology clinics of 4 public hospitals in Attica between June 2015 and October 2015.

This patient sample was a convenience one (convenience sample).

Inclusion criteria were (a) an established diagnosis of HF, (b) at least 2 days' hospitalization in cardiology clinics because of HF, and (c) sufficient understanding of the Greek language. Participation was anonymous and voluntary; however, patients were able to withdraw from the study at any moment.

Patients were excluded if they had a concurrent diagnosis of other life-threatening diseases (e.g., cancer) or a chronic severe psychiatric condition (e.g., psychosis), had a history of alcohol abuse in the past six months, or were unable to communicate with the researcher or to give their written consent.

The process of filling out the questionnaires took between 15 and 30 minutes.

Ethical Considerations. All participants gave their written informed consent. The study was approved by the Ethics Committee for Medical Research in each participating hospital and was conducted in accordance with the Declaration of Helsinki (1989) of the World Medical Association.

Data collection was performed by the method of the interview using a questionnaire developed by the researchers of the study so as to fully serve its purposes.

The data collected for each patient included sociodemographic characteristics (e.g., gender, age, education level, job, and residency) and characteristics concerning the state of health: (a) clinical characteristics (e.g., medication, other diseases, years of having the problem, prior hospitalization, frequency, and days of hospitalization) and (b) other self-report characteristics (e.g., level of information about the state of health, relations with the medical and nursing staff, considering themselves as anxious, and retirement or absence from work due to the cardiac problem).

2.2. Health Related Quality of Life (HRQOL) in HF Patients. The "Minnesota Living with Heart Failure" questionnaire (MLHFQ) was used to evaluate the health related quality of life (HRQOL) in hospitalized HF patients. It is the most widely known and used disease-specific instrument and has been translated in at least 34 languages with proven reliability and validity [11, 12].

This scale which was proposed in 1986 by the University of Minnesota [12] consists of 21 questions asking about how much the disease and its treatment had affected the patient's life in the last month (4 weeks). Respondents are able to answer each question in a Likert type scale (scores from 0: no effect to 5: very much).

The Minnesota Living with Heart Failure Questionnaire (MLHFQ) measures the total score of HRQOL and two separate dimensions of HRQOL: (a) the physical state of the patient and (b) the mental state of the patient. In more detail, from MLHFQ, three scores were calculated: (a) the physical state of the patients (range: 0–40), (b) the mental state of patients (range: 0–25), and (c) the total score of quality of life from all 21 questions (range: 0–105).

The score assigned to the questions is summed separately to questions that assess physical state, for those that assess mental state and all 21 questions together to an aggregate score, the total quality of life.

Higher values of scores indicate poorer quality of life.

2.3. Statistical Analysis. Categorical data are presented in absolute and relative (%) frequencies, whereas continuous data are presented with a median (interquartile range) if normality is not followed (the criterion was tested with Kolmogorov-Smirnov). The Kruskal-Wallis test was used to test the existence of association between the quality of life and a factor with more than two categories, while the Mann–Whitney test for the existence of association between the quality of life and a factor with two categories. Moreover, multiple linear regression was performed to conclude which independent statistically significant factors affect the quality of life. Results are presented as regression coefficients b (b-coefficients) and 95% confidence interval (95% CI). The statistically significant level of 5% was observed. All statistical analyzes were performed using the SPSS version 20 package (SPSS Inc., Chicago, Il, USA).

3. Results

3.1. Descriptive Results. In total, 300 hospitalized HF patients were enrolled in the study, of whom men constitute 55.7%, while 90% of the sample was aged over 60 years.

37.3% had a high school education, while 65% were pensioners. The majority of patients were leaving in Attica (43.7%) (Table 1).

28.7% and 4.7% of participants were receiving medication with anxiolytics and antidepressants, respectively.

In 42.7%, other diseases coexisted. Only one person had not been informed at all about the health problem. The majority of patients (34.7%) had the disease for 6–10 years, while 55% were hospitalized once a year because of the problem.

66.7% of the participants characterized themselves as anxious and the vast majority of the patients reported that they had good or very good relations with both the medical and nursing staff.

The median duration of hospitalization in the clinic was 5 days (Table 2).

Table 3 presents the results relating to participants' quality of life. It is observed that at least 50% of the patients had scores below 46 (median) *n* in the total score of quality of life and 22 and 6 in physical and mental score, respectively. These values indicate moderate effects of heart failure in the quality of life of patients.

TABLE 1: Patients characteristics ($N = 300$).

	N (%)
Sex	
Male	167 (55.7%)
Female	133 (44.3%)
Age	
30–39	7 (2.3%)
40–49	7 (2.3%)
50–59	17 (5.7%)
60–69	98 (32.7%)
≥70	171 (57%)
Education	
Primary	124 (41.3%)
Secondary	112 (37.3%)
University	56 (18.7%)
M.S., Ph.D.	8 (2.7%)
Job	
Unemployed	4 (1.3%)
Civil servant	16 (5.3%)
Private employee	34 (11.3%)
Freelancer	6 (2%)
Household	44 (14.7%)
Pensioner	195 (65%)
Other	1 (0.3%)
Residency	
Attica	131 (43.7%)
County capital	94 (31.3%)
Small town	28 (9.3%)
Rural	47 (15.7%)

3.2. Association between Quality of Life and Patients' Characteristics. Tables 4 and 5 present the associations between quality of life and patients' characteristics.

The total score for quality of life was statistically significantly associated with educational level ($p = 0.002$), job ($p < 0.001$), and place of residence ($p < 0.001$) (Table 4). More specific, patients with a high school education level (median 54) scored higher meaning that they had a worse quality of life in relation to the remaining patients. Also, employees (civil/private employees) had a worse quality of life (median 58.5). Finally, patients who resided in a county capital had higher scores (worse quality of life, median 54) compared to patients living in Attica or a small town.

Physical state was statistically significantly associated with educational level ($p = 0.003$) and job ($p = 0.007$). Specifically, patients with secondary educational level (median 25) and employees (civil/private employees) (median 26) scored higher meaning that they were in worse physical state in relation to the remaining patients.

Mental state was statistically significantly associated with age ($p < 0.001$), educational level ($p < 0.001$), job ($p < 0.001$), and place of residence ($p < 0.001$). Patients aged under 60 years had higher scores of mental state (worse mental state, median 11) compared to patients older than 60. Patients with high school educational level scored higher

meaning that they were in worse mental state (median 12) compared to patients with a lower level of education. Similarly for patients who were employees (civil/private employees) and those who were living in a county capital, they were also in worse mental state (median 12 and 11, resp.).

Table 5 presents the association between quality of life and patients' characteristics (clinical and self-report characteristics).

The total score of patients' quality of life was statistically significantly associated with the following: the medication with anxiolytics ($p < 0.001$) and antidepressants ($p < 0.001$), years of having the problem ($p < 0.001$), if they had been hospitalized before ($p = 0.005$), if they considered themselves anxious ($p < 0.001$), and if they were retired or absent from work because of the problem ($p < 0.001$ and $p < 0.001$, resp.). More specifically, it was found that patients taking antidepressants and anxiolytics had a worse quality of life (median 54 and 64, resp.); patients suffering from 6 to 10 years had also worse quality of life (median 54) and similarly the ones that had been hospitalized before (median 46) and those who had not retired or were not absent from work because of the problem (median 46 and 46, resp.).

Physical state was statistically significantly associated with the following: the medication with anxiolytics ($p < 0.001$) and antidepressants ($p < 0.001$), whether suffering from another disease ($p < 0.001$), the degree of information ($p = 0.031$), years of having the problem ($p < 0.001$), if the patient had been hospitalized before ($p = 0,001$), the frequency of hospitalization ($p = 0.035$), if patients considered themselves anxious ($p < 0.001$), and if they were retired or absent from work because of the problem ($p = 0.003$ and $p = 0.023$, resp.).

Specifically, patients who were taking anxiolytics and antidepressants, were suffering from another disease, were "a little" aware of their problem, were suffering the disease for 6–10 years, were hospitalized before, were considering themselves anxious, and had not been retired or absent from work because of the problem were in a worse physical state than other patients.

Mental state was statistically significantly associated with the following: the medication with anxiolytics ($p < 0.001$) and antidepressants ($p < 0.001$), years of having the problem ($p < 0.001$), if a relative suffered from heart problems ($p = 0.001$), hospitalization frequency ($p = 0.015$), if patients considered themselves anxious ($p < 0.001$), if they were retired or absent from work because of the problem ($p = 0.002$ and $p = 0.001$, resp.), and the relations with the medical staff ($p = 0.015$) and the nursing staff ($p < 0.001$). Specifically, patients who were taking anxiolytics and antidepressants, were suffering for 6–10 years from the problem, were considering themselves anxious, and had not retired or were absent from work because of the problem and those who reported having substandard relations with the medical and nursing staff were in a worse mental state than other patients.

3.3. Assessing the Effect of the Factors on Quality of Life. Multivariate linear regression was performed to check which independent factors affect the quality of life of HF patients. As

TABLE 2: Characteristics concerning the state of health of patients.

	N (%)
Medication with anxiolytics	
Yes	86 (28.7%)
No	214 (71.3%)
Medication with antidepressants	
Yes	14 (4.7%)
No	286 (95.3%)
Other diseases	
Yes	128 (42.7%)
No	172 (57.3%)
Informed about the state of health	
Very	90 (30%)
Enough	190 (63.3%)
A little	19 (6.3%)
Not at all	1 (0.3%)
Years of having the problem	
<1 year	40 (13.3%)
2–5	45 (15%)
6–10	104 (34.7%)
11–15	55 (18.3%)
>15	56 (18.7%)
Any family member that suffers from a disease of the circulatory system	
Yes	200 (66.7%)
No	100 (33.3%)
Have you ever been hospitalized for the same reason?	
Yes	246 (82%)
No	54 (18%)
Frequency of hospitalization	
1 per year	165 (55%)
2 per year	47 (15.7%)
3 per year	18 (6%)
>3 per year	38 (12.7%)
Consider yourself anxious?	
Yes	200 (66.7%)
No	100 (33.3%)
Did you retire because of your cardiac problem?	
Yes	21 (7%)
No	279 (93%)
Are you absent from work because of your cardiac problem?	
Yes	40 (13.3%)
No	260 (86.7%)
Relations with medical staff	
Very good	157 (52.3%)
Good	130 (43.3%)
Moderate	12 (4%)
Bad	0 (0%)
Very bad	1 (0.3%)

TABLE 2: Continued.

	N (%)
Relations with nursing staff	
Very good	176 (58.7%)
Good	109 (36.3%)
Moderate	13 (4.3%)
Bad	1 (0.3%)
Very bad	1 (0.3%)
	Median (IQR)
Days of hospitalization	5 (4–6)

TABLE 3: Measuring impact of heart failure on quality of life.

	Median (IQR)
Total score MINNESOTA (range 0–105)	46 (35–54)
Physical state (range 0–40)	22 (17–26)
Mental state (range 0–25)	6 (4–11)

independent variables in the model were entered, the factors that were statistically significant associated with the quality of life in the univariate analysis.

From Table 6, it is concluded that patients who were householders or had "other" professions had lower score of 17 points and therefore better quality of life in relation to patients who were civil/private employees ($p < 0.001$ and $p < 0.001$, resp.). Patients who did not take anxiolytics and antidepressants had lower quality of life scores of 6 and 15.5 points, respectively, compared to patients who did ($p = 0.003$ and $p < 0.001$, resp.). In addition, patients who had not been hospitalized before had lower score of 7 points compared to patients that had been hospitalized before ($p = 0.002$), whereas patients that were not retired due to the problem had higher score of 7 points ($p = 0.034$).

From Table 7 we conclude that patients who were householders, were pensioners, or had "other" professions had lower scores of 6.4, 4.7, and 9.2 points, respectively, and hence better levels of physical state in relation to the patients who were civil/private employees ($p < 0.001$, $p = 0.001$, and $p < 0.001$, resp.). Patients who did not take anxiolytics had lower score of physical state of 2.8 points than patients who did ($p = 0.005$). Patients who did not have other diseases had better physical state score of 3.6 points ($p < 0.001$). Patients who were enough or a little informed about their state of health had worse physical state score of 2.3 and 8.7 points, respectively, than those who were very informed ($p = 0.011$ and $p < 0.001$, resp.). Patients suffering for 6 to 10 years and 11–15 years from the problem had worse physical state score of 4.4 and 5 points, respectively, than those who suffered for less than a year ($p = 0.010$ and $p = 0.005$, resp.). In addition, patients who had not been hospitalized before had better physical state score of 5 points ($p = 0.001$), whereas patients that were hospitalized more than three times a year had worse physical state score of 6 points in relation to those who were hospitalized once a year ($p < 0.001$). Finally, patients who

had not retired because of the problem had worse physical state score of 3.8 points ($p = 0.024$).

Regarding mental state, patients aged 60–69 years had lower score of 1.9 points and therefore better mental state than patients aged <60 years ($p = 0.024$). Patients with secondary educational level had worse mental state score of 1.2 points than patients with primary educational level ($p = 0.042$). Patients who were householders, were pensioners, or had "other" professions had lower scores 6, 3, and 4.7 points, respectively, and hence better mental state in relation to patients who were civil/private employees ($p < 0.001$, $p = 0.002$, and $p < 0.001$, resp.). Patients living in a county capital had worse mental state score of 2.15 points than patients who lived in Attica ($p = 0.008$). Patients who did not take anxiolytics and antidepressants have lower mental state scores of 1.4 and 5.3 points, respectively, than patients who did ($p = 0.005$ and $p < 0.001$, resp.). Patients suffering for 2–5 years and 6–10 years from the problem had worse mental state score of 2.3 and 2.7 points, respectively, than those suffering for less than a year ($p = 0.008$ and $p = 0.002$, resp.). In addition, patients who were hospitalized more than 3 times a year had worse mental state score of 1.7 points than those who were hospitalized once a year ($p = 0.005$). Patients who characterized themselves anxious had better mental state score of 1.15 points. Finally, patients who had good or below moderate relationship with the medical staff had worse mental state score of 1.8 and 5 points, respectively, than patients who had very good relationship ($p = 0.013$ and $p < 0.001$, resp.).

4. Discussion

The results of the present study showed that patients who had high school education level, were employees (civil/private employees), and were residents in a county capital had worse quality of life.

Education level and its close association with socioeconomic status are predictive of reduced quality of life [4, 13]. A possible explanation is that low financial sources along with inability to understand medical instructions imply lack of adherence to treatment and, therefore, reduced effectiveness of disease management.

The finding of the present study that living in county capital was associated with reduced total quality of life is

TABLE 4: Associations between patients' characteristics and quality of life.

	Total median (IQR)	Physical state median (IQR)	Mental state median (IQR)
Age	$p = 0.301$	$p = 0.167$	**$p < 0.001$**
<60	53 (41–57)	20 (17–24)	11 (9–13)[*]
60–69	40 (35–64)	20,5 (17–28)	6 (4–12)
>69	46 (39–54)	23 (18–25)	6 (5–10)
Education	**$p = 0.002$**	**$p = 0.003$**	**$p < 0.001$**
Primary	46 (35–53)	22 (17–27)	5 (4–8)
Secondary	54 (35–62)[*]	25 (17–28)[*]	10 (4–12)[*]
University, M.S., Ph.D.	42,5 (32,5–52)	20 (16–23)	6 (4–11)
Job	**$p < 0.001$**	**$p = 0.007$**	**$p < 0.001$**
Civil/private employee	58,5 (51–66)[*]	26 (20–28)[**]	12 (11-12)[*]
Householder	54 (35–54)	25 (17–25)	11 (4–11)
Pensioner	45 (34–51)	22 (17–26)	5 (4–8)
Other	36 (22–52)	17 (7–20)	4 (2–11)
Residency	**$p < 0.001$**	$p = 0.096$	**$p < 0.001$**
Attica	41 (35–49)	21 (17–26)	6 (3–8)
County capital	54 (35–66)[*]	25 (17–28)	11 (4–12)[*]
Small town/ rural	46 (31–55)	22 (15–27)	5 (5–9)

[*]Statistically significant different score from other categories, after Bonferroni correction (multiple comparisons $p < 0.05$). [**]Statistically significant different score from category "other," after Bonferroni correction (multiple comparisons $p < 0.05$).

possibly attributed to the stressful everyday living. However, place of residency needs further scrutiny as it seems to influence quality of life, indirectly. For example, rural patients may have limited access to health care services including cardiac rehabilitation interventions and are more likely to be readmitted due to the exacerbations of disease [4].

Regarding age, the results revealed that HF patients aged under 60 years had worse mental state. Based on the knowledge that HF incidence increases with age, researchers would anticipate that older patients who experience several limitations such as cognitive impairment, loss of personal autonomy, or anxiety and depression may have poor quality of life. However, Erceg et al. [14] who also explored hospitalized patients found no correlation between age, gender, and quality of life. Moreover, the same researches showed the depressive symptoms, the higher NYHA class, the lower income, and the longer duration of heart failure as independent predictors of poor quality of life.

The finding that participants taking anxiolytics and antidepressants were in both physical and mental worse state is attributed to adverse outcomes of depression in HF patients' life. In more detail, depression involves physical impairment, limited social functioning, role restrictions or emotional distress, and high risk of hospitalization [15–18]. On the other end of the spectrum, HF patients need this medication to alleviate the emotional burden of this unpredictable disease and the shortened lifespan.

Also associated with both physical and mental worse state were the years of suffering from the disease (6–10 years) which may reflect symptoms' severity. HF patients often experience loss of functional independence in daily activities such as feeding, dressing, housekeeping, bathing, and walking [19]. The most common symptoms affecting quality of life are dyspnea at rest or on exertion, paroxysmal nocturnal dyspnea, orthopnea, and fatigue as well as lack of energy [20, 21].

It is noteworthy that evaluation is needed of all the changes that take place through years and that may exacerbate HF patients' quality of life such as inability to fulfill their prior role (social, professional, and family), diminished self-esteem, and distorted picture of themselves.

Data revealed that patients suffering from other diseases and those who had prior hospitalization were in a worse physical state. Comorbidities amongst HF patients, such as diabetes, peripheral vascular disease, and cerebrovascular disease, are responsible for poor performance in activities, for hospitalization, and for increased health care expenditures [20–23]. Unfortunately, in the present study, 42.7% suffered from another disease.

Interestingly, there is a high incidence of readmissions in HF patients with ≥50% of them to be readmitted to hospital within 6 months of discharge [24, 25]. Many reasons are held to be responsible for frequent rehospitalizations such as clinical and laboratory parameters, the overall disability, the inadequate self-monitoring, and treatment adherence failure [26–28]. Length of hospital stay is correlated inversely with overall quality of life [14]. In the present study, 82% of the participants had prior hospitalization due to the same reason.

Patients who considered themselves anxious were in a worse physical and mental state. Anxiety is characterized as a subjective unpleasant feeling emerging when anticipated events are experienced as a menace. Patients who characterize themselves as anxious usually perceive the disease and its inevitable consequences as a threat or as a loss of control on effects of the disease. Working individuals are socially active and do not easily accept the role of "patient." On the other hand, some individuals when performing occupational tasks may feel lack of energy or diminished level of functional

TABLE 5: Associations between patients characteristics concerning the state of health of patients and quality of life.

	Total median (IQR)	Physical state median (IQR)	Mental state median (IQR)
Medication with anxiolytics	**p < 0.001**	**p < 0.001**	**p < 0.001**
Yes	54 (50–66)	25 (24–28)	11 (9–12)
No	43 (35–50)	21 (17–24)	5 (4–8)
Medication with antidepressants	**p < 0.001**	**p < 0.001**	**p < 0.001**
Yes	64.5 (55–70)	28 (25–32)	14 (10–17)
No	46 (35–54)	22 (17–26)	6 (4–11)
Other diseases	*p = 0.792*	**p < 0.001**	*p = 0.130*
Yes	45 (37–55.5)	24 (19.5–28)	6 (5–9)
No	46 (35–54)	21.5 (17–25)	6.5 (4–12)
Informed about the state of health	*p = 0.224*	*p = 0.031*	*p = 0.542*
Very	46 (31–66)	24 (17–28)	6 (3–12)
Enough	46 (35–54)	22 (17–25)	6 (4–11)
A little/not at all	48 (43–57)	25 (18–31)*	10 (5–11)
Years of having the problem	**p < 0.001**	**p < 0.001**	**p < 0.001**
Less than two years	42.5 (28–53)	18.5 (14.5–30)	6 (3–8)
2–5	46 (36–54)	20 (17–22)	10 (5–12)
6–10	54 (41–64.5)*	25 (17–28)*	11 (4–12)*
11–15	46 (39–46)	22 (21–23)	5 (5–6)
>15	35 (29.5–52.5)	20.5 (16–26)	4 (3–6)
Any family member that suffers from a disease of the circulatory system	*p = 0.064*	*p = 0.603*	**p < 0.001**
Yes	46 (35–54.5)	22 (17–25)	7.5 (5–11)
No	44 (32.5–54)	23 (16–28)	5.5 (3–8)
Have you ever been hospitalized for the same reason?	**p = 0.005**	**p < 0.001**	*p = 0.702*
Yes	46 (35–56)	23 (17–27)	6 (4–11)
No	41.5 (31–50)	18 (15–22)	6 (4–10)
Frequency of hospitalization	*p = 0.795*	**p = 0.035**	**p = 0.015**
1 per year	48 (35–54)	23 (17–26)	8 (4–12)
2 per year	46 (35–50)	22 (20–22)*	5 (4–8)*
3 per year	41.5 (35–57)	23.5 (19–29)	6 (4–9)
>3 per year	45.5 (37–56)	24.5 (17–30)	6.5 (3–8)
Consider yourself anxious?	**p < 0.001**	**p < 0.001**	**p < 0.001**
Yes	46 (36.5–56.5)	23 (17–27)	7 (5–11)
No	41 (31–51)	20 (15.5–24)	5 (3–8)
Did you retire because of your cardiac problem?	**p < 0.001**	**p = 0.003**	**p = 0.003**
Yes	33 (25–37)	17 (15–20)	4 (3–6)
No	46 (35–55)	22 (17–27)	6 (4–11)
Are you absent from work because of your cardiac problem?	**p < 0.001**	**p = 0.023**	**p < 0.001**
Yes	35.5 (25–51)	19 (11.5–26)	4.5 (3–9)
No	46 (35–54.5)	22 (17–26.5)	6 (4–11)
Relations with medical staff	*p = 0.588*	*p = 0.889*	**p = 0.015**
Very good	46 (36–55)	22 (17–28)	6 (5–11)
Good	45 (35–54)	23 (17–25)	6.5 (4–11)
Below moderate	48 (46–57)	21 (18–23)	11 (10–13)*
Relations with nursing staff	*p = 0.053*	*p = 0.321*	**p < 0.001**

TABLE 5: Continued.

	Total median (IQR)	Physical state median (IQR)	Mental state median (IQR)
Very good	46 (37–54)	22.5 (18–26.5)	6 (5–11)
Good	41 (35–54)	20 (17–26)	5 (4–8)
Below moderate	52 (42–59)	22 (17–28)	11 (10–14)*
	Spearman's rho	*Spearman's rho*	*Spearman's rho*
Days of hospitalization	0.039 ($p = 0.497$)	0.059 ($p = 0.305$)	0.038 ($p = 0.513$)

*Statistically significant different score from other categories, after Bonferroni correction (multiple comparisons $p < 0.05$).

TABLE 6: Assessment of the effect of the factors on quality of life.

	Total β coef. (95% CI)	p value
Job		
Civil/private employee	Ref. Cat	
Householder	−17.6 (−23.15–−12.04)	**<0.001**
Pensioner	−4.63 (−10.75–1.5)	0.138
Other	−17.37 (−25.66–−9.08)	**<0.001**
Medication with anxiolytics		
Yes	Ref. Cat	
No	−5.93 (−9.82–−2.04)	**0.003**
Medication with antidepressants		
Yes	Ref. Cat	
No	−15.58 (−22.5–−8.66)	**<0.001**
Have you ever been hospitalized for the same reason?		
Yes	Ref. Cat	
No	−7.04 (−11.37–−2.71)	**0.002**
Did you retire because of your cardiac problem?		
Yes	Ref. Cat	
No	7.02 (0.53–13.51)	**0.034**

ability due to the disease which partially explains their worse physical and mental state [1, 29].

Also in a worse physical and mental state were patients who were absent or retired from work because of the problem. Theories about association between work and chronic illness are contradictory. On the one hand, individuals who are working are socially active and do not easily accept the role of "patient," while, on the other hand, they may face difficulties during performing occupational tasks due to the lack of energy or the diminished level of functional ability [30]. Therefore, this finding raises concern about the appropriate time to retire from work.

Participants being "a little" aware of their health were in worse physical state. Patients with a knowledge deficit about the disease may underestimate its magnitude or fail to adhere to the therapeutic regimen [5]. Functional and cognitive limitations are the most common barriers in terms of disease knowledge, while only well-informed patients may take control for their own health [31, 32].

On the basis of these findings, we seek to determine the crucial role of health professionals to provide accurate information. Lack of awareness about the disease among HF

patients and their families is not a rare issue since clinicians often (a) put more emphasis on therapy and have diminished available time for conversations with HF patients, (b) lack confidence to provide end life care, and (c) show reluctance to negotiate end-of-life issues or experience uncertainty whether patients wish to obtain an in-depth knowledge of the disease [33–36].

The key-factor in providing care of high quality to HF patients is constant assessment of their information needs which may vary in different stages of the disease. In more detail, elaborate information motivates individuals to seek help in the early stages of heart failure, whereas in advanced disease, patients' needs (physical, emotional, or practical) are frequently unmet as health professionals are unable to provide any further medical aid [37].

Clinical approaches will be most effective when tailored to patients' needs and preferences. Need for orientated approach is of fundamental importance, since, nowadays, it is widely acknowledged that the ultimate goal in HF treatment is not solely patients' survival but also improvement of their quality of life [38]. Other significant areas within the field of HF are to facilitate hospital to home transition by evaluating

TABLE 7: Assessment of the effect of the factors on quality of life (subscales).

	Physical State β coef. (95% CI)	p value	Mental state β coef. (95% CI)	p value
Age				
<60	—		Ref. Cat	
60–69	—		−1.91 (−3.57–−0.26)	**0.024**
>69	—		0.26 (−1.54–2.07)	0.776
Education				
Primary	Ref. Cat		Ref. Cat	
Secondary	1.86 (−0.54–4.26)	0.129	1.22 (0.04–2.4)	**0.042**
University, M.S., Ph.D.	0.01 (−2.37–2.4)	0.990	0.14 (−0.97–1.24)	0.810
Job				
Civil/private employee	Ref. Cat		Ref. Cat	
Householder	−6.43 (−9.49–−3.37)	**<0.001**	−6.06 (−7.71–−4.41)	**<0.001**
Pensioner	−4.74 (−7.63–−1.84)	**0.001**	−3.06 (−4.94–−1.18)	**0.002**
Other	−9.27 (−13.41–−5.12)	**<0.001**	−4.73 (−6.83–−2.63)	**<0.001**
Residency				
Attica	—		Ref. Cat	
County capital	—		2.15 (0.57–3.74)	**0.008**
Small town/rural	—		0.25 (−0.73–1.24)	0.615
Medication with anxiolytics				
Yes	Ref. Cat		Ref. Cat	
No	−2.86 (−4.84–−0.89)	**0.005**	−1.44 (−2.45–−0.44)	**0.005**
Medication with antidepressants				
Yes	Ref. Cat		Ref. Cat	
No	−2.8 (−6.58–0.98)	0.146	−5.28 (−7.13–−3.43)	**<0.001**
Other diseases				
Yes	Ref. Cat		—	
No	−3.61 (−5.51–−1.71)	**<0.001**	—	
Informed about the state of health				
Very	Ref. Cat		—	
Enough	2.38 (0.55–4.22)	**0.011**	—	
A little/not at all	8.72 (5.37–12.06)	**<0.001**	—	
Years of having the problem				
<1	Ref. Cat		Ref. Cat	
2–5	0.06 (−3.45–3.57)	0.972	2.34 (0.61–4.07)	**0.008**
6–10	4.43 (1.05–7.8)	**0.010**	2.69 (1.03–4.35)	**0.002**
11–15	5.06 (1.53–8.59)	**0.005**	0.97 (−0.76–2.7)	0.270
>15	−0.25 (−3.69–3.19)	0.888	1.15 (−0.54–2.84)	0.180

TABLE 7: Continued.

	Physical State β coef. (95% CI)	p value	Mental state β coef. (95% CI)	p value
Have you ever been hospitalized for the same reason?				
Yes	Ref. Cat		—	
No	−4.9 (−7.81−−1.98)	**0.001**	—	
Frequency of hospitalization				
1 per year	Ref. Cat		Ref. Cat	
2 per year	1.85 (−0.67−4.37)	0.149	0.49 (−0.77−1.74)	0.446
3 per year	3.16 (−0.09−6.4)	0.056	0.18 (−1.42−1.77)	0.828
>3 per year	6.16 (3.59−8.72)	**<0.001**	1.72 (0.52−2.93)	**0.005**
Consider yourself anxious?				
Yes	Ref. Cat		Ref. Cat	
No	0.63 (−1.21−2.47)	0.501	−1.15 (−2.15−−0.16)	**0.023**
Did you retire because of your cardiac problem?				
Yes	Ref. Cat		Ref. Cat	
No	3.8 (0.51−7.1)	**0.024**	−0.61 (−2.3−1.08)	0.479
Relations with medical staff				
Very good	—		Ref. Cat	
Good	—		1.79 (0.38−3.2)	**0.013**
Below moderate	—		5.01 (2.46−7.55)	**<0.001**

and meeting their needs, through multidisciplinary team approach including involvement of palliative care [39].

What is more intriguing is that data highlighted worse mental state in participants who reported having substandard relations with the medical and nursing staff. Poor communication between health professionals and patients is an obstacle to patients' effective self-care [40]. However, positive and therapeutic relations demand great effort. Though contact with a HF nurse is not associated with quality of life, it increases patients' satisfaction with treatment [41].

5. Study Limitations

The present study was cross-sectional and collected data at one point in time, thus not allowing for inferences or changes over time. A cross-sectional study does not allow the determination of a causal relation between quality of life and the sociodemographic and clinical variables.

The sampling method of the present study was a convenience one, which is not representative of HF patients in Greece, thus limiting the generalizability of the results. The strengths of the study include (a) the use of a wide spread instrument, (b) the number of HF patients, and (c) "hospitalization" as most research is conducted either in community or in outpatient department of hospital when they come for regular monitoring and follow-up.

6. Conclusions

Measuring health related quality of life is increasingly important in both clinical practice and research and constitutes a challenge for clinicians involved in the care of HF. Given the high incidence of comorbidities in heart failure, it is essential to provide multidisciplinary care involving other specialties apart from cardiologists.

Early assessment of factors affecting quality of life would have a positive effect on disease management and outcomes. The study findings underscore the importance of individualized care for HF patients and suggest future directions for research in this important area. Finally, clinicians should maintain focus on treating disease, maximizing life expectancy, and optimizing quality of life for HF patients at all disease stages.

Authors' Contributions

Georgia Audi, Aggeliki Korologou, and Maria Polikandrioti designed and performed the research, analyzed the data, and wrote the manuscript. Ioannis Koutelekos provided support for data selection. Georgios Vasilopoulos, Kostas Karakostas, and Kleanthi Makrygianaki provided support for data selection. All authors contributed substantially to drafts and revisions of the manuscript. They also approved the current revised version.

References

[1] M. Polikandrioti, J. Goudevenos, L. K. Michalis et al., "Factors associated with depression and anxiety of hospitalized patients with heart failure," *Hellenic Journal of Cardiology*, vol. 56, no. 1, pp. 26–35, 2015.

[2] V. L. Roger, "Heart Failure Compendium Epidemiology of Heart Failure," *Circulation Research*, vol. 113, no. 6, pp. 646–659, 2013.

[3] E. Braunwald, "Research advances in heart failure: A compendium," *Circulation Research*, vol. 113, no. 6, pp. 633–645, 2013.

[4] T. Nesbitt, S. Doctorvaladan, J. A. Southard et al., "Correlates of quality of life in rural patients with heart failure," *Circulation: Heart Failure*, vol. 7, no. 6, pp. 882–887, 2014.

[5] K. Klindtworth, P. Oster, K. Hager, O. Krause, J. Bleidorn, and N. Schneider, "Living with and dying from advanced heart failure: Understanding the needs of older patients at the end of life," *BMC Geriatrics*, vol. 15, no. 1, article no. 125, 2015.

[6] A. Mosterd and A. W. Hoes, "Clinical epidemiology of heart failure," *Heart*, vol. 93, no. 9, pp. 1137–1146, 2007.

[7] M. Gheorghiade, M. Vaduganathan, G. C. Fonarow, and R. O. Bonow, "Rehospitalization for heart failure: problems and perspectives," *Journal of the American College of Cardiology*, vol. 61, no. 4, pp. 391–403, 2013.

[8] A. P. Ambrosy, G. C. Fonarow, J. Butler et al., "The global health and economic burden of hospitalizations for heart failure," *Journal of the American College of Cardiology*, vol. 63, no. 12, pp. 1123–1133, 2014.

[9] J. P. Hellermann, T. Y. Goraya, S. J. Jacobsen et al., "Incidence of heart failure after myocardial infarction: is it changing over time?" *American Journal of Epidemiology*, vol. 157, no. 12, pp. 1101–1107, 2003.

[10] J. Coviello, "Heart failure: An update," *Home Healthcare Nurse*, vol. 27, no. 6, pp. 354–361, 2009.

[11] A. Bilbao, A. Escobar, L. García-Perez, G. Navarro, and R. Quirós, "The Minnesota living with heart failure questionnaire: comparison of different factor structures," *Health and Quality of Life Outcomes*, vol. 14, no. 1, article no. 23, 2016.

[12] T. S. Rector, S. H. Kubo, and J. N. Cohn, "Patients' self-assessment of their congestive heart failure. Part 2: Content, reliability and validity of a new measure, the Minnesota Living with Heart Failure Questionnaire," *Heart Failure*, vol. 3, no. 5, pp. 198–209, 1987.

[13] B. Carlson, B. Pozehl, M. Hertzog, L. Zimmerman, and B. Riegel, "Predictors of overall perceived health in patients with heart failure," *Journal of Cardiovascular Nursing*, vol. 28, no. 3, pp. 206–215, 2013.

[14] P. Erceg, N. Despotovic, D. P. Milosevic et al., "Health-related quality of life in elderly patients hospitalized with chronic heart failure," *Clinical Interventions in Aging*, vol. 8, pp. 1539–1546, 2013.

[15] R. A. Carels, "The association between disease severity, functional status, depression and daily quality of life in congestive heart failure patients," *Quality of Life Research*, vol. 13, no. 1, pp. 63–72, 2004.

[16] P. Johansson, U. Dahlström, and A. Broström, "Consequences and predictors of depression in patients with chronic heart failure: implications for nursing care and future research.," *Progress in cardiovascular nursing*, vol. 21, no. 4, pp. 202–211, 2006.

[17] E. K. Song, T. A. Lennie, and D. K. Moser, "Depressive symptoms increase risk of rehospitalisation in heart failure patients with preserved systolic function," *Journal of Clinical Nursing*, vol. 18, no. 13, pp. 1871–1877, 2009.

[18] A. Sherwood, J. A. Blumenthal, R. Trivedi et al., "Relationship of depression to death or hospitalization in patients with heart failure," *Archives of Internal Medicine*, vol. 167, no. 4, pp. 367–373, 2007.

[19] S. M. Dunlay, S. M. Manemann, A. M. Chamberlain et al., "Activities of daily living and outcomes in heart failure," *Circulation: Heart Failure*, vol. 8, no. 2, pp. 261–267, 2015.

[20] T. S. Rector, I. S. Anand, and J. N. Cohn, "Relationships between clinical assessments and patients' perceptions of the effects of heart failure on their quality of life," *Journal of Cardiac Failure*, vol. 12, no. 2, pp. 87–92, 2006.

[21] C. H. Zambroski, D. K. Moser, G. Bhat, and C. Ziegler, "Impact of symptom prevalence and symptom burden on quality of life in patients with heart failure," *European Journal of Cardiovascular Nursing*, vol. 4, no. 3, pp. 198–206, 2005.

[22] J. P. Barile, W. W. Thompson, M. M. Zack, G. L. Krahn, W. Horner-Johnson, and S. E. Bowen, "Multiple chronic medical conditions and health- related quality of life in older adults, 2004-2006," *Preventing Chronic Disease*, vol. 10, no. 9, Article ID 120282, 2013.

[23] M. Gott, S. Barnes, C. Parker et al., "Predictors of the quality of life of older people with heart failure recruited from primary care," *Age and Ageing*, vol. 35, no. 2, pp. 172–177, 2006.

[24] S. Chun, J. V. Tu, H. C. Wijeysundera et al., "Lifetime analysis of hospitalizations and survival of patients newly admitted with heart failure," *Circulation: Heart Failure*, vol. 5, no. 4, pp. 414–421, 2012.

[25] K. E. Joynt and A. K. Jha, "Who has higher readmission rates for heart failure, and why? implications for efforts to improve care using financial incentives," *Circulation: Cardiovascular Quality and Outcomes*, vol. 4, no. 1, pp. 53–59, 2011.

[26] S. Heo, D. K. Moser, B. Riegel, L. A. Hall, and N. Christman, "Testing a published model of health-related quality of life in heart failure," *Journal of Cardiac Failure*, vol. 11, no. 5, pp. 372–379, 2005.

[27] A. S. Desai and L. W. Stevenson, "Rehospitalization for heart failure: Predict or prevent?" *Circulation*, vol. 126, no. 4, pp. 501–506, 2012.

[28] S. R. Greysen, I. S. Cenzer, A. D. Auerbach, and K. E. Covinsky, "Functional impairment and hospital readmission in medicare seniors," *JAMA Internal Medicine*, vol. 175, no. 4, pp. 559–565, 2015.

[29] K. S. Johnson, J. A. Tulsky, J. C. Hays et al., "Which domains of spirituality are associated with anxiety and depression in patients with advanced illness?" *Journal of General Internal Medicine*, vol. 26, no. 7, pp. 751–758, 2011.

[30] L. A. Kaminsky and M. S. Tuttle, "Functional assessment of heart failure patients," *Heart Failure Clinics*, vol. 11, no. 1, pp. 29–36, 2015.

[31] A. Strömberg, "The crucial role of patient education in heart failure," *European Journal of Heart Failure*, vol. 7, no. 3, pp. 363–369, 2005.

[32] S. Unverzagt, G. Meyer, S. Mittmann, F.-A. Samos, M. Unverzagt, and R. Prondzinsky, "Improving treatment adherence in heart failure-a systematic review and meta-analysis of pharmacological and lifestyle interventions," *Deutsches Arzteblatt International*, vol. 113, no. 25, pp. 423–430, 2016.

[33] K. Wotton, S. Borbasi, and M. Redden, "When all else has failed: Nurses' perception of factors influencing palliative care for patients with end-stage heart failure.," *The Journal of cardiovascular nursing*, vol. 20, no. 1, pp. 18–25, 2005.

[34] E. L. Garland, A. Bruce, and K. Stajduhar, "Exposing barriers to end-of-life communication in heart failure: an integrative review," *Canadian Journal of Cardiovascular Nursing*, vol. 23, no. 1, pp. 12–18, 2013.

[35] N. C. Momen and S. I. G. Barclay, "Addressing 'the elephant on the table': Barriers to end of life care conversations in heart failure - A literature review and narrative synthesis," *Current Opinion in Supportive and Palliative Care*, vol. 5, no. 4, pp. 312–316, 2011.

[36] P. M. Davidson, "Difficult conversations and chronic heart failure: do you talk the talk or walk the walk?" *Current opinion in supportive and palliative care*, vol. 1, no. 4, pp. 274–278, 2007.

[37] M. Polikandrioti, J. Goudevenos, L. K. Michalis et al., "Association between characteristics of hospitalized heart failure patients with their needs," *Global Journal of Health Science*, vol. 8, no. 6, p. 95, 2015.

[38] M. Polikandrioti and M. Ntokou, "Needs of hopitalized patients," *Health Science Journal*, vol. 5, no. 1, pp. 15–22, 2011.

[39] S. M. Dunlay, J. L. Foxen, T. Cole et al., "A survey of clinician attitudes and self-reported practices regarding end-of-life care in heart failure," *Palliative Medicine*, vol. 29, no. 3, pp. 260–267, 2015.

[40] K. Currie, P. H. Strachan, M. Spaling, K. Harkness, D. Barber, and A. M. Clark, "The importance of interactions between patients and healthcare professionals for heart failure self-care: A systematic review of qualitative research into patient perspectives," *European Journal of Cardiovascular Nursing*, vol. 14, no. 6, pp. 1–11, 2014.

[41] R. Lucas, J. P. Riley, P. A. Mehta et al., "The effect of heart failure nurse consultations on heart failure patients' illness beliefs, mood and quality of life over a six-month period," *Journal of Clinical Nursing*, vol. 24, no. 1-2, pp. 256–265, 2015.

9

The Current Approach to Diagnosis and Management of Left Ventricular Noncompaction Cardiomyopathy

Courtney E. Bennett[1] and Ronald Freudenberger[2]

[1]Mayo Clinic, 200 First Street SW, Rochester, MN 55902, USA
[2]Lehigh Valley Health Network, 1250 S Cedar Crest Boulevard, Allentown, PA 18103, USA

Correspondence should be addressed to Courtney E. Bennett; courtneyellenbennett@gmail.com

Academic Editor: Hugo A. Katus

Isolated left ventricular noncompaction (LVNC) is a genetic cardiomyopathy characterized by prominent ventricular trabeculations and deep intertrabecular recesses, or sinusoids, in communication with the left ventricular cavity. The low prevalence of patients with this cardiomyopathy presents a unique challenge for large, prospective trials to assess its pathogenesis, management, and outcomes. In this paper we review the embryology and genetics of LVNC, the diagnostic approach, and propose a management approach based on the current literature available.

1. Introduction

Isolated left ventricular noncompaction (LVNC) is a genetic cardiomyopathy characterized by prominent ventricular trabeculations and deep intertrabecular recesses, or sinusoids, in communication with the left ventricular cavity [1]. The clinical sequelae of these deformities are the syndrome of heart failure and the risk for arrhythmias and stroke. Dusek first described the postnatal persistence of spongy myocardium in 1975 pathologically, but Engberding and Bender made the first clinical recognition with two-dimensional (2D) echocardiography in 1984 [2, 3]. Three decades later, with only morphologic assessment available and no definitive genetic pathway, isolated left ventricular noncompaction (LVNC) remains a diagnostic and management challenge. In this review, we wish to define a unified process for diagnosis and suggest a management approach with special attention to guidance for anticoagulation and prevention of sudden cardiac death (SCD).

2. Embryology

The pathologic theory of LVNC is the failure of compaction during fetal development. Cardiomyocytes form a tube in the midline of the embryo from the mesodermal primordia and differentiate into myocardium based on multiple genetic factors, including positive and negative gene regulators [4]. Ventricular myocardial trabeculations are evident in the human heart by the end of the first trimester and occur as protrusions from the endocardial layer. The trabeculations allow for a greater surface to volume ratio and increasing muscle mass before the establishment of the coronary arteries. The next step includes compaction of the trabecular layers. This begins in the human embryo by 10 to 12 weeks and by the fourth month of gestation the compacted myocardium composes the majority of the ventricular volume [4, 5]. Compaction continues into the postnatal period with continued growth and increasing systemic pressures. The final process is development of the spiral pattern of the myocardial fibers, which is responsible for the twisting nature of contraction. Without the completion of compaction, there is myocardial dysfunction secondary to the failure of the efficient rotational ventricular system to develop for contractile performance. This concept has been demonstrated by abnormal speckle tracking and is further discussed later [6].

TABLE 1: Echocardiographic diagnostic criteria.

Criteria	Chin	Jenni	Stöllberger
Description	(i) Prominent trabeculations with deep recesses (ii) Decrease in ratio from MV level to papillary muscle level of the distance from the epicardium to the trough of the trabeculations (X) to the epicardium to the peak of the trabeculations (Y) (iii) Increasing LV wall thickness from base to apex	(i) Bilayered myocardium with multiple, prominent trabeculations in end-systole (ii) NC/C ratio of >2:1 (iii) Communication with the intertrabecular space demonstrated with color Doppler (iv) Absence of coexisting cardiac abnormalities	(i) Two-layer myocardium in which the noncompacted layer is thicker than the compacted myocardium (ii) >3 prominent trabeculations protruding from the LV wall apical to the papillary muscles (iii) Perfused intertrabecular spaces
Phase	End-diastole	End-systole	N/A

3. Genetics

There are multiple genetic proposals for the phenotypic development of noncompaction [1, 7–12]. None of them have been consistently identified to be the single gene abnormality causing LVNC, but they are briefly included here for completeness (see the list below) [7]. It is established that a thorough, three-generational family history should be obtained for evaluation of genetic influence, which may also impact the screening of additional family members [1, 7, 8, 10]. A systematic review by Bhatia et al. identified a familial occurrence rate of 30% in family members that were screened based on an index case [13]. Oechslin and Jenni have proposed an acquired pathogenesis in patients with prior normal cardiac structure and function that develop LVNC later in life. This supports the hypothesis that LVNC may represent a morphologic continuum of genetic cardiomyopathies, including dilated and hypertrophic cardiomyopathies [14]. Sporadic occurrence is thought to account for up to 60–70% of the cases [12]. In addition, LVNC has association with Barth syndrome, mitochondrial disorders, and myotonic dystrophy [7].

Genes Identified. The identified genes are as follows:

Fbkp1a/Notch pathway.

G4.5 gene/TAZ protein.

14-3-3 deletion.

ZASP protein.

TNNT2 protein.

MYH7 protein.

TPM1 protein.

MYBPC3 protein.

ACTC1 protein.

The Heart Rhythm Society states that genetic testing is recommended (Class I) for relatives and appropriate family members when a mutation-specific gene has been identified in the index case [12]. The molecular genetics of inherited cardiomyopathies have been reviewed and the evidence to support routine genetic testing in all patients diagnosed with LVNC is not available [11, 12]. The current genes available for testing are variants of established dilated cardiomyopathy and hypertrophic cardiomyopathy genes [11].

4. Diagnostic Approach

There is much debate regarding the diagnostic criteria for LVNC and the predilection for overdiagnosis. One case report expresses the importance of not making the diagnosis of LVNC based purely on visualized estimate on echocardiography. It is important to consider the entire diagnostic criterion as described in this section to avoid overdiagnosis [15]. In this case report, a patient was diagnosed with LVNC based on prominent trabeculations and intertrabecular recesses, but there was a better explanation for the cardiomyopathy based on the patient's history, and acute myocarditis was confirmed with cardiac magnetic resonance imaging (CMR) and myocardial biopsy.

We will review the current diagnostic criteria available for two-dimensional echocardiography, cardiac magnetic resonance imaging (CMR), and computed tomography (CT) imaging. Multiple modalities may be required for complete assessment.

4.1. Two-Dimensional Echocardiography. The traditional diagnostic study for evaluation of LVNC is echocardiography [1, 16–19]. It is still the most common initial test that identifies the characteristic findings of LVNC and may lead to further evaluation. There are three proposed diagnostic criteria that are most utilized in the literature. These criteria are summarized in Table 1. Chin et al. are credited with the first attempt at defining specific criteria for the diagnosis of LVNC [20]. The evaluation includes left ventricular (LV) free-wall thickness at end-diastole, prominent trabeculations, and a progressive decrease in the ratio of myocardial thickness from the epicardial surface to the trough (X) and the epicardial surface to the peak (Y) of the trabeculations in the PSAX and apical views. Stöllberger and Finsterer refined the definition as >3 trabeculations protruding from the LV wall apical to the papillary muscles, perfused intertrabecular spaces, and a two-layered myocardium with the noncompacted layer usually thicker than the compacted myocardium in end-systole [21]. We feel that the Stöllberger criteria alone may lead to the overdiagnosis of LVNC because the inclusion criteria are less detailed than other criteria and they were largely extrapolated from a large postmortem study. Subsequent recent studies have used the Jenni criteria to evaluate the presence of LVNC [13, 16]. These criteria include a bilayered myocardium, a noncompacted to compacted ratio >2:1, communication with the intertrabecular space demonstrated by Doppler, absence of coexisting cardiac abnormalities, and presence of multiple prominent trabeculations in end-systole [22].

Many articles have attempted to narrow the evaluation of LVNC to either end-systole or end-diastole, but a recent refinement of the echographic criteria by Stöllberger et al. stressed the importance of including both in consideration of the diagnosis [17]. In their study, three experts with more than 17 years of experience with LVNC reviewed a total of 115 echocardiograms that were proposed for inclusion in a registry. There diagnostic criteria were as follows: (1) >3 prominent trabecular formations along the left ventricular endocardial border, which are visible in end-diastole, distinct from papillary muscles, false tendons, or aberrant bands, (2) trabeculations move synchronously with the compacted myocardium, (3) trabeculations form the noncompacted part of the two-layer myocardial structure, best visible at end-systole, and (4) perfusion of the intertrabecular spaces from the ventricular cavity is present at end-diastole on color-Doppler echocardiography or contrast echocardiography. They excluded 11 patients based on their review. All experts agreed that measurement of the myocardial layers is not feasible due to the lack of uniformly accepted standards for measurements. Paterick et al. suggest measuring the myocardial layers in end-diastole based on the American Society of Echocardiography Guidelines for Chamber Quantification, which suggests wall thickness be measured in end-diastole [23]. They suggest the images for evaluation focus on nontangential short-axis views of the LV apex with special attention to the apicolateral wall. We agree on using criteria that consider both end-systolic and end-diastolic parameters, but validation of this criterion is still needed. The reproducibility of the current criteria has been tested in a small case-control study in which two echocardiography observers were blinded to the index diagnosis and reviewed 104 studies of patients with LVNC. They were in agreement with the initial diagnosis of LVNC only 67% of the time [18].

There have been recent evaluations using speckle tracking echocardiography and real-time 3-dimensional imaging (RT3DE) [24]. Speckle tracking is able to identify the abnormal ventricular mechanics by demonstrating that the basal and apical rotations are in the same direction. Real-time 3DE is useful for evaluation of LV function and quantification of trabeculations. The number of trabeculations and LV mass has been underestimated using 2-dimensional imaging when compared to RT3DE. In a study comparing 60 patients with LVNC to age-matched controls, rigid body rotation was identified in 32 of the 60 patients with LVNC [6]. This was significantly more than the normal controls and the 28 patients with normal rotation still had significantly less twist than the control patients. The patients with LVNC and rigid body rotation had worse NYHA functional status as well. The studies using both of these modalities are limited so their incorporation into the diagnosis is unclear at this time but may be considered for guidance when the diagnosis is unclear.

There are some disadvantages when using echocardiography for the assessment of LVNC. These include the inaccuracy of off-axis or oblique image planes and the challenges of evaluating the apex. These are overcome with skilled sonographers obtaining standard chamber views and the addition of contrast when the apex is not will visualized.

4.2. Cardiac Magnetic Resonance Imaging (CMR). The high resolution imaging of cardiac magnetic resonance (CMR) has allowed improvement in differentiating the noncompacted and compacted myocardium. Key features of CMR in addition to the spatial resolution are the ability to image the apex well and the use of late gadolinium enhancement for the evaluation of fibrosis. A study of magnetic resonance imaging demonstrated that there are age- and sex-related differences in trabeculated and compacted myocardium of 120 normal volunteers that must be taken into consideration when making the diagnosis of LVNC [25]. They found that there is an increase in the compacted layer after the fourth decade, but a decrease in the trabecular layer. Kawel et al. analyzed the MRI findings of the 1000 participants of the Multiethnic Study of Atherosclerosis (MESA). They found that 43% of the patients without cardiac disease or hypertension had at least one of eight regions evaluated with trabeculated to compacted myocardial ratio >2.3 [26].

In 2005, Petersen et al. compared the noncompacted to compacted layers of myocardium on CMR of healthy volunteers and patients with hypertrophic cardiomyopathy, dilated cardiomyopathy, hypertensive heart disease, and aortic stenosis and patients previously diagnosed with LVNC based on other findings [27]. They found that pathological noncompaction had a NC/C >2.3 in end-diastole and that the specificity and negative predictive values were both 99%. Later in 2010, Jacquier et al. proposed that the trabeculated mass be taken into consideration when they found that the percentage of trabeculated mass was three times higher in patients with LVNC compared to other groups including controls [28]. LV trabecular mass >20% of the global mass predicted the diagnosis of LVNC with a sensitivity and specificity of 93.7%. An example of these findings is shown in Figure 1. The advantage of this later method is not depending on the evaluation of specific myocardial segments, but rather the entire mass. The patients in this study population were not provided in detail with demographic data and they note one limitation as needing to validate this method in other ethnic groups.

Dodd et al. performed a blinded, retrospective CMR review of patients with LVNC and control subjects to compare the extent and severity of noncompaction and the degree of late gadolinium enhancement (LGE) between the groups [29]. They found that the degree of delayed enhancement correlated significantly with the ejection fraction (EF). They also found that the severity of the delayed enhancement differed among patients with mild, moderate, and severe disease. This is supported in a study of patients with cardiomyopathy and progressive LV dysfunction, which correlated with a larger extent of LGE [30]. A case correspondence by Chaowu et al. correlated the late gadolinium enhancement on CMR with histopathological evidence of fibrosis in a 27-year-old patient with LVNC that underwent cardiac transplant [31]. In contrast to these findings, one study reviewed the CMR of 47 patients diagnosed with LVNC and found that the

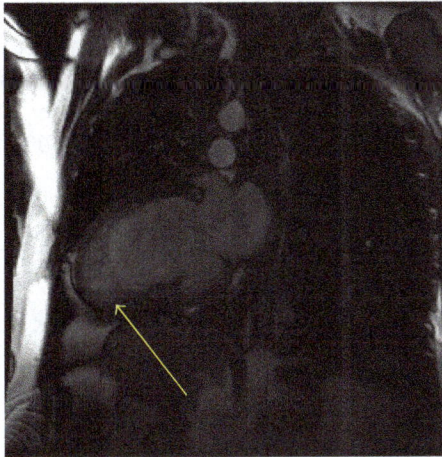

FIGURE 1: Cardiac magnetic resonance imaging (CMR) of a 38-year-old male that presented with a new cardiomyopathy and congestive heart failure. Note the prominent apical trabeculations compared to the compacted myocardium. Cardiac catheterization demonstrated no angiographic coronary disease and LVNC was the most likely diagnosis.

characteristics of LGE were heterogeneous [32]. Despite the nonspecific findings in the later study, the degree of LGE is significant because it is associated with the degree of LV reverse remodeling and LV dysfunction in patients with nonischemic cardiomyopathy [33].

Disadvantages of this modality include the availability of MRI and the time to complete the exam and required breath holding that pose challenges to the patients. There is also an inability to image patients with some devices/implants. We feel that CMR should play a major role in the evaluation of patients with LVNC when (1) the diagnosis by echocardiogram is not confirmed; (2) a good quality echocardiogram cannot be obtained; and/or (3) the degree of fibrosis may help delineate the severity of disease.

4.3. Cardiac Computed Tomography.
There have been case reports in the literature that identify the diagnosis of LVNC by cardiac computed tomography (CT) [34]. The spatial resolution for identification of LVNC is good with cardiac CT [34, 35]. CT imaging also allows for visualization of the coronary arteries and great vessels. There are studies demonstrating the high specificity and negative predictive value for exclusion of CAD [36]. An advantage of using CT is the capability to evaluate the presence of both CAD and LVNC in patient with new heart failure and low likelihood of CAD. The disadvantages of CT imaging are the high radiation exposure and reactions to the contrast dye, including renal failure. The standard use of cardiac CT in evaluation of LVNC is not yet established.

5. Management

Management of patients with LVNC is complicated because prospective studies of large cohorts do not exist. There is limited data prospectively assessing specific agents for long-term outcomes in LVNC. Beta-blocker therapy was evaluated in a small, retrospective study of patients with LVNC in which the LV mass was reduced on beta-blocker therapy compared to the patients that were not on beta-blocker therapy at approximately one-year follow-up [37]. All patients had reduced ejection fractions at baseline, which did not show significant improvement. In general, medications for LVNC should include evidence-based, guideline directed medical therapy for patients with cardiomyopathy [38]. The standard of care for patients with dilated cardiomyopathy has been extrapolated to LVNC patients with reduced ejection fraction, but there are a few management issues that are unique to LVNC patients, including anticoagulation and primary prevention of sudden cardiac death (SCD).

5.1. Anticoagulation.
The event rate of stroke in patients with LVNC is 1-2% per year or a total risk thromboembolism of 21–38% [39, 40]. In a review of 144 patients diagnosed with LVNC, 22 patients experienced stroke or embolism [40]. Sixty-four percent of these patients had reduced left ventricular function evaluated by echocardiogram, which suggests a higher risk of embolism in these patients. It is not clarified in the paper what is the percentage of patients with reduced EF who also had atrial fibrillation (AF), but 27% of the patients with an event also had AF. This identifies patients with reduced EF and AF as being at higher risk for stroke or embolism. Stöllberger et al. analyzed the risk of embolism or stroke in LVNC patients using the $CHADS_2$/$CHADS_2$-Vasc scores [41]. They found in their retrospective analysis that the patients with LVNC and a history of stroke or embolism had significantly higher $CHADS_2$/$CHADS_2$-Vasc scores. These patients also had a higher occurrence of atrial fibrillation, but it was not statistically significant. The $CHADS_2$/$CHADS_2$-Vasc score may play a role in decision-making regarding oral anticoagulation for patients with LVNC. Oral anticoagulation should be used when a definite left ventricular clot has been identified on imaging or the patient has documented atrial fibrillation. For the patients that do not fall into either of these categories, we suggest a risk assessment using the $CHADS_2$/$CHADS_2$-Vasc scores as guidance and a discussion with the patient regarding the risks and benefits of anticoagulation.

5.2. Primary Prevention of Sudden Cardiac Death.
One of the greatest challenges of managing LVNC patients is whether or not an internal cardiac defibrillator (ICD) should be placed for primary prevention. Many patients with LVNC present with reduced left ventricular function, but the guidelines for patients with decreased LV function excluded patients with LVNC. In 2011, Caliskan et al. evaluated the indications and outcomes in patients with LVNC [42]. They concluded that it is appropriate to apply the current guidelines for implantation of ICD for primary or secondary prevention to patients with LVNC. The challenge is that, as previously mentioned, CMR imaging has identified late gadolinium enhancement in patients with LVNC and histopathologic confirmation of fibrosis has been performed. In the situation of normal left ventricular function with fibrosis identified on CMR the question is whether or not to place an ICD. In the previously

mentioned study they required an additional risk factor for ICD implantation in patients with reduced ejection fraction (EF) and no clinical heart failure. They were family history of SCD, nonsustained VT (NSVT) on Holter monitoring, and/or self-reported history of syncope. Interestingly, 8% of the patients that received the ICD in the primary prevention group had NSVT on Holter monitoring compared to 7% of patients that received an ICD for secondary prevention of ventricular arrhythmias. This may suggest a role for applying Holter monitoring to patients with normal ejection fractions to assess the risk for SCD. One case report identified a 63-year woman with atrial tachycardia and monomorphic VT during exercise testing for evaluation of chest pain and CMR testing revealed the diagnosis of LVNC [43]. Her nuclear perfusion imaging was normal and her echocardiogram revealed only borderline left ventricular enlargement with normal left ventricular function. This supports the theory that these patients are at higher risk for SCD even with normal EF.

6. Summary

The overwhelming theme upon review of the current literature is that the exact method for diagnosis is still in progress, but what is clear is that the mortality of patients identified with LVNC is significant. Patients have a high incidence of NYHA III-IV heart failure, sudden cardiac death, and transplant [44–46]. It is important to take a comprehensive approach to evaluation and not rely on a single diagnostic study or parameter.

The initial study of choice remains echocardiography. Based on the current literature, we recommend the use of the Jenni criteria with consideration of both the end-diastolic and end-systolic myocardial layer thickness. As mentioned earlier, the Jenni criteria include a bilayered myocardium, a noncompacted to compacted ratio >2:1, communication with the intertrabecular space demonstrated by color Doppler, absence of coexisting cardiac abnormalities, and the presence of multiple prominent trabeculations in end-systole [22]. If the diagnosis is indeterminate based on the echocardiogram, then additional imaging modalities should be performed. Contrast echocardiography may be applied to further define the trabeculations and endocardium for accurate measurement of the myocardial layers. If more information is needed, then a CMR may be the reasonable next test. This will also allow for the assessment of fibrosis. If the patient is young with minimal risk for CAD and cardiac catheterization is being considered in evaluation of a new cardiomyopathy, then cardiac CT is reasonable.

Once the diagnosis has been made, then the next step is to define management goals based on the ejection fraction and degree of symptoms. If the patient meets the criteria for ICD based on reduced EF, then it is reasonable to proceed with this intervention [47]. If the patient has a normal EF, but a history of syncope, nonsustained ventricular tachycardia, or a family history of sudden cardiac death (SCD), then the clinician should review the risks and benefits of ICD therapy with the patient as an option for management. It is reasonable to take into consideration the degree of late gadolinium enhancement on MRI if this is known. For patients with reduced EF, there is evidence for the use of anticoagulation based on risk assessment with the $CHADS_2$-Vasc score. If the patient has a normal EF without atrial fibrillation or visible clot, then the benefit of anticoagulation has not yet been demonstrated.

As we increase recognition and further define this cardiomyopathy it will allow for additional prospective studies to improve management and outcomes of this population.

References

[1] B. J. Maron, J. A. Towbin, G. Thiene et al., "Contemporary definitions and classification of the cardiomyopathies: an American heart association scientific statement from the council on clinical cardiology, heart failure and transplantation committee; quality of care and outcomes research and functional genomics and translational biology interdisciplinary working groups; and council on epidemiology and prevention," *Circulation*, vol. 113, no. 14, pp. 1807–1816, 2006.

[2] J. Dusek, B. Ostadal, and M. Duskova, "Postnatal persistence of spongy myocardium with embryonic blood supply," *Archives of Pathology*, vol. 99, no. 6, pp. 312–317, 1975.

[3] R. Engberding and F. Bender, "Identification of a rare congenital anomaly of the myocardium by twodimensional echocardiography: persistence of isolated myocardial sinusoids," *The American Journal of Cardiology*, vol. 53, no. 11, pp. 1733–1734, 1984.

[4] D. Sedmera and T. McQuinn, "Embryogenesis of the heart muscle," *Heart Failure Clinics*, vol. 4, no. 3, pp. 235–245, 2008.

[5] D. J. Henderson and R. H. Anderson, "The development and structure of the ventricles in the human heart," *Pediatric Cardiology*, vol. 30, no. 5, pp. 588–596, 2009.

[6] F. Peters, B. K. Khandheria, E. Libhaber et al., "Left ventricular twist in left ventricular noncompaction," *European Heart Journal—Cardiovascular Imaging*, vol. 15, no. 1, pp. 48–55, 2014.

[7] J. Finsterer, "Cardiogenetics, neurogenetics, and pathogenetics of left ventricular hypertrabeculation/noncompaction," *Pediatric Cardiology*, vol. 30, no. 5, pp. 659–681, 2009.

[8] S. Probst, E. Oechslin, P. Schuler et al., "Sarcomere gene mutations in isolated left ventricular noncompaction cardiomyopathy do not predict clinical phenotype," *Circulation: Cardiovascular Genetics*, vol. 4, no. 4, pp. 367–374, 2011.

[9] J. A. Towbin, "Left ventricular noncompaction: a new form of heart failure," *Heart Failure Clinics*, vol. 6, no. 4, pp. 453–469, 2010.

[10] Y. M. Hoedemaekers, K. Caliskan, M. Michels et al., "The importance of genetic counseling, DNA diagnostics, and cardiologic family screening in left ventricular noncompaction cardiomyopathy," *Circulation: Cardiovascular Genetics*, vol. 3, no. 3, pp. 232–239, 2010.

[11] P. Teekakirikul, M. A. Kelly, H. L. Rehm, N. K. Lakdawala, and B. H. Funke, "Inherited cardiomyopathies: molecular genetics and clinical genetic testing in the postgenomic era," *The Journal of Molecular Diagnostics*, vol. 15, no. 2, pp. 158–170, 2013.

[12] M. J. Ackerman, S. G. Priori, S. Willems et al., "HRS/EHRA expert consensus statement on the state of genetic testing for

the channelopathies and cardiomyopathies this document was developed as a partnership between the Heart Rhythm Society (HRS) and the European Heart Rhythm Association (EHRA)," *Heart Rhythm*, vol. 8, no. 8, pp. 1308–1339, 2011.

[13] N. L. Bhatia, A. J. Tajik, S. Wilansky, D. E. Steidley, and F. Mookadam, "Isolated noncompaction of the left ventricular myocardium in adults: a systematic overview," *Journal of Cardiac Failure*, vol. 17, no. 9, pp. 771–778, 2011.

[14] E. Oechslin and R. Jenni, "Left ventricular non-compaction revisited: a distinct phenotype with genetic heterogeneity?" *European Heart Journal*, vol. 32, no. 12, pp. 1446–1456, 2011.

[15] M. Niemann, S. Störk, and F. Weidemann, "Left ventricular noncompaction cardiomyopathy: an overdiagnosed disease," *Circulation*, vol. 126, no. 16, pp. e240–e243, 2012.

[16] G. Habib, P. Charron, J.-C. Eicher et al., "Isolated left ventricular non-compaction in adults: clinical and echocardiographic features in 105 patients. Results from a French registry," *European Journal of Heart Failure*, vol. 13, no. 2, pp. 177–185, 2011.

[17] C. Stöllberger, B. Gerecke, J. Finsterer, and R. Engberding, "Refinement of echocardiographic criteria for left ventricular noncompaction," *International Journal of Cardiology*, vol. 165, no. 3, pp. 463–467, 2013.

[18] S. F. Saleeb, R. Margossian, C. T. Spencer et al., "Reproducibility of echocardiographic diagnosis of left ventricular noncompaction," *Journal of the American Society of Echocardiography*, vol. 25, no. 2, pp. 194–202, 2012.

[19] C. H. A. Jost and H. M. Connolly, "Left ventricular non-compaction: dreaming of the perfect diagnostic tool," *European Journal of Heart Failure*, vol. 14, no. 2, pp. 113–114, 2012.

[20] T. K. Chin, J. K. Perloff, R. G. Williams, K. Jue, and R. Mohrmann, "Isolated noncompaction of left ventricular myocardium. A study of eight cases," *Circulation*, vol. 82, no. 2, pp. 507–513, 1990.

[21] C. Stöllberger and J. Finsterer, "Left ventricular hypertrabec-ulation/noncompaction," *Journal of the American Society of Echocardiography*, vol. 17, no. 1, pp. 91–100, 2004.

[22] R. Jenni, E. Oechslin, J. Schneider, C. Attenhofer Jost, and P. A. Kaufmann, "Echocardiographic and pathoanatomical characteristics of isolated left ventricular non-compaction: a step towards classification as a distinct cardiomyopathy," *Heart*, vol. 86, no. 6, pp. 666–671, 2001.

[23] T. E. Paterick, M. M. Umland, M. F. Jan et al., "Left ventricular noncompaction: a 25-Year Odyssey," *Journal of the American Society of Echocardiography*, vol. 25, no. 4, pp. 363–375, 2012.

[24] A. Nemes, A. Kalapos, P. Domsik, and T. Forster, "Identification of left ventricular 'rigid body rotation' by three-dimensional speckle-tracking echocardiography in a patient with noncompaction of the left ventricle: a case from the MAGYAR-path study," *Echocardiography*, vol. 29, no. 9, pp. E237–E240, 2012.

[25] D. K. Dawson, A. M. MacEira, V. J. Raj, C. Graham, D. J. Pennell, and P. J. Kilner, "Regional thicknesses and thickening of compacted and trabeculated myocardial layers of the normal left ventricle studied by cardiovascular magnetic resonance," *Circulation: Cardiovascular Imaging*, vol. 4, no. 2, pp. 139–146, 2011.

[26] N. Kawel, M. Nacif, A. E. Arai et al., "Trabeculated (noncompacted) and compact myocardium in adults: the multi-ethnic study of atherosclerosis," *Circulation: Cardiovascular Imaging*, vol. 5, no. 3, pp. 357–366, 2012.

[27] S. E. Petersen, J. B. Selvanayagam, F. Wiesmann et al., "Left ventricular non-compaction: insights from cardiovascular magnetic resonance imaging," *Journal of the American College of Cardiology*, vol. 46, no. 1, pp. 101–105, 2005.

[28] A. Jacquier, F. Thuny, B. Jop et al., "Measurement of trabeculated left ventricular mass using cardiac magnetic resonance imaging in the diagnosis of left ventricular non-compaction," *European Heart Journal*, vol. 31, no. 9, pp. 1098–1104, 2010.

[29] J. D. Dodd, G. Holmvang, U. Hoffmann et al., "Quantification of left ventricular noncompaction and trabecular delayed hyperenhancement with cardiac MRI: correlation with clinical severity," *American Journal of Roentgenology*, vol. 189, no. 4, pp. 974–980, 2007.

[30] P. G. Masci, R. Schuurman, B. Andrea et al., "Myocardial fibrosis as a key determinant of left ventricular remodeling in idiopathic dilated cardiomyopathy: a contrast-enhanced cardiovascular magnetic study," *Circulation: Cardiovascular Imaging*, vol. 6, no. 5, pp. 790–799, 2013.

[31] Y. Chaowu, L. Li, and Z. Shihua, "Histopathological features of delayed enhancement cardiovascular magnetic resonance in isolated left ventricular noncompaction," *Journal of the American College of Cardiology*, vol. 58, no. 3, pp. 311–312, 2011.

[32] J. Wan, S. Zhao, H. Cheng et al., "Varied distributions of late gadolinium enhancement found among patients meeting cardiovascular magnetic resonance criteria for isolated left ventricular non-compaction," *Journal of Cardiovascular Magnetic Resonance*, vol. 15, article 20, 2013.

[33] K. Kida, K. Yoneyama, Y. Kobayashi, M. Takano, Y. J. Akashi, and F. Miyake, "Late gadolinium enhancement on cardiac magnetic resonance images predicts reverse remodeling in patients with nonischemic cardiomyopathy treated with carvedilol," *International Journal of Cardiology*, vol. 168, no. 2, pp. 1588–1589, 2013.

[34] M. M. Benjamin, R. A. Khetan, R. C. Kowal, and J. M. Schussler, "Diagnosis of left ventricular noncompaction by computed tomography," *Baylor University Medical Center Proceedings*, vol. 25, no. 4, pp. 354–356, 2012.

[35] R. T. Gandhi, G. Sarraf, and M. Budoff, "Isolated noncompaction of the left ventricular myocardium diagnosed upon cardiovascular multidetector computed tomography," *Texas Heart Institute Journal*, vol. 37, no. 3, pp. 374–375, 2010.

[36] P. Fazel, M. A. Peterman, and J. M. Schussler, "Three-year outcomes and cost analysis in patients receiving 64-slice computed tomographic coronary angiography for chest pain," *The American Journal of Cardiology*, vol. 104, no. 4, pp. 498–500, 2009.

[37] J. Li, J. Franke, R. Pribe-Wolferts et al., "Effects of beta-blocker therapy on electrocardiographic and echocardiographic characteristics of left ventricular noncompaction," *Clinical Research in Cardiology*, vol. 104, no. 3, pp. 241–249, 2015.

[38] C. W. Yancy, M. Jessup, B. Bozkurt et al., "2013 ACCF/AHA guideline for the management of heart failure: a report of the American college of cardiology foundation/american heart association task force on practice guidelines," *Journal of the American College of Cardiology*, vol. 62, no. 16, pp. e147–e239, 2013.

[39] C. Cevik, N. Shah, J. M. Wilson, and R. F. Stainback, "Multiple left ventricular: in a patient with left ventricular noncompaction," *Texas Heart Institute Journal*, vol. 39, no. 4, pp. 550–553, 2012.

[40] C. Stöllberger, G. Blazek, C. Dobias, A. Hanafin, C. Wegner, and J. Finsterer, "Frequency of stroke and embolism in left

ventricular hypertrabeculation/noncompaction," *The American Journal of Cardiology*, vol. 108, no. 7, pp. 1021–1023, 2011.

[41] C. Stöllberger, C. Wegner, and J. Finsterer, "CHADS$_2$- and CHA$_2$DS$_2$VASc scores and embolic risk in left ventricular hypertrabeculation/noncompaction," *Journal of Stroke and Cerebrovascular Diseases*, vol. 22, no. 6, pp. 709–712, 2013.

[42] K. Caliskan, T. Szili-Torok, D. A. M. J. Theuns et al., "Indications and outcome of implantable cardioverter-defibrillators for primary and secondary prophylaxis in patients with noncompaction cardiomyopathy," *Journal of Cardiovascular Electrophysiology*, vol. 22, no. 8, pp. 898–904, 2011.

[43] S. Seethala, F. Knollman, D. McNamara et al., "Exercise-induced atrial and ventricular tachycardias in a patient with left ventricular noncompaction and normal ejection fraction," *Pacing and Clinical Electrophysiology*, vol. 34, no. 10, pp. e94–e97, 2011.

[44] T. Tian, Y. Liu, L. Gao et al., "Isolated left ventricular noncompaction: clinical profile and prognosis in 106 adult patients," *Heart and Vessels*, vol. 29, no. 5, pp. 645–652, 2013.

[45] J. L. Jefferies, J. D. Wilkinson, L. A. Sleeper et al., "Cardiomyopathy phenotypes and outcomes for children with left ventricular myocardial noncompaction: results from the pediatric cardiomyopathy registry," *Journal of Cardiac Failure*, 2015.

[46] F. Peters, B. K. Khandheria, F. Botha et al., "Clinical outcomes in patients with isolated left ventricular noncompaction and heart failure," *Journal of Cardiac Failure*, vol. 20, no. 10, pp. 709–715, 2014.

[47] C. W. Yancy, M. Jessup, B. Bozkurt et al., "2013 ACCF/AHA guideline for the management of heart failure: a report of the American college of cardiology foundation/American heart association task force on practice guidelines," *Journal of the American College of Cardiology*, vol. 62, no. 16, pp. e147–e239, 2013.

10

Progenitor Hematopoietic Cells Implantation Improves Functional Capacity of End Stage Coronary Artery Disease Patients with Advanced Heart Failure

Yoga Yuniadi,[1] Yuyus Kusnadi,[2] Lakshmi Sandhow,[2] Rendra Erika,[2] Dicky A. Hanafy,[1] Caroline Sardjono,[2] R. W. M. Kaligis,[1] Manoefris Kasim,[1] and Ganesja M. Harimurti[1]

[1]Department of Cardiology and Vascular Medicine, Faculty of Medicine,
 University of Indonesia and National Cardiovascular Center Harapan Kita, Jakarta 11420, Indonesia
[2]Stem Cell and Cancer Institute, Jakarta 13210, Indonesia

Correspondence should be addressed to Yoga Yuniadi; yogay136@gmail.com

Academic Editor: Terrence D. Ruddy

Background. Proangiogenic Hematopoietic Cells (PHC) which comprise diverse mixture of cell types are able to secrete proangiogenic factors and interesting candidate for cell therapy. The aim of this study was to seek for benefit in implantation of PHC on functional improvement in end stage coronary artery disease patients with advanced heart failure. *Methods.* Patients with symptomatic heart failure despite guideline directed medical therapy and LVEF less than 35% were included. Peripheral blood mononuclear cells were isolated, cultivated for 5 days, and then harvested. Flow cytometry and cell surface markers were used to characterize PHC. The PHC were delivered retrogradely via sinus coronarius. Echocardiography, myocardial perfusion, and clinical and functional data were analyzed up to 1-year observation. *Results.* Of 30 patients (56.4 ± 7.40 yo) preimplant NT proBNP level is 5124.5 ± 4682.50 pmol/L. Harvested cells characterized with CD133, CD34, CD45, and KDR showed 0.87 ± 0.41, 0.63 ± 0.66, 99.00 ± 2.60, and 3.22 ± 3.79%, respectively. LVEF was improved (22 ± 5.68 versus 26.8 ± 7.93, $p < 0.001$) during short and long term observation. Myocardial perfusion significantly improved 6 months after treatment. NYHA Class and six-minute walk test are improved during short term and long term follow-up. *Conclusion.* Expanded peripheral blood PHC implantation using retrograde delivery approach improved LV systolic function, myocardial perfusion, and functional capacity.

1. Introduction

Heart failure is one of the major health problems worldwide [1]. Myocardial cells damage during myocardial infarction results in the reduction of left ventricle systolic function which leads to heart failure [2]. Even in this era of advanced heart failure treatment, its survival rate remains low estimated at 50% and 10% in 5 and 10 years, respectively [3–5]. Furthermore, there was only about 12 percent decrease in death rate from heart failure per decade over the past fifty years [6, 7].

Cell therapy has been used as regenerative therapy in acute myocardial infarction and heart failure patient with promising results [8–10]. Myocardial regeneration potentially improves heart failure prognosis by increasing the number of functioning myocytes and enhances angiogenesis as well as the role of paracrine effects. Most clinical stem cell studies to date have been performed by using total bone marrow mononuclear cells which comprise hematopoietic progenitor cells, mesenchymal stem cells, and monocytes.

Endothelial progenitor cells (EPCs) have been a candidate that shows a therapeutic capacity to help treat heart failure. However, the identification of EPC remains controversial due to lack of firm consensus on its definition and classification. In most recent publication, EPCs are classified into Proangiogenic Hematopoietic Cells (PHC) and Endothelial Colony Forming Cells (ECFC) [11]. Proangiogenic Hematopoietic Cells which comprise diverse mixture of cell types including monocytes, macrophages, and hematopoietic progenitor cells are able to secrete proangiogenic factors. This study is aimed at seeking benefit of implantation of PHC derived from peripheral blood to induce functional improvement in end stage coronary artery disease patients with advanced heart failure and no other therapeutic option.

2. Methods

2.1. Patients. Thirty patients, aged from 18 to 75 years, with advanced heart failure participated in this study. All patients were still symptomatic (New York Heart Association [NYHA] Class of II or more) despite the guideline directed medical therapy (GDMT). To be included in this study patient must have left ventricle ejection fraction (LVEF) of 35% or less as measured by echocardiography. Patients with acute heart failure as well as cardiogenic shock, kidney, or liver failure were excluded from this study. Exclusion criteria also included past history of neoplasm or malignancies. Female patients must not be pregnant or lactating. Those who fulfilled the requirements would need to complete the patients consent form. The study was conducted in compliance with regulations by the ethics committee.

2.2. Preimplant Examination. Preimplant examination comprised assessment of left ventricle systolic function with Simpson's method of echocardiography examination, assessment of myocardial perfusion with Technetium (Tc) 99M Sestamibi scanning, assessment of heart failure biomarker, and assessment of functional status with NYHA classification and standard six-minute walk test.

2.3. Follow-Up. Data were collected based on short term (up to three months) and long term (up to one year) follow-up following PHC implantation. Repeat assessment of echocardiography and six-minute walk test are performed any time during short and long term follow-up. Perfusion scanning is performed only before and 6 months after stem cell implantation.

2.4. Collection of Peripheral Blood Sample. To avoid hemodynamic compromise, peripheral blood sample is collected in three divided times on three consecutive days. Only 80 mL of blood is collected at each time. An additional volume of 35 mL of peripheral blood was also taken on the first day to obtain the serum required as component of the growth medium of cells. Blood sample was then transported to the laboratory where isolation of mononuclear cells and cultivation of PHC would be performed.

2.5. Isolation, Cultivation, and Preparation of PHC. Mononuclear cells were isolated ex vivo out of 80 mL of peripheral blood each day by Ficoll density-gradient centrifugation as previously described [12, 13]. These cells were suspended in growth medium consisting of X-Vivo-15 (Lonza), 20% patient's serum, 1 ng/mL human recombinant vascular endothelial growth factor (VEGF) (R&D), and 0.1 μmol/L atorvastatin (Pfizer). Cells were subsequently seeded at a density of 5.8×10^5 cells/cm^2 for the first day of blood collection and at a density of 8.7×10^5 cells/cm^2 for

the second and third day of blood collection, in 2 self-coated fibronectin culture plates. The isolated mononuclear cells were also grown in 96-well plates under identical conditions to be used in the characterization of cells on the harvesting day.

On the fifth day after the first blood collection, adherent cells were harvested. Adherent cells were detached using 0.5 mmol/L ethylenediaminetetraacetic acid (EDTA). The harvested cells were then washed twice and resuspended in X-Vivo-10 to reach a final volume of 10 mL. This ready-to-use suspension contains heterogeneous population of progenitor cells which was then transported back to the hospital for implantation.

2.6. Characterization of PHC

2.6.1. Immunophenotyping. Flow cytometry with combinations of antibody for cell surface markers including CD34, CD45, CD133, and kinase insert domain receptor (KDR) was used to characterize PHC. The following approach was used: 1 million cells were set aside from the total harvested cells and transported to the analytical laboratory. These cells were then washed with 10 mL PBS/2% FBS twice before being resuspended in the same solution and added with FcR blocker. Following 15 minutes of incubation at room temperature, cells were treated with different combinations of antibodies which would be the marker of the flow cytometry analysis performed afterwards. All reactions were carried out on ice.

2.6.2. Functional Assays. As an alternative approach to determine the phenotype of PHC, functional assay was performed. Adherent cells from 96-well plate were added with DiI-acetylated-LDL, fixated with 3% paraformaldehyde, treated with UEA-1 lectin, and subjected to staining with DAPI consecutively with appropriate incubation and washing with PBS in-between staining. Fluorescence was observed with fluorescence microscope in the dark.

2.7. Retrograde Delivery Approach. The progenitor cell solution was delivered into the heart via sinus coronarius tributaries. Cannulation of coronary sinus was performed using Attain Command™ sheath (Medtronic) via right subclavian or internal jugular vein. As the majority of patients suffered from anterior myocardial infarction, posterolateral or anterolateral vein was the target site selected for progenitor cell implantation. Target vein was wired using soft tip angioplasty wire. The vein branch without collateral to other veins (end vessel) was chosen. The particular vein branch was selected by injection of contrast media through OTW (over the wire) balloon to visualize whether collateral existed or not (Figure 1). After the completion of stem cell injection, the balloon remained inflated (6-7 atmosphere) up to fifteen minutes.

2.8. Perfusion Scanning. Technetium (Tc) 99m Sestamibi tracer is used to examine myocardial perfusion before and

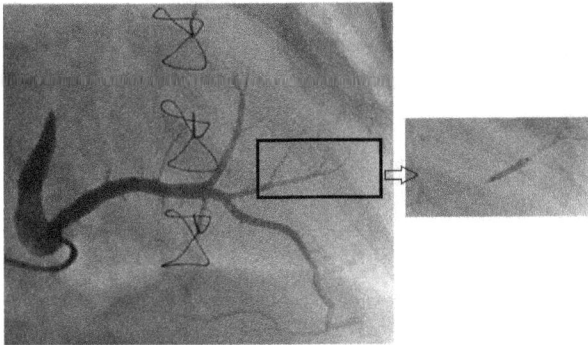

FIGURE 1: Retrograde delivery. Coronary sinus is cannulated using AL-1 catheter. Venogram shows anterolateral vein branches associated with infarcted area. The vein branch which is end vessel is selected as target vein. End vessel is confirmed by contrast injection through inflation over the wire balloon which shows no collateral (inset). Stem cells were delivered via the same balloon which is kept inflated for 15 minutes afterward.

TABLE 1: Clinical characteristics.

Variable	Results
Age (years)	56.4 ± 7.40
Sex M/F (n)	25/1
Angiography [n (%)]	
One VD	4 (15)
Two VD	3 (12)
Three VD ± LMD	19 (73)
Myocardial infarction [n (%)]	17 (65)
Diabetes mellitus [n (%)]	15 (58)
Creatinine	1.2 ± 0.29
Hemoglobin	12.7 ± 3.13
Hematocrit	37.8 ± 9.23
Leukocyte	6748 ± 1959.48
hsCRP	7.5 ± 8.39
NT proBNP	5124.5 ± 4682.50

VD: vessel disease, hsCRP: high sensitive C reactive protein, and NT proBNP: N-terminal prohormone of brain natriuretic peptide, LMD: left main disease.

after eEPCs implantation. Using a score that represents perfusion for each of the multiple segments of the myocardium visual analysis is performed semiquantitatively. A segmentation model has been standardized for this approach by dividing the myocardium into 17 segments on the basis of three short axis slices and a representative long axis slice to depict the apex [14]. Perfusion was graded within each segment on a scale of 0 to 4, with 0 representing normal perfusion and 4 representing a very severe perfusion defect. Scores for all 17 segments were added to create a "summed" score. The sum of the segmental scores from the stress images (the Summed Stress Score (SSS)) represents the extent as well as the severity of stress perfusion abnormality and the magnitude of perfusion defects related to both ischemia and infarction. The sum of the 17 segmental scores from the rest images (the Summed Rest Score (SRS)) represents the extent of infarction. The summed difference score (SDS) was derived by subtracting the SRS from the SSS and represents the extent and severity of stress-induced ischemia [15].

2.9. Statistical Analysis. Clinical data collected for four weeks and three months after treatment were combined and analyzed as one variable which was called short term. Meanwhile, those obtained in six months and one year after injection were categorized as long term. Continuous variables were tested for normal distribution using Kolmogorov-Smirnov test and expressed as mean ± SD. Comparisons of normalized data between different times points were performed using paired Student's t-test while those without normal distribution were analyzed with nonparametric Wilcoxon test. Chi-squared test was used for categorical variables. Comparisons between different patient categories were done by using independent sample Student's t-test. SPSS Version 19.0 (SPSS Inc., Chicago, IL) was used to perform all statistical analysis. A p value of less than 0.05 was considered to be statistically significant.

3. Results

3.1. Clinical Characteristics. The data reported in this study consisted of results from 26 patients whose data were sufficiently complete to establish meaningful conclusions. All patients suffered from ambulatory heart failure as indicated by high NT proBNP level. Majority of subjects have severe three-vessel disease and suffered from diabetes mellitus (Table 1). Based on their clinical history, 9 patients were identified to suffer from coronary artery disease (CAD) while the remaining 15 were grouped under myocardial infarction (MCI) category. Baseline comparison between these two groups showed homogeneity in almost all variables except that for hsCRP which were significantly higher in MCI group. Sixteen patients who were diagnosed with diabetes mellitus showed no significant difference of clinical characteristics compared to those without diabetes mellitus, except for NT proBNP which was higher in diabetes group (1682.75 ± 789.255 versus 6501.2 ± 4908.402, $p = 0.013$).

3.2. Cellular Characteristics. Average total cell counts after 5-day expansion were more than 16 million cells with more than 92% of cells viability. CD45 was expressed by approximately 99.0 ± 2.60% of total population, making it the most dominantly expressed marker. Meanwhile, the other markers were low (0.87 ± 0.41%, 0.63 ± 0.66%, and 3.22 ± 3.79% for CD133, CD34, and KDR, resp.). The described cell marker proportion indicates that the cells possessed characteristic of hematopoietic cells. There was no difference in total cell number between CAD and MCI groups and between those with and without diabetes mellitus.

On day 5 of culturing, three characteristics changes are observed. The first change is some PBMNCs morphology changed to more spindle-shaped cells which resembled more of eEPCS (Figure 2). The second change is functional assays result that revealed ability to uptake DiI-acetylated LDL and

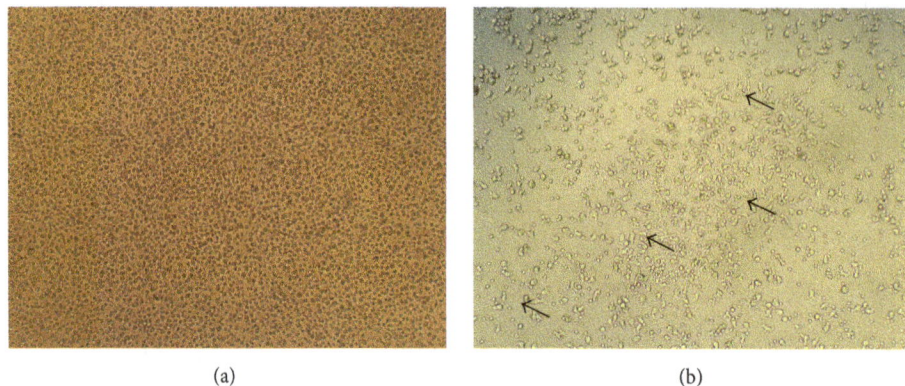

(a)   (b)

FIGURE 2: Observation of the cultured PMNCs. On day 1, the cells still display morphology resembling mononuclear cells (a). After 5-day culture, some of the cells exhibit spindle-like morphology (arrow), indicating that the cells are becoming more eEPCs like (b). Original magnification 100x.

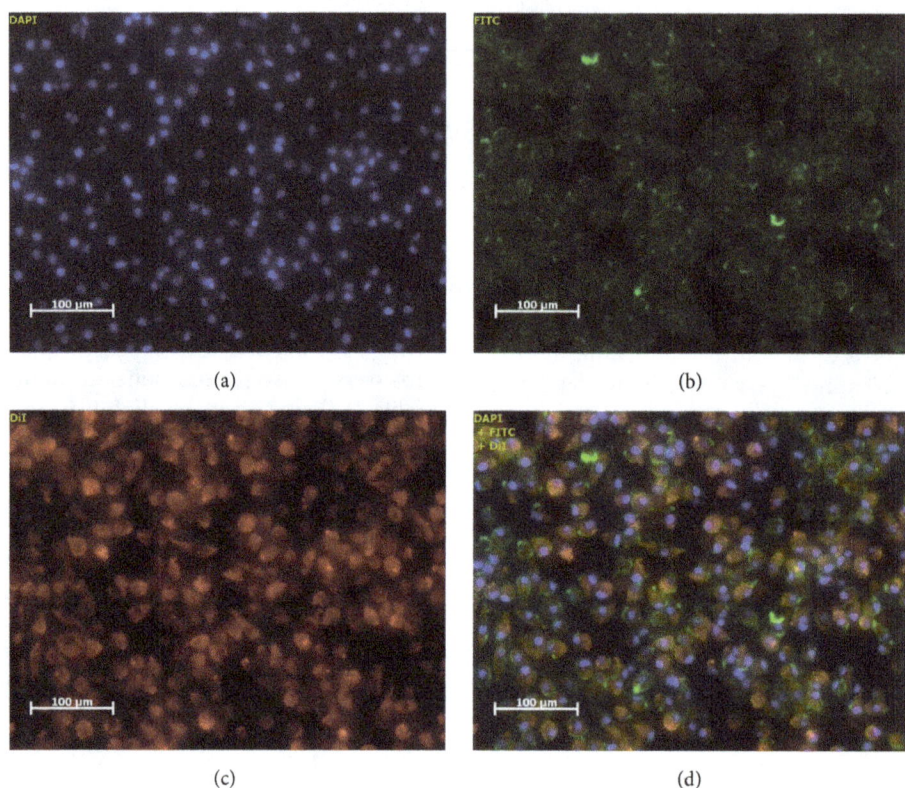

(a)   (b)

(c)   (d)

FIGURE 3: After 5 days of culture in the presence of VEGF and statin, the cells were stained with DAPI (a), UEA-1 lectin (b), Dil-acetylated LDL (c), and merge image (d). The cells exhibit the ability to bind lectin and uptake ac-LDL, one of the characteristics of eEPCs. Original magnification ×100.

to bind to FITC-labeled lectin (UEA-1) favor of endothelial characteristic. The third change is cell's nuclei visible in blue-colored fluorescent of DAPI stain (Figure 3). Cells showing all the above three properties represent the phenotype found in endothelial cells, indicating the possibility that these cells have proangiogenic ability.

3.3. Follow-Up Data.

Short and long term clinical data obtained during the scheduled follow-up sessions were compared with pretreatment data. It has been shown that there were significant improvements in echocardiography parameters that included both left and right ventricle systolic function as measured by LVEF and TAPSE (Table 2). The improvements of functional capacity are represented by increasing distance during the six-minute walk test and decreasing NYHA functional classification (Table 3). NT proBNP and hsCRP were reduced during short and long term observation but did not reach statistical significance (Table 4).

TABLE 2: Echocardiography parameters.

Parameters	Baseline	Short term	Long term	p value (baseline to short term)	p value (baseline to long term)	p value (short to long term)
LV EF (%)	22 ± 5.68	26.8 ± 7.93	26.9 ± 10.72	<0.001	0.014	0.983
LV EDD (mm)	66.0 ± 8.60	64.8 ± 8.10	66.0 ± 9.28	0.331	0.975	0.302
LV ESD (mm)	58.7 ± 9.74	56.1 ± 9.79	57.4 ± 18.76	0.079	0.408	0.373
TAPSE	1.3 ± 0.41	1.5 ± 0.42	1.6 ± 0.44	0.018	<0.001	0.019

LV: left ventricle, EF: ejection fraction, EDD: end diastolic dimension, ESD: end systolic dimension, EDV: end diastolic volume, ESV: end systolic volume, and TAPSE: tricuspid annular presystolic excursion.

TABLE 3: Functional capacity parameters.

Parameters	Baseline	Short term	Long term	p value (baseline to short term)	p value (baseline to long term)	p value (short to long term)
NYHA Class	2.16 ± 0.69	1.2 ± 0.38	1.2 ± 0.34	<0.001	<0.001	0.327
6 WT						
(i) Distance	297.8 ± 91.63	345 ± 73.94	351.9 ± 89.77	0.006	0.006	0.519
(ii) METS	5.2 ± 1.74	6.0 ± 1.46	6.2 ± 1.79	0.012	0.004	0.130

NYHA Class: New York Heart Association Classification and 6 WT: six-minute walk test.

TABLE 4: Laboratory parameters.

Parameters	Baseline	Short term	Long term	p value (baseline to short term)	p value (baseline to long term)	p value (short to long term)
NT proBNP	5124.5 ± 4682.50	3235.1 ± 2190.74	3092 ± 2079.75	0.101	0.087	0.858
hsCRP	7.5 ± 8.39	7.1 ± 9.33	5.3 ± 8.53	0.877	0.084	0.142

hsCRP: high sensitive C reactive protein and NT proBNP: N-terminal prohormone of brain natriuretic peptide.

TABLE 5: Perfusion data.

	SSS	SRS	PDSS	PDSR
Before	26.6 ± 12.45	26.2 ± 11.507	53.88 ± 19.32	50.16 ± 18.929
6 months	18.32 ± 16.09	17.8 ± 15.521	34.8 ± 29.165	33.28 ± 28.6
p value	0.007	0.006	0.003	0.004

PDSR: Perfusion Defect Score Rest; PDSS: Perfusion Defect Score Stress; SRS: Summed Rest Score; SSS: Summed Stress Score.

However, the long term values were not significantly different from the short term values in all above parameters except for TAPSE.

Myocardial perfusion scanning study using Technetium (Tc) 99M Sestamibi was performed before and six months after stem cell implantation. All perfusion data of automated quantification either at resting state or under stress showed significant improvement (Table 5). Visual perfusion improvement was showed in Figure 4. Reduction of Summed Stress Score (SSS) and Perfusion Defect Size Stress (PDSS) after stem cell implantation indicated improvement of myocardial perfusion and reduction of perfusion defect. Reduction of Summed Rest Score (SRS) and Perfusion Defect Size Rest (PDSR) indicated reduction of nonviable tissue or increasing of viable tissue.

There were no significant differences of biomarker, echocardiography parameters, perfusion scan, and functional improvement between CAD and MCI groups. Comparing subjects with and without diabetes mellitus also shows no significant difference of the above-mentioned parameters, except for short term hsCRP marker which was lower in nondiabetic subjects.

There were total of 32 hospitalizations a year before study enrollment which reduced to only totally 6 hospitalizations during one-year follow-up. There was no death during one-year follow-up as well.

4. Discussion

This study showed that PHC implantation using retrograde delivery approach improved the LV systolic function, myocardial perfusion, and functional capacity. These promising results might give additional therapeutic alternative in symptomatic ischemic cardiomyopathy patients who have no other feasible therapeutic option.

4.1. PHC Characteristics. Our FACS results showed a low expression of EPC marker such as KDR, CD34, and CD133 but a high expression of CD45 indicating hematopoietic cells. However, our cells also exhibit positive results for ac-LDL uptake and lectin binding which implies the phenotype of endothelial cells. The low expression of EPCs markers on the positive ac-LDL uptake and lectin binding shows that these cells may be more resembling PHC instead of ECFC. Proangiogenic Hematopoietic Cells mainly comprise

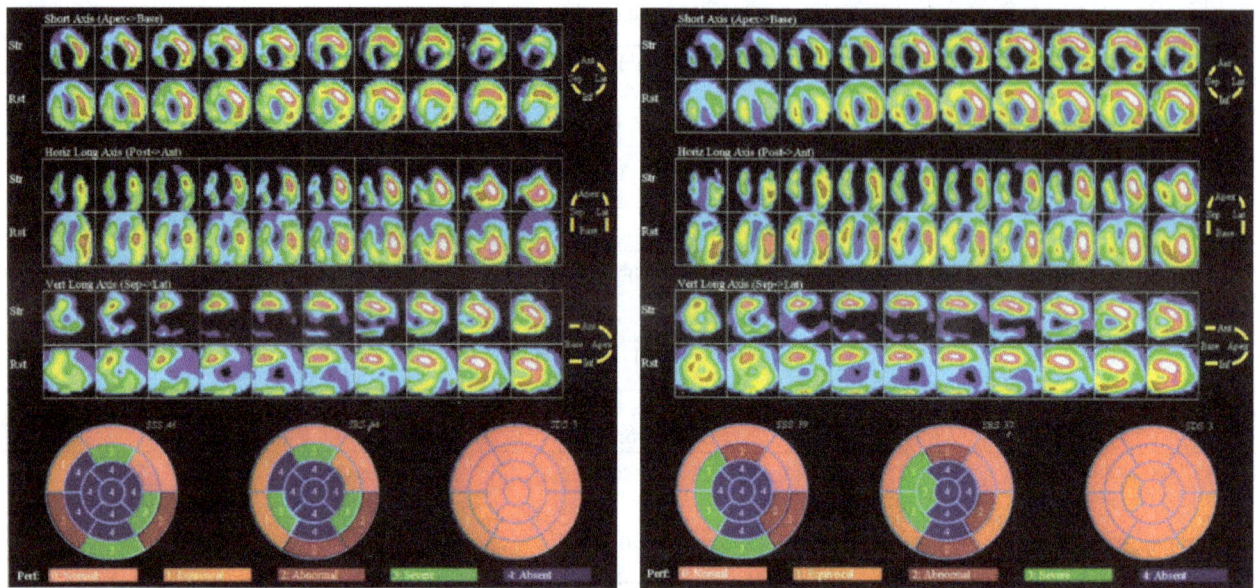

FIGURE 4: Myocardial perfusion. Left and right panel represent pre- and post-stem cell implantation status, respectively. Upper panels are visual interpretation that comprise short axis view, horizontal long axis view, and vertical long axis view during stress (Str) and rest (Rst). Lower panels are semiquantitative interpretation. Post-stem cell implantation shows more massive perfused myocard as presented with green and yellow color. Semiquantitative interpretation shows less area with score of 4 meaning less area with absent perfusion or nonviable cells. The Summed Stress Score (SSS) and Summed Rest Score (SRS) reduced after stem cell implantation.

monocyte/macrophage derived cells but they possibly contained small proportion of true stem/progenitor cells and endothelial cells [11, 16, 17]. Proangiogenic Hematopoietic Cells promote angiogenesis via paracrine effects, in contrast to ECFC which have the capability to form new endothelium. Proangiogenic Hematopoietic Cells which comprise diverse mixture of cell types including monocytes, macrophages, and hematopoietic progenitor cells are similar to early EPCs characterized by Yoder from adherent cells in petri dish [18].

Surprisingly, autologous stem cells derived from peripheral blood of patients with advanced heart failure with severe coronary artery disease and multiple risk factors resulted in significant improvement of clinical parameters. The composition of medium used for ex vivo cultivation of cells and duration of culture influence the surface profiling of cells produced. In our protocol where statin was incorporated into the growth medium continuously, the number of endothelial progenitor colonies isolated from mononuclear cells was expected to improve [19]. The mechanisms of statin related stem cell functions improvement are increasing number of EPCs, accelerating reendothelialization, and reducing neointimal formation [19–21]. Ex vivo culturing of EPCs led to "uncapping" of telomeres, indicated by the loss of TRF2. Statin cotreatment of EPCs prevents impairment of their functional capacity by a TRF2-dependent, posttranscriptional mechanism [19].

4.2. Retrograde Approach.

The delivery route of stem cell implantation might be another important key of beneficial effect in this study. Using retrograde approach through coronary vein system, stem can be delivered adjacent to infarcted area without facing any of the resistance from arteriole in scar area. In contrast to the transendocardial approach, in which cells are injected perpendicularly into the left ventricular wall, the transcoronary venous approach allowed parallel cell injection, which might result in greater cell retention [22]. This delivery method did not produce hemodynamic changes and reported enhanced angiogenesis and observed autologous bone marrow stem cells in the myocardium [23–25].

4.3. On Short versus Long Term Data.

Significant improvement of functional capacity and LV systolic function was achieved during short term follow-up and persisted during long term follow-up. However, there was no significant difference between short and long term improvement. Using autologous bone marrow mononuclear cells previous studies showed similar results of improved quality of life and exercise capacity during short and long term follow-up [26, 27]. The pattern of clinical improvements consists of peak initial short term improvement which is maintained during long term observation [27]. The persistent beneficial hemodynamic effects in the long term justified the assumption that PHC implantation might overcome the possible detrimental effects of ventricular remodelling [27].

During one-year follow-up, hospitalization rate was significantly reduced and no death was observed in our patients. Similar to our results, recent meta-analysis of thirteen trials reported no death during their follow-up and five trials reported significant lower rehospitalization rate due to worsening of heart failure among patients receiving cell therapy [28].

4.4. *Myocardial Perfusion*. Significant improvement of myocardial perfusion had been shown six months after stem cell implantation. Technetium (Tc) 99M Sestamibi was used to examine myocardial perfusion and viability. Technetium (Tc) 99M Sestamibi is a cationic Tc 99M complex which has been found to accumulate in viable myocardial tissue with less soft-tissue attenuation, better counting statistics, and improved image quality with single-photon emission CT (SPECT) [29]. This study utilized automated quantification of myocardial perfusion and showed that SSS, SRS, PDSS, and PDSR value were improved after stem cell implantation. Reduction of SSS and PDSS after stem cell implantation indicates improvement of myocardial perfusion and reduction of perfusion defect. Reduction of SRS and PDSR indicates reduction of nonviable tissue or increasing of viable tissue. These findings employ therapeutic nature of ex vivo cultivated PHC in the treatment of cardiovascular diseases. The perfusion improvement may not be achieved by incorporation of PHC to form new endothelium but is more likely due to proangiogenic factors secreted by implanted PHC such as vascular endothelial growth factor (VEGF), hepatocyte growth factor (HGF), granulocyte colony stimulating factor (GCSF), and granulocyte-macrophage colony stimulating factor (GMCSF) [16]. This secretome then helps the recruitment of native EPCs and maintains their proliferation and survival. Moreover, although it is not proven in this study, there might be a very small population of ECFC in our culture that may contribute to vasculogenesis [16, 17].

4.5. *Limitation*. Our study used a simple FACS panel to characterize PHC and the growth factors secreted by our cells were not analyzed. Further studies should apply a more comprehensive FACS panel to make sure what kind of cells are cultured and a range of growth factors ought to be assessed to measure the proangiogenic capacity of PHC.

In this pre-post study, control group and experimental group were of same patients. Even though all patients were in stable condition with fixed GDMT before study enrollment, some changes might happen during the course of study.

5. Conclusion

Implantation of peripheral blood PHC resulted in clinical and functional improvement in end stage coronary artery disease with advanced heart failure patients. The study shows potential clinical efficacy and gives a basis for future studies with a larger number of patients.

Abbreviations

CHF: Chronic heart failure
LVEF: Left ventricle ejection fraction
CAD: Chronic artery disease
MI: Myocardial infarction
EDTA: Ethylenediaminetetraacetic acid
FBS: Fetal bovine serum
GDMT: Guideline directed medical therapy

LDL: Low density lipoprotein
DiI: 1,1′-Dioctadecyl-3,3,3′3′-tetramethylindocarbocyanine perchlorate
UEA-1: Ulex Europaeus Agglutinin-1
eEPCs: Early Endothelial Progenitor Cells
VD: Vessel disease
EF: Ejection fraction
METS: Metabolic equivalents
TAPSE: Tricuspid annular plane systolic excursion
hsCRP: High sensitivity C reactive protein
SCD: Sudden cardiac death
KDR: Kinase insert domain receptor
DAPI: 4′6-Diamidino-2-phenylindole
PBS: Phosphate buffered saline
PDSR: Perfusion Defect Score Rest
PDSS: Perfusion Defect Score Stress
PMNCs: Peripheral mononuclear cells
VEGFR: Vascular endothelial growth factor receptor
SRS: Summed Rest Score
SSS: Summed Stress Score.

Competing Interests

The authors declare that they have no competing interests.

References

[1] V. L. Roger, "Epidemiology of heart failure," *Circulation Research*, vol. 113, no. 6, pp. 646–659, 2013.

[2] V. Dzau and E. Braunwald, "Resolved and unresolved issues in the prevention and treatment of coronary artery disease: a workshop consensus statement," *American Heart Journal*, vol. 121, no. 4, article 1, pp. 1244–1263, 1991.

[3] M. R. Cowie, D. A. Wood, A. J. S. Coats et al., "Survival of patients with a new diagnosis of heart failure: a population based study," *Heart*, vol. 83, no. 5, pp. 505–510, 2000.

[4] K. MacIntyre, S. Capewell, S. Stewart et al., "Evidence of improving prognosis in heart failure: trends in case fatality in 66 547 patients hospitalized between 1986 and 1995," *Circulation*, vol. 102, no. 10, pp. 1126–1131, 2000.

[5] A. Mosterd, B. Cost, A. W. Hoes et al., "The prognosis of heart failure in the general population: the Rotterdam Study," *European Heart Journal*, vol. 22, no. 15, pp. 1318–1327, 2001.

[6] D. Levy, S. Kenchaiah, M. Glarson et al., "Long-term trends in the incidence of and survival with heart failure," *The New England Journal of Medicine*, vol. 347, no. 18, pp. 1397–1402, 2002.

[7] V. L. Roger, S. A. Weston, M. M. Redfield et al., "Trends in heart failure incidence and survival in a community-based population," *Journal of the American Medical Association*, vol. 292, no. 3, pp. 344–350, 2004.

[8] B. J. Gersh, R. D. Simari, A. Behfar, C. M. Terzic, and A. Terzic, "Cardiac cell repair therapy: a clinical perspective," *Mayo Clinic Proceedings*, vol. 84, no. 10, pp. 876–892, 2009.

[9] R. Mingliang, Z. Bo, and W. Zhengguo, "Stem cells for cardiac repair: status, mechanisms, and new strategies," *Stem Cells International*, vol. 2011, Article ID 310928, 8 pages, 2011.

[10] J. Bartunek, A. Behfar, D. Dolatabadi et al., "Cardiopoietic stem cell therapy in heart failure: the C-CURE (cardiopoietic stem

cell therapy in heart failURE) multicenter randomized trial with lineage-specified biologics," *Journal of the American College of Cardiology*, vol. 61, no. 23, pp. 2329–2338, 2013.

[11] J. A. Rose, S. Erzurum, and K. Asosingh, "Biology and flow cytometry of proangiogenic hematopoietic progenitors cells," *Cytometry A*, vol. 87, no. 1, pp. 5–19, 2014.

[12] M. K. Bach and J. R. Brashler, "Isolation of subpopulations of lymphocytic cells by the use of isotonically balanced solutions of ficoll. I. Development of methods and demonstration of the existence of a large but finite number of subpopulations," *Experimental Cell Research*, vol. 61, no. 2-3, pp. 387–396, 1970.

[13] M. Fotino, E. J. Merson, and F. H. Allen Jr., "Micromethod for rapid separation of lymphocytes from peripheral blood," *Annals of Clinical Laboratory Science*, vol. 1, no. 2, pp. 131–133, 1971.

[14] M. D. Cerqueira, N. J. Weissman, V. Dilsizian et al., "Standardized myocardial sementation and nomenclature for tomographic imaging of the heart: a Statement for Healthcare Professionals from the Cardiac Imaging Committee of the Council on Clinical Cardiology of the American Heart Association," *Circulation*, vol. 105, no. 4, pp. 539–542, 2002.

[15] J. E. Udelson, V. Dilsizian, and R. O. Bonow, "Nuclear cardiology," in *Braunwald's Heart Disease*, R. O. Bonow, Ed., pp. 293–336, Saunders, 9th edition, 2011.

[16] J. Rehman, J. Li, C. M. Orschell, and K. L. March, "Peripheral blood 'endothelial progenitor cells' are derived from monocyte/macrophages and secrete angiogenic growth factors," *Circulation*, vol. 107, no. 8, pp. 1164–1169, 2003.

[17] J. Hur, C.-H. Yoon, H.-S. Kim et al., "Characterization of two types of endothelial progenitor cells and their different contributions to neovasculogenesis," *Arteriosclerosis, Thrombosis, and Vascular Biology*, vol. 24, no. 2, pp. 288–293, 2004.

[18] M. C. Yoder, "Editorial: Early and late endothelial progenitor cells are miR-tually exclusive," *Journal of Leukocyte Biology*, vol. 93, no. 5, pp. 639–641, 2013.

[19] I. Spyridopoulos, J. Haendeler, C. Urbich et al., "Statins enhance migratory capacity by upregulation of the telomere repeat-binding factor TRF2 in endothelial progenitor cells," *Circulation*, vol. 110, no. 19, pp. 3136–3142, 2004.

[20] B. Assmus, C. Urbich, A. Aicher et al., "HMG-CoA reductase inhibitors reduce senescence and increase proliferation of endothelial progenitor cells via regulation of cell cycle regulatory genes," *Circulation Research*, vol. 92, no. 9, pp. 1049–1055, 2003.

[21] J.-H. Zhu, Q.-M. Tao, J.-Z. Chen, X.-X. Wang, J.-H. Zhu, and Y.-P. Shang, "Statins contribute to enhancement of the number and the function of endothelial progenitor cells from peripheral blood," *Sheng Li Xue Bao*, vol. 56, no. 3, pp. 357–364, 2004.

[22] C. C. Sheng, L. Zhou, and J. Hao, "Current stem cell delivery methods for myocardial repair," *BioMed Research International*, vol. 2013, Article ID 547902, 15 pages, 2013.

[23] J. Vicario, J. Piva, A. Pierini et al., "Transcoronary sinus delivery of autologous bone marrow and angiogenesis in pig models with myocardial injury," *Cardiovascular Radiation Medicine*, vol. 3, no. 2, pp. 91–94, 2002.

[24] J. Vicario, C. Campo, J. Piva et al., "One-year follow-up of transcoronary sinus administration of autologous bone marrow in patients with chronic refractory angina," *Cardiovascular Revascularization Medicine*, vol. 6, no. 3, pp. 99–107, 2005.

[25] S.-I. Yokoyama, N. Fukuda, Y. Li et al., "A strategy of retrograde injection of bone marrow mononuclear cells into the myocardium for the treatment of ischemic heart disease," *Journal of Molecular and Cellular Cardiology*, vol. 40, no. 1, pp. 24–34, 2006.

[26] E. C. Perin, G. V. Silva, T. D. Henry et al., "A randomized study of transendocardial injection of autologous bone marrow mononuclear cells and cell function analysis in ischemic heart failure (FOCUS-HF)," *American Heart Journal*, vol. 161, no. 6, pp. 1078–1087.e3, 2011.

[27] B.-E. Strauer, M. Yousef, and C. M. Schannwell, "The acute and long-term effects of intracoronary Stem cell Transplantation in 191 patients with chronic heARt failure: the STAR-heart study," *European Journal of Heart Failure*, vol. 12, no. 7, pp. 721–729, 2010.

[28] S. A. Fisher, C. Doree, A. Mathur, and E. Martin-Rendon, "Meta-analysis of cell therapy trials for patients with heart failure," *Circulation Research*, vol. 116, no. 8, pp. 1361–1377, 2015.

[29] J. Maddahi, H. Kiat, K. F. Van Train et al., "Myocardial perfusion imaging with technetium-99m sestamibi SPECT in the evaluation of coronary artery disease," *The American Journal of Cardiology*, vol. 66, no. 13, pp. E55–E62, 1990.

11

Aerobic Training Intensity for Improved Endothelial Function in Heart Failure Patients

M. J. Pearson and N. A. Smart

School of Science and Technology, University of New England, Armidale, NSW 2351, Australia

Correspondence should be addressed to N. A. Smart; nsmart2@une.edu.au

Academic Editor: Stephan von Haehling

Objective. Flow-mediated dilation (FMD) is widely utilised to assess endothelial function and aerobic exercise improves FMD in heart failure patients. The aim of this meta-analysis is to quantify the effect of aerobic training intensity on FMD in patients with heart failure. *Background.* A large number of studies now exist that examine endothelial function in patients with heart failure. We sought to add to the current literature by quantifying the effect of the aerobic training intensity on endothelial function. *Methods.* We conducted database searches (PubMed, Embase, ProQuest, and Cochrane Trials Register to June 30, 2016) for exercise based rehabilitation trials in heart failure, using search terms exercise training, endothelial function, and flow-mediated dilation (FMD). *Results.* The 13 included studies provided a total of 458 participants, 264 in intervention groups, and 194 in nonexercising control groups. Both vigorous and moderate intensity aerobic training significantly improved FMD. *Conclusion.* Overall both vigorous and moderate aerobic exercise training improved FMD in patients with heart failure.

1. Introduction

Results of numerous studies and meta-analyses have now shown that exercise training is not only safe but is associated with a range of physiological, functional, and clinical benefits in patients with heart failure (HF) [1–3]. While exercise interventions in HF patients have utilised a range of training modalities, aerobic or endurance training is the most investigated and has been shown to improve a range of parameters in HF patients [1, 4], including endothelial function [5]. Endothelial dysfunction is associated with the pathogenesis and progression of HF [6] and flow-mediated dilation (FMD), a noninvasive assessment of endothelial function, has been shown to be predictive of deterioration and death [7] in HF patients. Aerobic exercise training improves endothelial dependent vasodilation primarily by improving nitic oxide (NO) bioavailability [8].

Despite a large number of exercise training studies it was not until 2011 that a consensus document by the Heart Failure Association (HFA) and European Association for Cardiovascular Prevention and Rehabilitation (EACPR) provided a detailed and comprehensive guideline for exercise training in HF patients [9]. However, while aerobic exercise is now a feature of cardiac rehabilitation guidelines around the world, training program characteristics still vary considerably and the focus of current and emerging research is on identifying the exercise modality, dose, and intensity that will deliver optimal benefits [10–13]. While all training characteristics will likely influence results to some degree, the role of exercise intensity in cardiac rehabilitation is considered a key issue [14]. As the pattern of blood flow and amount of shear stress [8] that occur during exercise may be related to the specific training characteristics, including training intensity, ascertaining an optimal training protocol is important.

A meta-analysis in HF patients by Ismail and colleagues (2013) [12] demonstrated that as exercise intensity increases the magnitude of change in $VO_{2\,peak}$ also increases. In addition, a considerable body of evidence is mounting in relation to aerobic intermittent or interval training in clinical populations including HF patients [15, 16], and more specifically in relation to high-intensity interval training (HIIT) [15] for improving a range of physiological, functional and clinical parameters, including vascular function [5].

While exercise intensity is associated with the magnitude of change in $VO_{2\,peak}$ in HF patients [12], the relationship between aerobic intensity and endothelial function is not clear. In healthy men, high-intensity exercise has been shown to increase oxidative stress reducing the bioavailability of NO and possibly negating the positive effect of exercise induced shear stress on endothelial function [17]. However, increases in antioxidant levels and greater improvements in FMD from HIIT compared to moderate intensity continuous training (MICT) in heart failure patients [5] suggest that intensity may have a role in the endothelial response to exercise in this population.

In a range of clinical populations both moderate [18] and high-intensity [19, 20] aerobic training have significantly improved FMD. A recent meta-analysis [21] across a diverse population reported a significant improvement in FMD from aerobic exercise and a significant dose-response relationship between intensity and FMD. In addition, Ramos and colleagues (2015) [22] examined the effects of high-intensity training, specifically HIIT compared to MICT across a diverse population, demonstrating HIIT to be more effective for improving FMD [22].

A number of aerobic exercise training studies have now investigated FMD in HF patients and therefore the primary aim of our paper was to conduct a systematic review and meta-analysis to investigate if training intensity reflects the magnitude of change in FMD.

2. Methods

2.1. Search Strategy. Potential studies were identified by conducting systematic searches of PubMed, Embase, CINAHL, SPORTDiscus, and the Cochrane Library of Controlled Trials up until 30 June 30, 2016. Searches included a mix of MeSH and free text terms related to the key concepts of heart failure, exercise training, endothelial function, and flow-mediated dilation. Additionally, systematic reviews, meta-analyses, and reference lists of papers were hand searched for additional studies. One reviewer (MJP) conducted the search; and full articles were assessed for eligibility by two reviewers (MJP and NAS). Two authors were contacted to provide additional information; one author did not respond and the second responded but was unable to provide any further details.

2.2. Study Selection. Randomised controlled trials and controlled trials of aerobic exercise training in heart failure patients with reduced ejection fractions (HFrEF) were included. Studies included in the review compare an aerobic training intervention to a no exercise or usual care control group or compared continuous aerobic training with interval or intermittent aerobic training. Only studies that measured endothelial function by flow-mediated dilation (FMD) measured via ultrasound reported as relative FMD% or absolute FMD (mm or μm) in either the brachial or radial artery were included.

2.3. Data Extraction and Outcome Measures. Data were extracted by one reviewer (MJP). The primary outcome measure was flow-mediated dilation (FMD% or FMD absolute (mm)). Where FMD was reported as FMD% and FMD (mm), FMD% was utilised in the analysis.

2.4. Data Synthesis. Statistical analyses were performed using Revman 5.3 (The Nordic Cochrane Centre, Copenhagen, Denmark). The individual meta-analyses were completed for continuous data by using the change in the mean and standard deviation (SD). The primary outcome measure was FMD%. Where the change in mean and SD were not reported, the change in mean was calculated by subtracting the preintervention mean form the postintervention mean, and Revman 5.3 enabled calculations of SD using number of participants in each group, within or between group p values or 95% CI. In cases where exact p values were not provided, we used default values; for example, $p < 0.05$ becomes $p = 0.049$, $p < 0.01$ becomes $p = 0.0099$, and $p =$ not significant becomes $p = 0.051$. Data not provided in main text or tables were extracted from figures. A random effects inverse variance was used with the effects measure of standardised mean difference (SMD). We utilised the widely accepted guideline for SMD interpretation [23], with 0.2 defined as small, 0.5 medium, and 0.8 as large. Where a study included multiple intervention groups and a control group, the sample size of the control group was divided by the number of intervention groups to eliminate over inflation of the sample size. We used a 5% level of significance and a 95% CI to report change in outcome measures. Aerobic intensity was defined and classified according to the ACSM (2011) [24]. Where prescribed intensity overlapped between two intensity classifications an additional analysis was conducted by reallocation of the studies to the alternative classification.

2.5. Heterogeneity and Publication Bias. Heterogeneity was quantified using the I^2 test [25]. Values range from 0% (homogeneity) to 100% (highly heterogeneity) [25]. Egger tests and funnel plots [26] were provided to assess risk of publication bias.

2.6. Study Quality. Study quality was assessed by using the TESTEX, the tool for assessment of study quality and reporting, designed specifically for use in exercise training studies [27]. This is a 15-point scale that assesses study quality (maximum 5 points) and reporting (maximum 10 points). Two reviewers (MJP and NAS) conducted quality assessment.

3. Results

The initial search identified 485 manuscripts. After removal of duplicates and exclusion of articles based on abstract and title, 26 full-text articles remained for screening. Full screening resulted in 13 articles meeting the stated inclusion criteria (Figure 1 PRISMA statement). The aerobic exercise intervention characteristics of the 13 studies in the meta-analysis are included in Table 1. Details of full-text articles reviewed but excluded are provided in Supplementary Table S1 in Supplementary Material available online at https://doi.org/10.1155/2017/2450202. Full participant details are provided in Supplementary Table S2.

3.1. Study Characteristics. Thirteen [5, 28–39] studies provided a total of 458 participants diagnosed with HFrEF, 264 exercising participants, and 194 nonexercising control

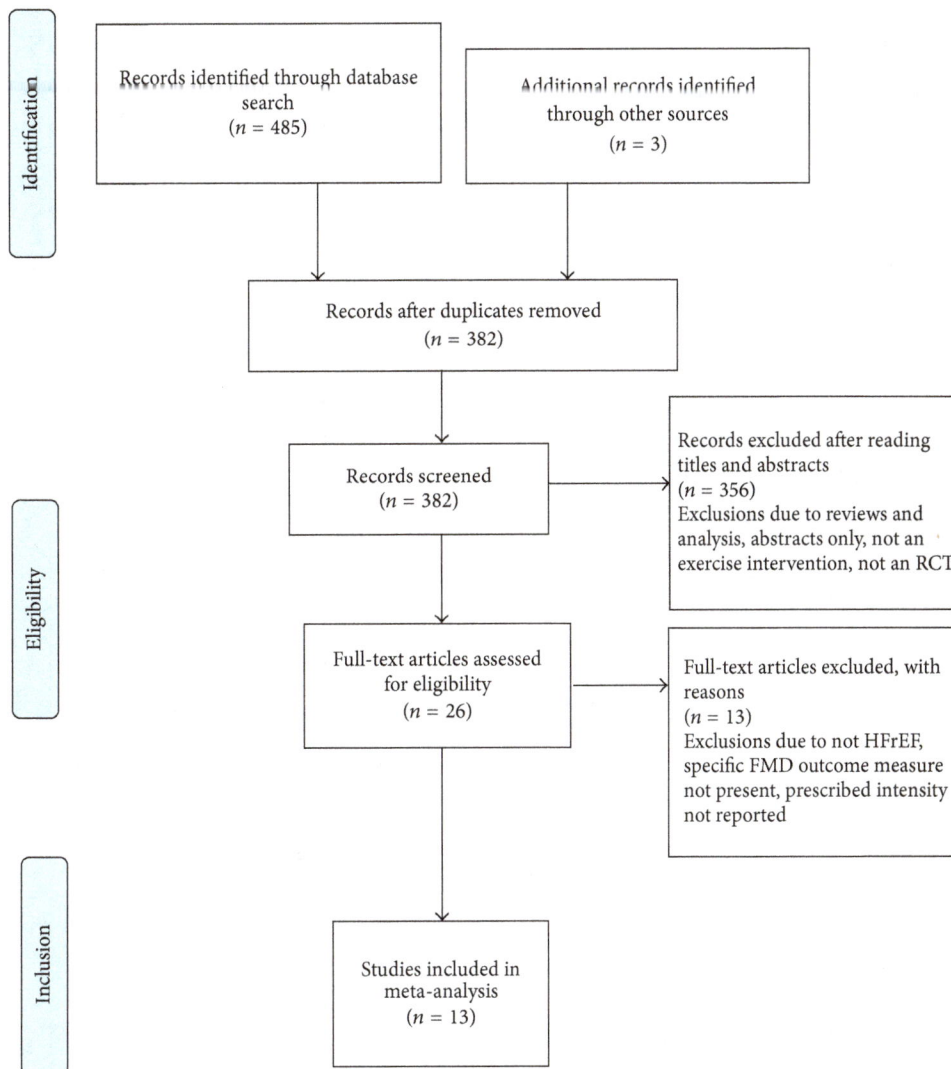

FIGURE 1: PRISMA flow diagram.

subjects. Twelve studies [5, 28–37, 39] included a usual care control group, of these, two studies [5, 28] included two different aerobic intervention groups. One study [38] did not include a control group and only compared intervention groups undertaking different aerobic exercise protocols. Ten studies [5, 29–33, 35–38] randomised participants, two studies were nonrandomised controlled trials [34, 39], and one study randomised participants between two exercise interventions but the control group was nonrandomised [28]. The average age of participants ranged between 49 ± 5 yrs and 76 ± 13 yrs and sex distribution was predominantly male. Brachial baseline FMD% ranged from ~3% to >7% and reported that baseline radial FMD% ranged from ~6% to >12% (Supplementary Table S2).

3.2. Intervention Details. Intervention duration ranged from 4 weeks to 6 months, the frequency of sessions ranged from 2 days per week to daily, and the duration of exercise sessions ranged from 10 to 60 minutes. All studies performed

an exercise test from which training intensity was prescribed and cycling was the most common mode of aerobic exercise. For pooled analysis, aerobic training intensity was classified according to ACSM (2011) [24]. The training protocol of four studies [5, 28, 34, 38] utilised interval/intermittent training and of these, three [5, 28, 34] utilised a training intensity deemed as high-intensity interval training (HIIT). Two [28, 38] studies employed short to moderate length intervals [40] and two [5, 34] utilised long length [40] intervals classified as a 4 × 4 HIIT protocol, but with different intensities. Seven [5, 28, 31, 34, 35, 37, 38] studies reported on how intensity was monitored, but only four [5, 28, 31, 34] studies reported actual or perceived (RPE) training intensity of participants and only one [32] reported actual energy expenditure (Supplementary Table S3). Seven [5, 28, 30–32, 34, 37] studies reported session attendance percentages and 11 studies [5, 28–35, 37, 38] reported on the occurrence of any adverse events (Supplementary Table S4). The assessment of FMD varied between studies (Supplementary Table S5) and

TABLE 1: Aerobic exercise characteristics of studies included in meta-analysis.

Study	Study design	Sample size (completed/analysed)	Intervention duration (weeks)	Training modality	Frequency (per wk.)	Session duration	Prescribed exercise intensity
Benda et al. (2015) [28]	Non-RCT[1]	29	12	Cycle	2	35 min (HIIT) 30 min (CT) plus 10 min warm-up, 5 min cooldown each group	HIIT: 10 × 1 min @ 90% max. workload (RPE 15-17) separated by 2.5 min @ 30% max. workload CT: @60-75% max. workload (RPE 12-14) warm-up @ 40% max. Workload & cooldown @ 30% max. workload
Belardinelli et al. (2006) [29]	RCT	52	8	Cycle	3	40 min plus 15 min warm-up stretch, 5 min cooldown	60% VO_{2peak}
Belardinelli et al. (2005) [30]	RCT	59	8	Cycle	3	40 min plus 15 min warm-up stretch, 5 min cooldown	60% VO_{2peak}
Eleuteri et al. (2013) [31]	RCT	21	12	Cycle	5	30 min plus 5 min warm-up, 5 min cooldown	HR & power @ VAT (cycle @ 60 RPM) (VAT ~ 60% VO_{2max})[1]
Erbs et al. (2010) [32]	RCT	34	12	Cycle 1 × GS*	Daily +1 GS wk.	20–30 min (plus 1 × 60 min GS/wk.)	HR @ 60% VO_{2max}
Guazzi et al. (2004) [33]	RCT	31	8	Cycle	4	30 min plus 5 min warm-up, 5 min cooldown	60% HRR wk. 1-2, ↑ 80% HRR @ wk. 3
Isaksen et al. (2015) [34]	Non-RCT	35	12	Cycle or treadmill	3	25 min plus 15 min warm-up, 5 min cooldown, 15 min strength/stretch	4 × 4 HIIT @ 85% HR_{max} (~RPE 15-17) separated by 3 min recovery @ 60–70% HR_{max}, warm-up @ 60–70% HR_{max}
Kobayashi et al. (2003) [35]	RCT	28	12	Cycle	2-3 (2x day)	2 × 15 min session/day (30 min/day total)	HR @ VAT (~60–70% VO_{2max})
Linke et al. (2001) [36]	RCT	22	4	Cycle	daily (6x per day)	10 min (60 min/day total)	70% VO_{2peak}
Sandri et al. (2015) [37]	RCT	60	4	Cycle 1 × GS*	5 (4x per weekday)	15–20 min (~60 min/day total) plus 5 min warm-up and cooldown (plus 1 × 60 min GS per/wk.)	70% of symptom limited VO_{2max}
Smart and Steele (2012) [38]	RCT	23	16	Cycle	3	60 min (INT) 30 min (CONT)	INT: work:rest (60 s:60 s) @ 60–70% VO_{2peak} CT: 60–70% VO_{2peak} (cycle @ 60 RPM)
Van Craenenbroeck et al. (2010) [39]	Non-RCT	38	26	Ambulatory base	3	60 min	90% HR @ respiratory compensation point
Wisloff et al. (2007) [5]	RCT	26	12	Treadmill/home walking	3	28 min (AIT) plus 10 min warm-up 47 min (MICT)	AIT: 4 min × 4 @ 90–95% HR_{max}, separated by 3 min @ 50–70% HR_{max}, MICT: @ 70–75% HR_{max}

AIT: aerobic interval training, Con: control, CT: continuous training, GS: group session, HIIT: high intensity interval training, HR: heart rate, HR_{max}: maximum heart rate, HR_{peak}: peak heart rate, HRR: heart rate reserve, MIACT: moderate intensity aerobic training, MICT: moderate continuous training, non-RCT: nonrandomised controlled trial, RCT: randomised controlled trial, RPE: rating of perceived exertion, RPM: revolutions per minute, VAT: ventilatory anaerobic threshold, VO_{2peak}: peak oxygen uptake, and VO_{2max}: maximal oxygen uptake. [1]Two exercise groups randomised, but control group not randomised. [1]VO_2 @ VT/VO_{2peak} = 8.8/14.8 = 59.5% of VO_{2peak}. * 1 group session per week composed of walking, calisthenics, and ball games.

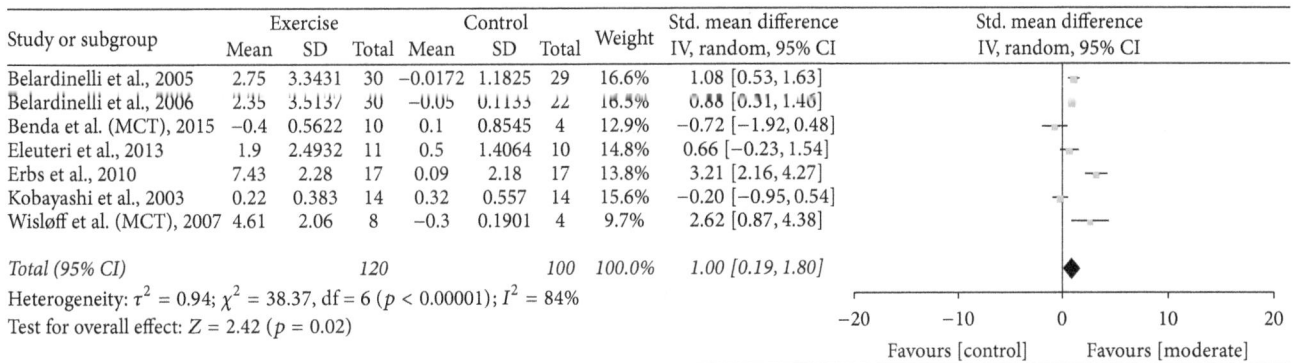

(a)

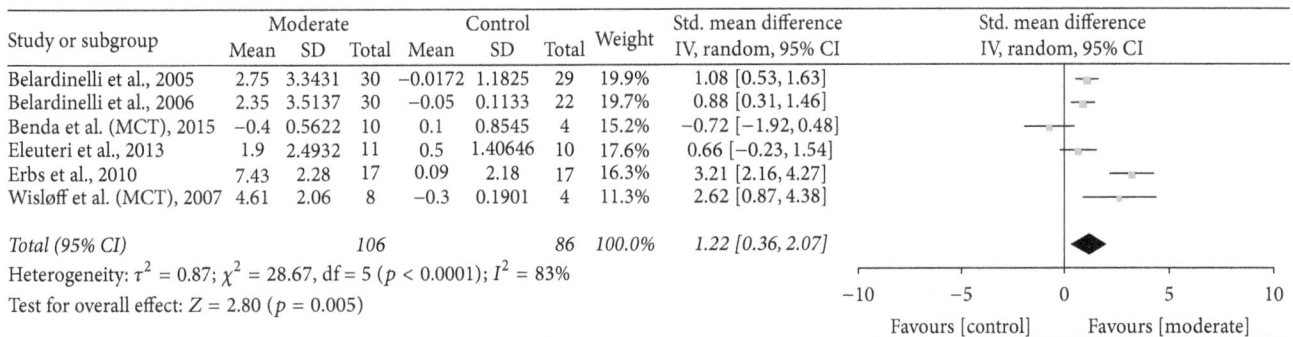

(b)

FIGURE 2: (a) FMD: moderate aerobic training versus control. (b) FMD: moderate aerobic training versus control (removal of Kobayashi study from moderate intensity).

10 studies [5, 28–31, 33–35, 38, 39] assessed FMD in the Brachial Artery (BA), with the Radial Artery utilised in three studies [32, 36, 37].

4. Outcome Measures

4.1. Flow-Mediated Dilation (FMD)

4.1.1. Moderate Aerobic Intensity versus Control. Pooled data from seven studies [5, 28–32, 35] that utilised moderate intensity demonstrated a significant improvement in FMD, exercise versus control, SMD of 1.00 (95% CI 0.19 to 1.80, $p = 0.02$) (Figure 2(a)). The significance level increased with removal of the one non-RCT [28], SMD of 1.24 (95% CI 0.42 to 2.06, $p = 0.003$). One [35] study prescribed an intensity range that incorporates both the moderate and vigorous intensity definition, and removal of the study resulted in an increased SMD of 1.22 (95% CI 0.36 to 2.07, $p = 0.005$) (Figure 2(b)), which increased further with removal of the one non-RCT [28] [SMD of 1.53 (95% CI 0.72 to 2.35, $p = 0.0002$)].

4.1.2. Vigorous Aerobic Intensity versus Control. Pooled data from seven studies [5, 28, 33, 34, 36, 37, 39] utilising vigorous intensity demonstrated a significant improvement in FMD, SMD of 1.21 (95% CI 0.60 to 1.82, $p = 0.0001$) (Figure 3(a)). Removal of the three non-RCTs [28, 34, 39] increased the

significance, SMD of 1.69 (95% CI 0.97 to 2.40, $p < 0.00001$). Reclassification of the one [35] study that straddled both moderate and vigorous intensity decreased SMD to 1.05 (95% CI 0.43 to 1.68, $p = 0.001$) (Figure 3(b)); however with removal of the three non-RCTs [28, 34, 39] SMD increased to 1.43 (95% CI 0.56 to 2.30, $p = 0.001$).

4.1.3. Aerobic Interval/Intermittent versus Continuous. Pooled data from three studies [5, 28, 38] demonstrated a nonsignificant change in FMD with interval training versus control; SMD of 0.56 (95% CI −0.49 to 1.61, $p = 0.30$) (Supplementary Figure S1). With removal of the one non-RCT [28] the change in FMD increased but remained nonsignificant [SMD of 1.00 (95% CI −0.33 to 2.33, $p = 0.14$)]. One [38] study utilised a moderate intensity, with the remaining two studies [5, 28] utilising a high intensity. With removal of the one [38] moderate intensity study the result remained nonsignificant for HIIT versus continuous [SMD of 0.70 (95% CI −1.27 to 2.69, $p = 0.49$)].

4.1.4. HIIT versus Control. Pooled data from three studies [5, 28, 34] that included a HIIT and control group, indicated a trend toward improvement with HIIT in FMD; however this was not significant, SMD of 1.80 (95% CI −0.69 to 4.29, $p = 0.16$) (Supplementary Figure S2). Two [28, 34] of the three studies were however non-RCTs.

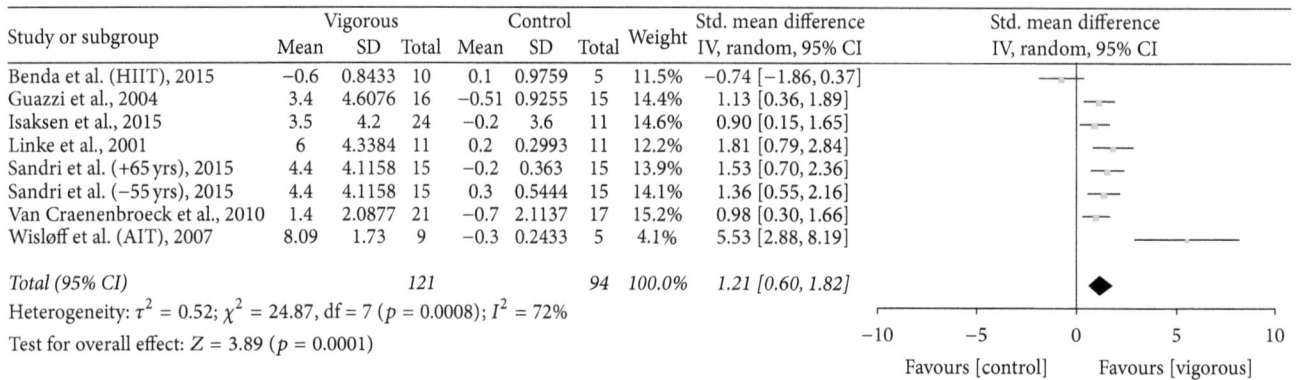

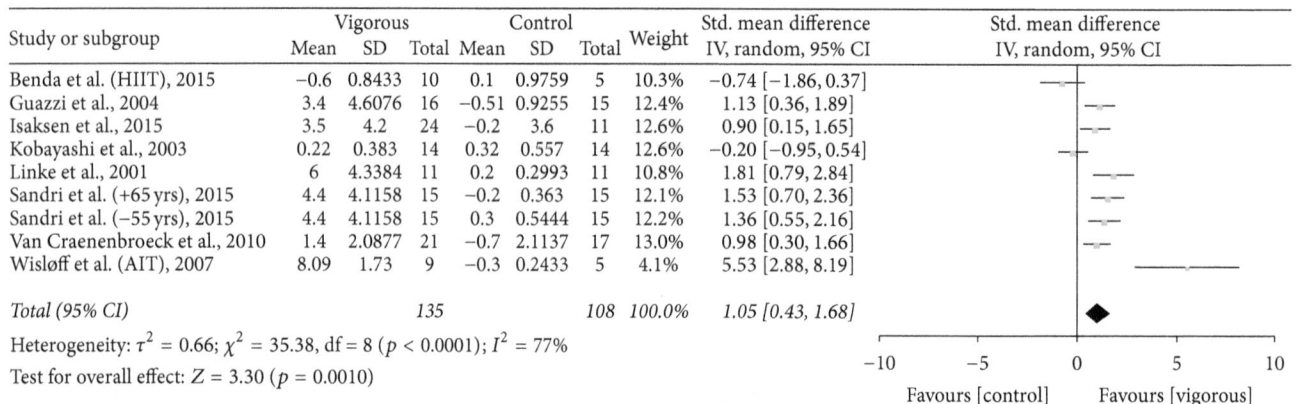

FIGURE 3: (a) FMD: vigorous aerobic training versus control. (b) FMD: vigorous aerobic training versus control (reallocation of Kobayashi from moderate to vigorous intensity).

4.2. Endothelial-Independent Dilation. Six [28–30, 33, 34, 36] of the included studies noted the assessment of endothelial-independent vasodilation. Five studies [28–30, 33, 34] provided relative% change in arterial diameter, while one study [36] provided both absolute and relative% change. The endothelial-independent response did not differ significantly between exercise and control, SMD of −0.02 (95% CI −0.85 to 0.82, $p = 0.97$) (Supplementary Figure S3).

4.3. Study Quality Assessment. The median TESTEX score was 9 (Supplementary Table S6). While RCTs noted participant randomisation, specific details were lacking from the majority of studies. The majority of studies lost points in the areas of allocation concealment and activity monitoring in the control group.

4.4. Heterogeneity and Publication Bias. All analyses demonstrated moderate to high heterogeneity. Funnel plots demonstrated some evidence of publication bias.

5. Discussion

This work analysed the effects of aerobic training intensity on FMD in patients with chronic heart failure. Our primary finding shows that aerobic exercise training significantly improves endothelial function, assessed via FMD, in patients with heart failure. Our pooled data failed to find a significant change in endothelial-independent vasodilation, indicating that the improvement occurred at the level of the endothelium [41]. All but two [28, 35] of the studies included in our analysis found improvements in brachial or radial artery FMD. Interestingly, while Kobayashi et al. (2003) [35] failed to find any improvement in upper limb FMD they did report a significant improvement in lower limb artery FMD (posterior tibial artery).

Training intensity is considered a key component in determining optimal outcomes in cardiac rehabilitation [14] and our analysis demonstrated that both moderate and vigorous intensity, defined according to ACSM (2011) [24], significantly improved FMD of the brachial or radial artery. However, whether or not the magnitude of improvement increased with intensity remains unclear. As only four studies reported actual training intensities, our analysis of intensity was based on the prescribed training intensity for the exercise intervention. Whether or not vigorous or moderate intensity provided greater improvements in FMD was dependent upon the allocation of one [35] study, which prescribed a training intensity range that fell within both moderate and vigorous categories. Two analyses were therefore conducted to ascertain the effect of this study, and due to the nonsignificant finding of the study, reallocation demonstrated contrasting results. Based on the analysis we therefore cannot conclude that the magnitude of the improvement in FMD increases with intensity as was recently reported in the case of $VO_{2\,peak}$ by Ismail and colleagues [12]. Additionally, it is likely that the result would also vary depending on the actual definition or range of a particular intensity adopted, which varies between organization [24, 42], and whether or not the actual training intensities were as prescribed.

Since the impressive findings of Wisløff et al. (2007) [5] there has been an increased interest in aerobic intermittent/interval training and some guidelines [9] now advocate for this as a form of aerobic training in stable HF patients, although the actual prescribed intensity of the intervals still vary. We therefore conducted an analysis of HIIT compared to MICT. Our analysis of FMD indicated a trend toward interval or HIIT providing a greater improvement than MICT; however, the pooled results were not significant. Only the study of Wisløff et al. [5] demonstrated HIIT as significantly superior to MICT. However, only two [5, 38] of the three studies included in our analysis were RCTs and while the RCT of Smart and Steele (2012) [38] utilised interval training, the intensity of the intervals did not fall within the definition of HIIT [40]. Interval or intermittent training can be performed at any intensity; however, HIIT has been shown to invoke more significant improvements in $VO_{2\,peak}$ compared to MICT in HF patients [15, 16].

The broad definition of HIIT also means that a range of protocols are employed in both research and practice and a large number of variables can be manipulated in prescribing HIIT [43]. All three studies in our analysis of HIIT versus MICT utilised different protocols, with only Wisløff et al. (2007) [5] employing a long interval (4×4) protocol, which may account for some of the contrasting results between studies. Different interval/HIIT protocols may have different physiological responses and may impact the amount of shear stress [5, 22, 28]. For this reason a long HIIT protocol may be more effective [22]. Interestingly the participants in the Wisløff et al. [5] study also had lower baseline FMD% (<4%) than participants in the other two studies [28, 38] and therefore could provide a further explanation of the contrasting results, as lower baseline FMD% is one factor suggested as differentiating FMD responders from nonresponders [44]. Our nonsignificant finding is in contrast to the significant and superior improvement in FMD after HIIT compared to MICT in studies across a diverse population [22], although in CAD patients the recent SAINTEX-CAD study [45] reported significant improvements in FMD from HIIT and MICT with no difference between groups. Recently it was demonstrated in obese adults that HIIT and MICT may result in different vascular adaptations with HIIT improving FMD and MICT improving resting brachial diameter [46]. However, no studies in our review reported a significant change in resting arterial diameter after MICT. Interestingly, a recent meta-analysis that compared HIIT to MICT to investigate other clinical parameters in heart failure patients (not FMD) revealed mixed findings [13], while data from

previous meta-analyses have shown HIIT more effective than MICT in improving $VO_{2\,peak}$ [12, 15].

In our pooled analysis of HIIT compared to no training, despite a trend toward HIIT, we failed to find a significant change in FMD. However, two of the three studies were non-RCTs [28, 34]. Of the three included studies, the non-RCT of Isaksen et al. (2015) [34] and RCT of Wisløff et al. (2007) [5] both reported a significant change in FMD in training groups after intervention with no change in controls, and interestingly both studies utilised a 4×4 HIIT protocol, which may be a more optimal protocol to improve vascular function [22]. Interestingly, a short duration HIIT interval (30 seconds work; 60 seconds rest) utilised by Anagnostakou et al. [47] in a comparison of HIIT to combined HIIT and resistance training failed to elicit a significant improvement in FMD in a HIIT only training group. However, FMD improved in a combined HIIT and resistance training group. Of particular interest is that, in the Isaksen et al. [34] study, while HR data was not stored for intensity analysis on any variables, they do note that, in a separate analysis on $VO_{2\,peak}$, the improvement in $VO_{2\,peak}$ was almost doubled in patients who reported an average RPE ≥ 16, and while no details are provided on FMD, one can question whether this may have occurred with FMD, indicating the role of intensity.

As there are still unanswered questions in relation to the role of endothelial dysfunction in the development and symptoms of HF patients with preserved ejection fractions [48] our analysis only included patients with reduced ejection fractions. Therefore our analysis cannot be generalised to HFpEF patients. Additionally, only minimal studies to date exist that have utilised aerobic training and investigated FMD. Kitzman and colleagues (2013) [49] failed to find any significant change in FMD following 16 weeks of high-intensity aerobic training (70% $VO_{2\,max}$), while more recently Angadi et al. (2015) [50] in a relatively small, short duration (4 weeks) study compared HIIT and MICT and failed to find a significant change in FMD in either group.

Strengths and Limitations in the Systematic Review and Meta-Analysis. To the best of our knowledge this is the first meta-analysis that provides analysis on aerobic training intensity and endothelial function in heart failure patients. The major limitation of the review is the high level of heterogeneity among studies. Differences in the methodological assessment of FMD and medication use may have contributed to the level of heterogeneity. Another limitation of the review is the classification of exercise intensity. We classified aerobic intensity according to the ACSM (2011) guidelines [24], which provides intensity ranges based on % HRR or VO_2 reserve (VO_2R), $VO_{2\,max}$, HR_{max}, RPE, or Metabolic Equivalent of Task (METS). Over the years these ranges have changed which would change the classification of studies. Additionally, intensity ranges defined by other organizations [42] differ from the ACSM [24]. As the majority of studies did not report on the actual training intensities of the sessions, whether or not the mean training intensity was firstly within the prescribed intensity range for the duration of the intervention and secondly whether the mean training intensity was closer to the upper or lower end of the prescribed ranges could not be ascertained. We were unable to conduct an analysis according to different intensity domains and thresholds, as opposed to ranges, as suggested by Mezzani et al. (2012) [14], as the relevant information could not be extracted from all studies. In regard to data pooling, we measured the difference between preintervention and postintervention means; however, in cases where exact p values, within groups or between groups, or 95% CI were not available, default values for p were utilised and this may introduce errors. Additionally, data from some studies was extracted from figures; this in itself has the potential to introduce errors.

6. Conclusion

This meta-analysis found that both vigorous and moderate aerobic exercise training improves endothelial function, assessed by FMD, in heart failure patients with reduced ejection fractions. Future studies investigating FMD responses to different training intensities including high-intensity training protocols will further assist in providing more evidence as to optimal aerobic training intensity prescription to elicit superior improvements in endothelial function as well as other physiological and clinically relevant endpoints.

Disclosure

This work received no financial support and has no relationship to industry. The authors take responsibility for all aspects of the reliability and freedom from bias of the data presented and their discussed interpretation.

Competing Interests

The authors report no relationships that could be construed as a conflict of interests.

References

[1] M. J. Haykowsky, Y. Liang, D. Pechter, L. W. Jones, F. A. McAlister, and A. M. Clark, "A meta-analysis of the effect of exercise training on left ventricular remodeling in heart failure patients: the benefit depends on the type of training performed," *Journal of the American College of Cardiology*, vol. 49, no. 24, pp. 2329–2336, 2007.

[2] N. A. Smart, T. Meyer, J. A. Butterfield et al., "Individual patient meta-analysis of exercise training effects on systemic brain natriuretic peptide expression in heart failure," *European Journal of Preventive Cardiology*, vol. 19, no. 3, pp. 428–435, 2012.

[3] G. Dieberg, H. Ismail, F. Giallauria, and N. A. Smart, "Clinical outcomes and cardiovascular responses to exercise training in heart failure patients with preserved ejection fraction: a systematic review and meta-analysis," *Journal of Applied Physiology*, vol. 119, no. 6, pp. 726–733, 2015.

[4] G. Cipriano Jr., V. T. F. Cipriano, V. Z. Maldaner Da Silva et al., "Aerobic exercise effect on prognostic markers for systolic heart failure patients: a systematic review and meta-analysis," *Heart Failure Reviews*, vol. 19, no. 5, pp. 655–667, 2014.

[5] U. Wisløff, A. Støylen, J. P. Loennechen et al., "Superior cardiovascular effect of aerobic interval training versus moderate continuous training in heart failure patients: a randomized study," *Circulation*, vol. 115, no. 24, pp. 3086–3094, 2007.

[6] C. N. Marti, M. Gheorghiade, A. P. Kalogeropoulos, V. V. Georgiopoulou, A. A. Quyyumi, and J. Butler, "Endothelial dysfunction, arterial stiffness, and heart failure," *Journal of the American College of Cardiology*, vol. 60, no. 16, pp. 1455–1469, 2012.

[7] B. Meyer, D. Mörtl, K. Strecker et al., "Flow-mediated vasodilation predicts outcome in patients with chronic heart failure: comparison with B-type natriuretic peptide," *Journal of the American College of Cardiology*, vol. 46, no. 6, pp. 1011–1018, 2005.

[8] D. J. Green, "Exercise training as vascular medicine: direct impacts on the vasculature in humans," *Exercise and Sport Sciences Reviews*, vol. 37, no. 4, pp. 196–202, 2009.

[9] M. F. Piepoli, V. Conraads, U. CorrÁ et al., "Exercise training in heart failure: From theory to practice. A consensus document of the heart failure association and the european association for cardiovascular prevention and rehabilitation," *European Journal of Heart Failure*, vol. 13, no. 4, pp. 347–357, 2011.

[10] T. Vromen, J. J. Kraal, J. Kuiper, R. F. Spee, N. Peek, and H. M. Kemps, "The influence of training characteristics on the effect of aerobic exercise training in patients with chronic heart failure: a meta-regression analysis," *International Journal of Cardiology*, vol. 208, pp. 120–127, 2016.

[11] H. Ismail, J. R. McFarlane, G. Dieberg, and N. A. Smart, "Exercise training program characteristics and magnitude of change in functional capacity of heart failure patients," *International Journal of Cardiology*, vol. 171, no. 1, pp. 62–65, 2014.

[12] H. Ismail, J. R. McFarlane, A. H. Nojoumian, G. Dieberg, and N. A. Smart, "Clinical Outcomes and cardiovascular responses to different exercise training intensities in patients with heart failure. A systematic review and meta-analysis," *JACC: Heart Failure*, vol. 1, no. 6, pp. 514–522, 2013.

[13] J. Cornelis, P. Beckers, J. Taeymans, C. Vrints, and D. Vissers, "Comparing exercise training modalities in heart failure: a systematic review and meta-analysis," *International Journal of Cardiology*, vol. 221, pp. 867–876, 2016.

[14] A. Mezzani, L. F. Hamm, A. M. Jones et al., "Aerobic exercise intensity assessment and prescription in cardiac rehabilitation: a joint position statement of the European Association for Cardiovascular Prevention and Rehabilitation, the American Association of Cardiovascular and Pulmonary Rehabilitation and the Canadian Association of Cardiac Rehabilitation," *European Journal of Preventive Cardiology*, vol. 20, no. 3, pp. 442–467, 2013.

[15] M. J. Haykowsky, M. P. Timmons, C. Kruger, M. McNeely, D. A. Taylor, and A. M. Clark, "Meta-analysis of aerobic interval training on exercise capacity and systolic function in patients with heart failure and reduced ejection fractions," *The American Journal of Cardiology*, vol. 111, no. 10, pp. 1466–1469, 2013.

[16] N. A. Smart, G. Dieberg, and F. Giallauria, "Intermittent versus continuous exercise training in chronic heart failure: a meta-analysis," *International Journal of Cardiology*, vol. 166, no. 2, pp. 352–358, 2013.

[17] C. Goto, Y. Higashi, M. Kimura et al., "Effect of different intensities of exercise on endothelium-dependent vasodilation in humans: role of endothelium-dependent nitric oxide and oxidative stress," *Circulation*, vol. 108, no. 5, pp. 530–535, 2003.

[18] M. Vona, G. M. Codeluppi, T. Iannino, E. Ferrari, J. Bogousslavsky, and L. K. Von Segesser, "Effects of different types of exercise training followed by detraining on endothelium-dependent dilation in patients with recent myocardial infarction," *Circulation*, vol. 119, no. 12, pp. 1601–1608, 2009.

[19] T. S. Hermann, C. H. Dall, S. B. Christensen, J. P. Goetze, E. Prescott, and F. Gustafsson, "Effect of high intensity exercise on peak oxygen uptake and endothelial function in long-term heart transplant recipients," *American Journal of Transplantation*, vol. 11, no. 3, pp. 536–541, 2011.

[20] P. S. Munk, E. M. Staal, N. Butt, K. Isaksen, and A. I. Larsen, "High-intensity interval training may reduce in-stent restenosis following percutaneous coronary intervention with stent implantation: a randomized controlled trial evaluating the relationship to endothelial function and inflammation," *American Heart Journal*, vol. 158, no. 5, pp. 734–741, 2009.

[21] A. W. Ashor, J. Lara, M. Siervo et al., "Exercise modalities and endothelial function: a systematic review and dose-response meta-analysis of randomized controlled trials," *Sports Medicine*, vol. 45, no. 2, pp. 279–296, 2015.

[22] J. S. Ramos, L. C. Dalleck, A. E. Tjonna, K. S. Beetham, and J. S. Coombes, "The impact of high-intensity interval training versus moderate-intensity continuous training on vascular function: a systematic review and meta-analysis," *Sports Medicine*, vol. 45, no. 5, pp. 679–692, 2015.

[23] J. Cohen, *Statistical Power Analysis for the Behavioral Sciences*, Lawrence Erlbaum Associates, Hillside, NJ, USA, 1988.

[24] C. E. Garber, B. Blissmer, M. R. Deschenes et al., "Quantity and quality of exercise for developing and maintaining cardiorespiratory, musculoskeletal, and neuromotor fitness in apparently healthy adults: guidance for prescribing exercise," *Medicine and Science in Sports and Exercise*, vol. 43, no. 7, pp. 1334–1359, 2011.

[25] J. P. T. Higgins, S. G. Thompson, J. J. Deeks, and D. G. Altman, "Measuring inconsistency in meta-analyses," *British Medical Journal*, vol. 327, no. 7414, pp. 557–560, 2003.

[26] M. Egger, G. D. Smith, M. Schneider, and C. Minder, "Bias in meta-analysis detected by a simple, graphical test," *British Medical Journal*, vol. 315, no. 7109, pp. 629–634, 1997.

[27] N. A. Smart, M. Waldron, H. Ismail et al., "Validation of a new tool for the assessment of study quality and reporting in exercise training studies: TESTEX," *International Journal of Evidence-Based Healthcare*, vol. 13, no. 1, pp. 9–18, 2015.

[28] N. M. M. Benda, J. P. H. Seeger, G. G. C. F. Stevens et al., "Effects of high-intensity interval training versus continuous training on physical fitness, cardiovascular function and quality of life in heart failure patients," *PLoS ONE*, vol. 10, no. 10, Article ID e0141256, 2015.

[29] R. Belardinelli, F. Capestro, A. Misiani, P. Scipione, and D. Georgiou, "Moderate exercise training improves functional capacity, quality of life, and endothelium-dependent vasodilation in chronic heart failure patients with implantable cardioverter defibrillators and cardiac resynchronization therapy," *European Journal of Cardiovascular Prevention and Rehabilitation*, vol. 13, no. 5, pp. 818–825, 2006.

[30] R. Belardinelli, F. Lacalaprice, E. Faccenda, A. Purcaro, and G. Perna, "Effects of short-term moderate exercise training on sexual function in male patients with chronic stable heart failure," *International Journal of Cardiology*, vol. 101, no. 1, pp. 83–90, 2005.

[31] E. Eleuteri, A. Mezzani, A. Di Stefano et al., "Aerobic training and angiogenesis activation in patients with stable chronic heart failure: a preliminary report," *Biomarkers*, vol. 18, no. 5, pp. 418–424, 2013.

[32] S. Erbs, R. Höllriegel, A. Linke et al., "Exercise training in patients with advanced chronic heart failure (NYHA IIIb) promotes restoration of peripheral vasomotor function, induction of endogenous regeneration, and improvement of left ventricular function," *Circulation: Heart Failure*, vol. 3, no. 4, pp. 486–494, 2010.

[33] M. Guazzi, G. Reina, G. Tumminello, and M. D. Guazzi, "Improvement of alveolar-capillary membrane diffusing capacity with exercise training in chronic heart failure," *Journal of Applied Physiology*, vol. 97, no. 5, pp. 1866–1873, 2004.

[34] K. Isaksen, P. S. Munk, T. Valborgland, and A. I. Larsen, "Aerobic interval training in patients with heart failure and an implantable cardioverter defibrillator: a controlled study evaluating feasibility and effect," *European Journal of Preventive Cardiology*, vol. 22, no. 3, pp. 296–303, 2015.

[35] N. Kobayashi, Y. Tsuruya, T. Iwasawa et al., "Exercise training in patients with chronic heart failure improves endothelial function predominantly in the trained extremities," *Circulation Journal*, vol. 67, no. 6, pp. 505–510, 2003.

[36] A. Linke, N. Schoene, S. Gielen et al., "Endothelial dysfunction in patients with chronic heart failure: systemic effects of lower-limb exercise training," *Journal of the American College of Cardiology*, vol. 37, no. 2, pp. 392–397, 2001.

[37] M. Sandri, M. Viehmann, V. Adams et al., "Chronic heart failure and aging—effects of exercise training on endothelial function and mechanisms of endothelial regeneration: results from the Leipzig Exercise Intervention in Chronic heart failure and Aging (LEICA) study," *European Journal of Preventive Cardiology*, vol. 23, no. 4, pp. 349–358, 2016.

[38] N. A. Smart and M. Steele, "A Comparison of 16 weeks of continuous vs intermittent exercise training in chronic heart failure patients," *Congestive Heart Failure*, vol. 18, no. 4, pp. 205–211, 2012.

[39] E. M. Van Craenenbroeck, V. Y. Hoymans, P. J. Beckers et al., "Exercise training improves function of circulating angiogenic cells in patients with chronic heart failure," *Basic Research in Cardiology*, vol. 105, no. 5, pp. 665–676, 2010.

[40] T. Guiraud, A. Nigam, V. Gremeaux, P. Meyer, M. Juneau, and L. Bosquet, "High-intensity interval training in cardiac rehabilitation," *Sports Medicine*, vol. 42, no. 7, pp. 587–605, 2012.

[41] A. Barac, U. Campia, and J. A. Panza, "Methods for evaluating endothelial function in humans," *Hypertension*, vol. 49, no. 4, pp. 748–760, 2007.

[42] K. Norton, L. Norton, and D. Sadgrove, "Position statement on physical activity and exercise intensity terminology," *Journal of Science and Medicine in Sport*, vol. 13, no. 5, pp. 496–502, 2010.

[43] M. Buchheit and P. B. Laursen, "High-intensity interval training, solutions to the programming puzzle: part I: cardiopulmonary emphasis," *Sports Medicine*, vol. 43, no. 5, pp. 313–338, 2013.

[44] D. J. Green, T. Eijsvogels, Y. M. Bouts et al., "Exercise training and artery function in humans: nonresponse and its relationship to cardiovascular risk factors," *Journal of Applied Physiology*, vol. 117, no. 4, pp. 345–352, 2014.

[45] V. M. Conraads, N. Pattyn, C. De Maeyer et al., "Aerobic interval training and continuous training equally improve aerobic exercise capacity in patients with coronary artery disease: The SAINTEX-CAD Study," *International Journal of Cardiology*, vol. 179, pp. 203–210, 2015.

[46] B. J. Sawyer, W. J. Tucker, D. M. Bhammar, J. R. Ryder, K. L. Sweazea, and G. A. Gaesser, "Effects of high-intensity interval training and moderate-intensity continuous training on endothelial function and cardiometabolic risk markers in obese adults," *Journal of Applied Physiology*, vol. 121, no. 1, pp. 279–288, 2016.

[47] V. Anagnostakou, K. Chatzimichail, S. Dimopoulos et al., "Effects of interval cycle training with or without strength training on vascular reactivity in heart failure patients," *Journal of Cardiac Failure*, vol. 17, no. 7, pp. 585–591, 2011.

[48] D. W. Kitzman and M. J. Haykowsky, "Vascular dysfunction in heart failure with preserved ejection fraction," *Journal of Cardiac Failure*, vol. 22, no. 1, pp. 12–16, 2016.

[49] D. W. Kitzman, P. H. Brubaker, D. M. Herrington et al., "Effect of endurance exercise training on endothelial function and arterial stiffness in older patients with heart failure and preserved ejection fraction: a randomized, controlled, single-blind trial," *Journal of the American College of Cardiology*, vol. 62, no. 7, pp. 584–592, 2013.

[50] S. S. Angadi, F. Mookadam, C. D. Lee, W. J. Tucker, M. J. Haykowsky, and G. A. Gaesser, "High-intensity interval training vs. moderate-intensity continuous exercise training in heart failure with preserved ejection fraction: a pilot study," *Journal of Applied Physiology*, vol. 119, no. 6, pp. 753–758, 2015.

12

Incidence and Factors Predicting Skin Burns at the Site of Indifferent Electrode during Radiofrequency Catheter Ablation of Cardiac Arrhythmias

Hussain Ibrahim,[1] Bohuslav Finta,[2] and Jubran Rind[1]

[1]Grand Rapids Medical Education Partners, Michigan State University, Grand Rapids, MI 49503, USA
[2]Spectrum Health Medical Group Cardiovascular Services, Grand Rapids, MI 49503, USA

Correspondence should be addressed to Hussain Ibrahim; hussain.ibrahim12@gmail.com

Academic Editor: Yi-Gang Li

Radiofrequency catheter ablation (RFA) has become a mainstay for treatment of cardiac arrhythmias. Skin burns at the site of an indifferent electrode patch have been a rare, serious, and likely an underreported complication of RFA. The purpose of this study was to determine the incidence of skin burns in cardiac RFA procedures performed at one institution. Also, we wanted to determine the factors predicting skin burns after cardiac RFA procedures at the indifferent electrode skin pad site. *Methods.* A retrospective case control study was performed to compare the characteristics in patients who developed skin burns in a 2-year period. *Results.* Incidence of significant skin burns after RFA was 0.28% (6/2167). Four of the six patients were female and all were Caucasians. Four controls for every case were age and sex matched. Burn patients had significantly higher BMI, procedure time, and postprocedure pain, relative to control subjects ($p < 0.05$, one-tailed testing). No one in either group had evidence of dispersive pad malattachment. *Conclusions.* Our results indicate that burn patients had higher BMI and longer procedure times compared to control subjects. These findings warrant further larger studies on this topic.

1. Introduction

Radiofrequency catheter ablation (RFA) has become a mainstay for treatment of cardiac arrhythmias. It is considered a highly effective treatment modality with a low complication rate [1, 2]. Up to 3% of patients undergoing radiofrequency catheter ablation develop major complications from the procedure. These complications include AV block, cardiac tamponade, coronary artery spasm, thrombosis, pericarditis, vascular injury, thromboembolism, TIA or stroke, pulmonary hypertension, pneumothorax, left atrial-esophageal fistula, and phrenic nerve paralysis [3]. Skin burns at the site of an indifferent electrode patch have been a rare, serious, and likely an underreported complication of RFA [4, 5]. Although different studies have looked at incidence and factors that have led to skin burns at the site of skin pad attachment while performing hepatic tumor ablative procedures, [6, 7] literature related to this complication is scant in cardiac

arrhythmia ablative procedures. Incidence of skin burns at the site of the indifferent electrode is currently low but it is likely going to increase in future as higher power settings and multiple ablations are more frequently used for ablation of cardiac arrhythmias [8]. Only case reports and case series have been published in the past. This study aims to determine the incidence and different factors predicting possible skin burns at the site of an indifferent electrode patch while performing these cardiac arrhythmia ablative procedures.

2. Methods

A retrospective case control study design was used to examine the characteristics in patients who developed skin burns related to the radiofrequency ablation, compared to those who did not develop this complication during the procedure. All patients ≥18 years of age who underwent cardiac RFA procedures from 4/1/2012 to 3/31/2014 that developed skin

TABLE 1: Comparisons for nominal variables between the cases (burn patients) and the controls[1].

Characteristic	Cases (%)	Controls (%)	p value
Hypertension	5/6 (83.3%)	20/24 (83.3%)	0.746
Diabetes	2/6 (33.3%)	5/24 (20.8%)	0.433
Postprocedure pain	4/6 (67.7%)	0/24 (0%)	0.001
Type of skin patch			0.545
3M stockert skin patch	4/6 (66.7%)	14/24 (58.3%)	
Valley Lab skin patch	2/6 (33.3%)	10/24 (41.7%)	
General anesthesia	4/6 (66.7%)	13/24 (54.2%)	0.469

[1] The one-tailed Fisher's exact test was used for the analyses.

TABLE 2: Comparisons for quantitative variables between the cases (burn patients) and the controls[1].

Characteristic	Cases (%)	Controls (%)	p value
BMI	36.6 (27.7–65.0)	30.6 (17.6–52.6)	0.044
Procedure time (min)	224.5 (63–332)	122.5 (23–357)	0.035
Maximum temperature (°C)	55.0 (50.0–65.0)	50.0 (40.0–70.0)	0.078
Maximum current (watts)	60.0 (35.0–70.0)	50.0 (35.0–100.0)	0.325

BMI: body mass index.
[1] The one-tailed Mann-Whitney U test was used for the analyses.

burns at the site of the indifferent electrode skin patch were included in the review. Controls, defined as patients >18 years of age who underwent cardiac RFA procedures and did not develop skin burns, were randomly selected from the same time frame and matched on age and sex.

Data collected included patient demographics, patient's past medical history (e.g., hypertension and diabetes), height, weight, and BMI. Procedure details (including diagnosis for ablation, type of sedation used, total procedure time, type of generator, maximum temperature reached, and maximum power in watts) were also obtained. Impedance data were not recorded for this patient population and were not included in our study. Indifferent electrode skin patch characteristics (e.g., type, area of attachment, and evidence of malattachment of skin pad at the end of procedure) were collected, as were data related to the characteristics of the burns (e.g., patient complains of pain or not and burn degree (redness, second-degree skin burns, and third-degree skin burns)). Length of hospital management for the burn was also recorded.

Incidence of skin burns from RFA was determined using a query of all patients who underwent cardiac RFA procedures. There were a total of six patients who developed a burn during the study time frame. For the sample size determination, we assumed an odds ratio of 6.0 as clinically important, with 20% of the controls exposed to the risk factor and with $\alpha = 0.05$ and $\beta = 0.20$. We planned to be able to detect a statistically significant effect with four control patients for every burn patient, using a one-tailed test. The records from 24 control patients and six burn patients were reviewed for this study.

Data were analyzed using IBM SPSS Statistics v 21.0. (Armonk, NY). Quantitative data were analyzed using the Mann-Whitney U test and are shown as the mean ± SD. Nominal data were analyzed using Fisher's exact test and are shown as percentages. Significance was assessed at $p < 0.05$, using one-tailed testing.

3. Results

Incidence of the significant skin burns after the RFA ablation procedure was found to be 0.28% (6/2167) during the study period. Two of our six burn subjects were males and all were Caucasians. Eight of the 16 control subjects were males, 22/24 were Caucasian, and their age (63.7 ± 8.6 years, mean ± SD) was similar to that of the burn patients (63.7 ± 8.1 years). No significant difference was present between cases and controls with regard to hypertension, diabetes, skin pad, or type of sedation (Table 1). Postprocedure pain was predictably present in significantly more cases compared to controls.

No patient in either group had evidence of dispersive pad malattachment and none of the patients' hair was removed at the site of attachment. Subjects with burns had significantly greater BMI and total procedure time, relative to the control subjects (Table 2). There were no statistically significant differences between the cases and controls with regard to maximum temperature reached or maximum current in watts.

4. Discussion

Radiofrequency ablation of cardiac arrhythmias uses low voltage and high frequency electrical energy. During the management of nonarrhythmic conditions like radiofrequency ablation of hepatic tumors, increased level of radiofrequency energy is frequently used, causing higher incidence of potential complications including skin burns at the site of the indifferent electrode patch [9]. Severe skin burns occur in 0.1%–3% of patients undergoing RF ablation of solid abdominal tumors while mild skin burns occur in up to 33% of such patients [6, 10]. This high rate is postulated to be secondary to high power settings and prolonged procedure times during these ablations [11].

Tissue temperature increases with the passage of electric current, with the greatest increase in temperature being at the site of catheter tip, while the temperature increase is attenuated at the site of indifferent electrode site with the help of dispersive skin patches. Increase of temperature at the catheter tip is the foundation of the therapy with RFA as it causes the local destruction of the tissue. Dispersive skin pads at the site of the indifferent electrode function to disperse the electrical energy exiting the body and thus prevent the occurrence of skin burns by spreading the energy over a larger surface area [3]. In prior studies, it has been predicted that the temperature rises to 45–47°C. At the indifferent electrode site, there is a risk factor for development of skin burns [12].

Malattachment of dispersive pads, presence of hair at the site of pad attachment, and increased amount of subdermal fat have been described as known risk factors for development of skin burns. Fat tissue acts like an insulator and increases the temperature secondary to increase in the resistance [9]. Dysfunction of the skin pad by either malattachment or physical damage concentrates the exiting current's available area, resulting in increased tissue temperature and higher risk for development of skin burns.

Our results showed that there was a low incidence of burns at the indifferent electrode skin pad during RFA ablation procedures for cardiac arrhythmias. Nevertheless, this can be a potentially serious complication, as two of our patients developed third-degree burns requiring increased burn care. All of our six burn patients were Caucasians, indicating that there might be a predisposition to develop the skin burns secondary to skin characteristics. However, 22 of our 24 controls were also Caucasians, thus making this association weaker as Caucasian patients seem to be the predominant ethnic group who underwent the RFA procedures at our institution.

BMI is an important factor which can be helpful in predicting the patients' risk of developing skin burns. It is expected that, with increased body weight, there would be more impedance during the RFA procedure, resulting in an increased incidence of the skin burns at the site of the indifferent electrode. Our results indicated that burn patients had significantly higher BMI relative to our control subjects. We suggest that care should be taken in patients who have increased BMI while performing the RFA procedures.

Hair was not removed at the site of the indifferent electrode in our patients, as this might lead to the malattachment of the dispersive skin pad, increased resistance, and thus increased incidence of skin burns which can be associated with it. There was no evidence of malattachment of the indifferent electrode in either the cases or the controls. Another interesting finding was that all patients who had burns had the indifferent electrode applied to the left flank. Among the controls, 12 out of 24 patients had the indifferent electrode attached in the left flank. One patient from the controls had the placement on the left leg, five had it on the right leg, and six controls had the indifferent electrode placed in the right flank region. In a previous study, risk of development of skin burns was found to be lower in patients with the dispersive skin pad attached to the thigh as compared to other body parts [13]. Optimal position of the dispersive

skin pad needs to be studied further as it seems to be an important risk factor that is easily modifiable.

Four out of our six cases with the skin burns complained of the pain at the site of indifferent electrode placement. Further, these patients had developed second- and third-degree skin burns. Pain assessment at the end of the procedure for the patients who are under conscious sedation and at the time of becoming conscious for those who undergo the procedure under general anesthesia can be helpful for actively looking for the skin lesions in a timely manner.

Total procedure time was significantly higher in burn patients relative to control subjects, suggesting that it may be a clinically important factor of predicting skin burns. Increased total procedure time indicates technical difficulty of the procedure, patient characteristics that are unfavorable, and/or a difficult to treat arrhythmia requiring increased duration of the procedure to achieve adequate ablation.

Maximum temperature reached during the procedure did not seem to have a major impact on our study sample. This points towards the fact that sustained ablation for longer period of time is more likely to cause the skin burns than higher temperature for shorter periods of time. Thus, one of the important steps in reduction of the post-RFA ablation skin burns is to not prolong the ablation procedure.

Impedance is an important factor in radiofrequency ablation procedures and its monitoring can be helpful in predicting development of skin burns. It is the weighted average of electrical resistivity of all the tissues between the ablation catheter and the indifferent electrode patch. Regions closer to the radiofrequency ablation catheter have the highest weightage in determination of impedance because of high electrical density [14].

Important determinants of impedance include increased body surface area, blood flow to the tissues, coagulum, and char formation. Volume of resistive medium between the two electrodes is proportional to the impedance. Thus, obesity and larger body surface area result in high impedance as subdermal fat acts as an insulator. Power used in radiofrequency ablation of cardiac arrhythmias is proportional to the voltage and inversely proportional to the system impedance [15]. Thus, if impedance increases, in order to deliver the same amount of energy to the cardiac tissue, higher power settings are needed. As studies have found that high power and prolonged periods of cardiac ablation are associated with higher incidence of skin burns, [9] it can be concluded that the high impedance is a risk factor for development of skin burns and would be interesting factor to look at in future studies.

Steam popping is another important phenomenon. During the generation of resistive heat during radiofrequency ablation of the cardiac arrhythmias, cardiac tissue fluid can vaporize, forming steam bubbles which can potentially burst open with an audible pop with continued ablation (generally occurs at tissue temperatures above 100°C). An important potential complication associated with this phenomenon is cardiac perforation. Steam popping and vaporization have been associated with a drop in the impedance [16, 17]. The frequency of the steam pops has been noted to be high with higher power [18]. Theoretically, steam popping can be used as a predictor of skin burns which also can occur at high power settings. This has not been described in the literature before and can be looked at in future studies as a potential predictor.

Further studies are needed to assess other possible predictors including impedance and voltage and for confirmation of our results. Establishment of these predictors would help decrease this possible complication, which can be a major issue in many patients.

5. Limitations

An important limitation of the study is its small sample size. Another important limitation is the fact that we did not have the complete records of the important possible predictor of voltage used during the procedure. Therefore, we could not assess any association with it. We used a case control study design, which could raise concerns as to whether there might be other differences between the cases and controls which could be driving the significant differences seen in this study. Finally, a decision was made at the time of writing the protocol to use one-tailed testing for all of the statistical analyses.

6. Conclusion

This is the first comparative study reporting on skin burns following RFA. Although the sample size was small, burn patients had significantly higher BMI, procedure times, and postprocedure pain relative to control subjects. While larger studies are needed to confirm these findings, these results should be kept in mind when planning to perform RFA.

Competing Interests

The authors declare that there are no competing interests regarding the publication of this paper.

References

[1] G. Hindricks, "The Multicentre European Radiofrequency Survey (MERFS): complications of radiofrequency catheter ablation of arrhythmias," *European Heart Journal*, vol. 14, no. 12, pp. 1644–1653, 1993.

[2] T. Rostock, T. Risius, R. Ventura et al., "Efficacy and safety of radiofrequency catheter ablation of atrioventricular nodal reentrant tachycardia in the elderly," *Journal of Cardiovascular Electrophysiology*, vol. 16, no. 6, pp. 608–610, 2005.

[3] S. R. Vanga, M. Biria, L. Berenbom, J. Vacek, and D. R. Lakkireddy, "Skin burns at the site of indifferent electrode after radiofrequency catheter ablation of AV node for atrial fibrillation," *Journal of Atrial Fibrillation*, vol. 1, no. 2, pp. 11–14, 2008.

[4] P. S. Dhillon, H. Gonna, A. Li, T. Wong, and D. E. Ward, "Skin burns associated with radiofrequency catheter ablation of cardiac arrhythmias," *Pacing and Clinical Electrophysiology*, vol. 36, no. 6, pp. 764–767, 2013.

[5] A. Goette, S. Reek, H. U. Klein, and J. Christoph Geller, "Case report: severe skin burn at the site of the indifferent electrode after radiofrequency catheter ablation of typical atrial flutter," *Journal of Interventional Cardiac Electrophysiology*, vol. 5, no. 3, pp. 337–340, 2001.

[6] H. Rhim, K.-H. Yoon, J. M. Lee et al., "Major complications after radio-frequency thermal ablation of hepatic tumors: spectrum of imaging findings," *Radiographics*, vol. 23, no. 1, pp. 123–136, 2003.

[7] T. de Baère, O. Risse, V. Kuoch et al., "Adverse events during radiofrequency treatment of 582 hepatic tumors," *American Journal of Roentgenology*, vol. 181, no. 3, pp. 695–700, 2003.

[8] S. J. Trivedi, T. W. Lim, M. A. Barry et al., "Clinical evaluation of a new technique to monitor return electrode skin temperature during radiofrequency ablation," *Journal of Interventional Cardiac Electrophysiology*, vol. 36, no. 3, pp. 307–314, 2013.

[9] K. Steinke, S. Gananadha, J. King, J. Zhao, and D. L. Morris, "Dispersive pad site burns with modern radiofrequency ablation equipment," *Surgical Laparoscopy, Endoscopy & Percutaneous Techniques*, vol. 13, no. 6, pp. 366–371, 2003.

[10] S. Mulier, P. Mulier, Y. Ni et al., "Complications of radiofrequency coagulation of liver tumours," *British Journal of Surgery*, vol. 89, no. 10, pp. 1206–1222, 2002.

[11] J. Machi, "Prevention of dispersive pad skin burns during RFA by a simple method," *Surgical Laparoscopy, Endoscopy and Percutaneous Techniques*, vol. 13, no. 6, pp. 372–373, 2003.

[12] J. A. Pearce, L. A. Geddes, J. F. van Vleet, K. Foster, and J. Allen, "Skin burns from electrosurgical current," *Medical Instrumentation*, vol. 17, no. 3, pp. 225–231, 1983.

[13] S. Nath, J. P. DiMarco, R. G. Gallop, I. D. McRury, and D. E. Haines, "Effects of dispersive electrode position and surface area on electrical parameters and temperature during radiofrequency catheter ablation," *American Journal of Cardiology*, vol. 77, no. 9, pp. 765–767, 1996.

[14] D. Haemmerich, "Biophysics of radiofrequency ablation," *Critical Reviews in Biomedical Engineering*, vol. 38, no. 1, pp. 53–63, 2010.

[15] M. Borganelli, R. El-Atassi, A. Leon et al., "Determinants of impedance during radiofrequency catheter ablation in humans," *The American Journal of Cardiology*, vol. 69, no. 12, pp. 1095–1097, 1992.

[16] J. Seiler, K. C. Roberts-Thomson, J.-M. Raymond, J. Vest, E. Delacretaz, and W. G. Stevenson, "Steam pops during irrigated radiofrequency ablation: feasibility of impedance monitoring for prevention," *Heart Rhythm*, vol. 5, no. 10, pp. 1411–1416, 2008.

[17] H. Iida, T. Aihara, S. Ikuta, and N. Yamanaka, "Effectiveness of impedance monitoring during radiofrequency ablation for predicting popping," *World Journal of Gastroenterology*, vol. 18, no. 41, pp. 5870–5878, 2012.

[18] C. Theis, T. Rostock, H. Mollnau et al., "The incidence of audible steam pops is increased and unpredictable with the Thermo-Cool® surround flow catheter during left atrial catheter ablation: a prospective observational study," *Journal of Cardiovascular Electrophysiology*, vol. 26, no. 9, pp. 956–962, 2015.

13

The Modification Effect of Influenza Vaccine on Prognostic Indicators for Cardiovascular Events after Acute Coronary Syndrome: Observations from an Influenza Vaccination Trial

Apirak Sribhutorn,[1,2] Arintaya Phrommintikul,[3] Wanwarang Wongcharoen,[3] Usa Chaikledkaew,[4] Suntara Eakanunkul,[5] and Apichard Sukonthasarn[3]

[1]*Ph.D. Program in Clinical Epidemiology, Faculty of Medicine, Chiang Mai University, Chiang Mai 50200, Thailand*
[2]*Department of Pharmacy Practice, School of Pharmaceutical Sciences, University of Phayao, Phayao 56000, Thailand*
[3]*Cardiology Division, Department of Internal Medicine, Faculty of Medicine, Chiang Mai University, Chiang Mai 50200, Thailand*
[4]*Social and Administrative Pharmacy Excellence Research (SAPER) Unit, Department of Pharmacy, Faculty of Pharmacy,*
 Mahidol University, Bangkok 10400, Thailand
[5]*Department of Pharmaceutical Sciences, Faculty of Pharmacy, Chiang Mai University, Chiang Mai 50200, Thailand*

Correspondence should be addressed to Arintaya Phrommintikul; arintayap@gmail.com

Academic Editor: Mariantonietta Cicoira

Introduction. The prognosis of acute coronary syndrome (ACS) patients has been improved with several treatments such as antithrombotics, beta-blockers, and angiotensin-converting enzyme inhibitors (ACEI) as well as coronary revascularization. Influenza vaccination has been shown to reduce adverse outcomes in ACS, but no information exists regarding the interaction of other treatments. *Methods.* This study included 439 ACS patients from Phrommintikul et al. A single dose of inactivated influenza vaccine was given by intramuscular injection in the vaccination group. The cardiovascular outcomes were described as major cardiovascular events (MACEs) which included mortality, hospitalization due to ACS, and hospitalization due to heart failure (HF). The stratified and multivariable Cox's regression analysis was performed. *Results.* The stratified Cox's analysis by influenza vaccination for each cardiovascular outcome and discrimination of hazard ratios showed that beta-blockers had an interaction with influenza vaccination. Moreover, the multivariable hazard ratios disclosed that influenza vaccine is associated with a significant reduction of hospitalization due to HF in patients who received beta-blockers (HR = 0.05, 95% CI = 0.004–0.71, $P = 0.027$), after being adjusted for prognostic indicators (sex, dyslipidemia, serum creatinine, and left ventricular ejection fraction). *Conclusions.* The influenza vaccine was shown to significantly modify the effect of beta-blockers in ACS patients and to reduce the hospitalization due to HF. However, further study of a larger population and benefits to HF patients should be investigated.

1. Introduction

Influenza vaccination in the community can significantly reduce influenza infection [1] and incidence of influenza-like illness among the elderly [2], as well as hospitalization and death due to pneumonia, influenza [3–7], or cardiovascular diseases [1, 3–8]. Furthermore, randomized controlled studies have demonstrated benefits in reducing major adverse cardiovascular events among patients with coronary artery diseases (CAD) [9–13]. For this reason, the American Heart Association and American College of Cardiology recommend influenza vaccination as a secondary prevention intervention in patients with CAD and atherosclerotic vascular diseases [14, 15] and those with ST-segment elevation myocardial infarction (STEMI) [16] and unstable angina/non-STEMI [17] as well as a plan of care for patients with chronic heart failure [18].

Nonetheless, the evidence-based recommendations and benefits of influenza vaccination have been shown in CAD; the mechanisms of its benefit have not yet been defined, as well as some queries on the vaccine immunological response in patients with various clinical characteristics, such as impaired renal function or concurrent medications [19–22]. The study of prognostic indicators and patients' clinical characteristics may describe the benefits of influenza vaccine for cardiovascular outcomes.

An annual influenza vaccination can prevent influenza virus infection and relieve the symptoms of acute infection. In fact, an annual influenza vaccination can prevent influenza infection and also decrease the results from acute infection, where it promotes inflammation and the progression of atherosclerosis and it serves as a trigger for acute myocardial infarction [23–29]. Consequently, the administration of influenza vaccine may reveal an influence on some prognostic indicators for cardiovascular outcomes, compared with patients not receiving the vaccination.

Therefore, this study aimed to explore the effects of the influenza vaccine through the prognostic indicators for each cardiovascular outcome among ACS patients.

2. Patients and Methods

2.1. Data Sources and Data Collection. This observational study was based on a prospective, randomized open with blinded endpoint study from Phrommintikul et al. [9], which enrolled 439 patients who had been admitted due to ACS and were older than 50 years old. Patients were excluded if they had hemoglobin level lower than 10 g/dL, elevated serum creatinine (SCr) level more than 2.5 mg/dL, well-established liver disease, cancer or life expectancy less than one year, and contraindications to, or previous, influenza vaccination. All patients were given standard treatment by their primary cardiologist in the tertiary care hospital of Chiang Mai University.

2.2. Definition. The ACS patients were classified into three groups. These included the following: (1) patients with an acute ST-segment elevation myocardial infarction (STEMI) described as a chest pain lasting longer than 20 minutes with ST-segment elevation of electrocardiograph (EKG) in two consecutive leads or more, (2) patients with chest pain lasting longer than 20 minutes, with rising of cardiac troponin or CK-MB and without ST-segment elevation EKG, defined as non-ST-segment elevation myocardial infarction (NSTEMI), and (3) patients with chest pain at rest without rising of cardiac troponin or CK-MB, diagnosed as an unstable angina (UA), whereas NSTEMI and UA were defined as non-ST-segment elevation ACS (NSTE-ACS).

The studied patients' characteristics included age, sex, concurrent comorbidities, that is, hypertension (HT); diabetes mellitus (DM); dyslipidemia; chronic obstructive pulmonary disease (COPD); smoking; prior myocardial infarction (MI); chronic kidney disease (CKD), SCr, type of ACS, revascularization procedure, left ventricular ejection fraction (LVEF), and medications.

The main cardiovascular outcomes of interest were defined as (1) major adverse cardiovascular events (MACEs), a composite of all cardiovascular events, (2) all causes of mortality, (3) hospitalization due to acute coronary syndrome

(ACS), (4) hospitalization due to heart failure (HF), and (5) composite outcomes of hospitalization (ACS, HF, or stroke). These outcomes were verified by cardiologists during the follow-up of 12 months. Survival status of patients lost to follow-up was determined by telephone.

2.3. Data Analysis. The patients' characteristics were compared among five types of adverse cardiovascular outcomes and each outcome-free group, using Fisher's exact test, where multiple imputations were manipulated for missing data management.

Prognostic indicators for each cardiovascular outcome were stratified by influenza vaccine groups and analyzed as multivariable hazard ratio by the stratified Cox regression.

The Z-test was performed to demonstrate significant discrimination of hazard ratio between influenza vaccination groups [30].

Multivariable Cox's regression was conducted to present the results, subsequently adjusted for independent prognostic indicators of each cardiovascular outcome.

This study was approved by the Ethics Committee, Faculty of Medicine, Chiang Mai University.

3. Results

3.1. Patients' Characteristics. In this observational study, data of 439 ACS patients were collected. Half of the patients were older than 65 years old and 56.7% of the patients (249) were males (Table 1). HT was present among 265 (60.4%); DM, 134 (30.5%); dyslipidemia, 206 (46.9%); COPD, 13 (3.0%); and CKD, 20 (4.56%). Regarding the index ACS, STEMI and NSTE-ACS were present among 159 (36.2%) and 280 (63.8%) of the patients, respectively. The majority of STEMI patients (79.25%) received reperfusion therapy and more than a half of the NSTE-ACS patients (53.21%) received coronary revascularization. Aspirin, beta-blockers, and statin were received among 427 (97.3%), 325 (74.0%), and 293 (66.7%) patients, respectively.

3.2. Prognostic Indicators of Adverse Outcomes. The characteristics of ACS patients with and without MACEs were not significantly different, except for dyslipidemia, LVEF, receiving angiotensin-converting enzyme inhibitors (ACE-I) or angiotensin receptor blockers (ARB), and influenza vaccination (Table 1). Patients with MACEs had higher proportion of dyslipidemia (61.3% versus 44.6%, $P = 0.019$) but a lower proportion of receiving ACE-I/ARB (45.2% versus 60.7%, $P = 0.026$) and influenza vaccination (33.9% versus 53.1%, $P = 0.006$). The MACEs-free patients also had a great proportion of preserved LVEF (LVEF > 40%) (70.8% versus 51.6%, $P = 0.005$) (Table 1).

Regarding the causes of death, patients who survived were younger (age 65 ± 9.17 versus 73.0 ± 9.29 years, $P = 0.0014$). The other clinical characteristics did not significantly differ between two groups (Table 1).

When comparing between patients with composite outcomes of hospitalization due to ACS, HF, or stroke and those who were not hospitalized (Table 2), patients with these events had a higher proportion of dyslipidemia (63.3% versus

TABLE 1: Patients' characteristics for MACEs and death.

Characteristics	Total (n = 439)		Event-free (A) (n = 377)		MACEs (n = 62)		P value	Survived (n = 421)		Death (n = 18)		P value
	n	%	n	%	n	%		n	%	n	%	
Age (year)												
≤65	219	49.9	194	51.5	25	40.3	0.131	216	51.3	3	16.7	0.006
>65	220	50.1	183	48.5	37	59.7		205	48.7	15	83.3	
Male	249	56.7	218	57.8	31	50.0	0.270	243	57.7	6	33.3	0.052
HT	265	60.4	222	58.9	43	69.4	0.126	252	59.9	13	72.2	0.336
DM	134	30.5	113	30.0	21	33.8	0.553	127	30.2	7	38.9	0.440
Dyslipidemia	206	46.9	168	44.6	38	61.3	0.019	197	46.8	9	50.0	0.814
COPD	13	3.0	11	2.9	2	3.2	1.000	13	3.1	0	0.0	1.000
Smoking	48	11.0	45	11.9	3	4.8	0.123	48	11.4	0	0.0	0.241
Prior MI	18	4.1	15	4.0	3	4.8	0.729	18	4.3	0	0.0	1.000
CKD	20	4.6	15	3.9	5	8.1	0.181	20	4.8	0	0.0	1.000
SCr (mg/dL)												
≤1.1	221	50.3	194	51.5	27	43.6	0.274	212	50.4	9	50.0	1.000
>1.1	218	49.7	183	48.5	35	56.5		209	49.6	9	50.0	
Type of ACS												
NSTEMI & UA	280	63.8	242	64.2	38	61.3	0.671	272	64.6	8	44.4	0.130
STEMI	159	36.2	135	35.8	24	38.7		149	35.4	10	55.6	
Reperfusion or revascularization												
No	164	37.4	141	37.4	23	37.1	1.000	158	37.3	6	33.3	0.808
Yes	275	62.6	236	62.6	39	62.9		263	62.5	12	66.7	
LVEF (%)												
>40	299	68.1	267	70.8	32	51.6	0.005	290	68.9	9	50.0	0.120
≤40	140	31.9	110	29.2	30	48.4		131	31.1	9	50.0	
Medication												
Aspirin	427	97.3	366	97.1	61	98.4	1.000	409	97.2	18	100.0	1.000
β-blocker	325	74.0	281	74.5	44	71.0	0.536	311	73.9	14	77.8	1.000
CCB	72	16.4	63	16.7	9	14.5	0.853	69	16.4	3	16.7	1.000
ACE-I/ARB	257	58.5	229	60.7	28	45.2	0.026	250	59.4	7	38.9	0.093
Statin	293	66.7	252	66.8	41	66.1	1.000	283	67.2	10	55.6	0.315
Influenza vaccination	221	50.3	200	53.1	21	33.9	0.006	215	51.1	6	33.3	0.156

DM, diabetes mellitus; HT, hypertension; COPD, chronic obstructive pulmonary disease; MI, myocardial infarction; CKD, chronic kidney disease; SCr, serum creatinine; ACS, acute coronary syndrome; STEMI, ST-segment elevation myocardial infarction; NSTEMI, non-ST-elevation myocardial infarction; UA, unstable angina; LVEF, left ventricular ejection fraction; CCB, calcium channel blocker; ACE-I, angiotensin-converting enzyme inhibitor; ARB, angiotensin II receptor blocker; MACEs, major adverse cardiovascular events; event-free (A), free events from MACEs.

44.9%, $P = 0.022$) and impaired LVEF (LVEF < 40%) (49.0% versus 29.7%, $P = 0.009$). They also had low proportion of influenza vaccination (32.7% versus 52.6%, $P = 0.010$) (Table 2).

The comparison of three outcomes among those hospitalized due to ACS, HF, and event-free patients revealed significant differences in proportion of dyslipidemia (58.9%, 78.6%, and 44.8%, resp., $P = 0.017$), CKD (2.9%, 28.6%, and 3.8%, resp., $P = 0.004$), impaired LVEF (35.3%, 78.6%, and 29.9%, resp., $P = 0.001$), and influenza vaccination (32.35%, 28.57%, and 52.69%, resp., $P = 0.020$) (Table 2). Interestingly, patients hospitalized due to HF had a high proportion of

dyslipidemia (78.6%, $P = 0.017$), presented CKD (28.6%, $P = 0.004$), and impaired LVEF (78.6%, $P = 0.001$) but revealed a lower proportion of receiving influenza vaccination (28.6%, $P = 0.020$).

When stratified Cox's regression analysis by influenza vaccine group was performed for each cardiovascular outcome (Table 3), the significant protective indicator was receiving ACE-I/ARB, while impaired LVEF, age above 65 years, and CKD presented poor indicators in the nonvaccination group.

The impaired LVEF variables were shown as poor prognostic indicators in both groups of patients with similar

TABLE 2: Patients' characteristics of composite outcomes of hospitalization (ACS, HF, or stroke), hospitalization due to ACS, and hospitalization due to HF.

Characteristics	Event-free (B) (n = 390)		Composite hospitalization (n = 49)		P value	Event-free (C) (n = 391)		Hospitalization due to ACS (n = 34)		Hospitalization due to HF (n = 14)		P value
	n	%	n	%		n	%	n	%	n	%	
Age (year)												
≤65	196	50.3	23	46.9	0.762	197	50.4	17	50.0	5	35.7	0.616
>65	194	49.7	26	53.1		194	49.6	17	50.0	9	64.3	
Male	223	57.2	26	53.1	0.647	224	57.3	20	58.8	5	35.7	0.306
HT	231	59.2	34	69.4	0.215	232	59.3	23	67.7	10	71.4	0.495
DM	116	29.7	18	36.7	0.326	116	29.7	11	32.4	7	50.0	0.242
Dyslipidemia	175	44.9	31	63.3	0.022	175	44.8	20	58.8	11	78.6	0.017
COPD	11	2.8	2	4.1	0.646	12	3.1	0	0.0	1	7.1	0.286
Smoking	45	11.5	3	6.1	0.335	45	11.5	3	8.8	0	0.0	0.491
Prior MI	15	3.9	3	6.1	0.439	15	3.8	1	2.9	2	14.3	0.147
CKD	15	3.9	5	10.2	0.060	15	3.8	1	2.9	4	28.6	0.004
SCr (mg/dL)												
≤1.1	201	51.5	20	40.8	0.174	202	51.7	16	47.1	3	21.4	0.077
>1.1	189	48.5	29	59.2		189	48.3	18	52.9	11	78.6	
Type of ACS												
NSTEMI & UA	247	63.3	33	37.4	0.639	248	63.4	22	64.7	10	71.4	0.907
STEMI	143	36.7	16	32.7		143	36.6	12	35.3	4	28.6	
Reperfusion or revascularization												
No	146	37.4	18	36.7	1.000	146	37.3	9	26.5	9	64.3	0.054
Yes	244	62.6	31	63.3		245	62.7	25	73.5	5	35.7	
LVEF (%)												
>40	274	70.3	25	51.0	0.009	274	70.1	22	64.7	3	21.4	0.001
≤40	116	29.7	24	49.0		117	30.0	12	35.3	11	78.6	
Medication												
Aspirin	379	97.2	48	98.0	1.000	380	97.2	33	97.1	14	100.0	1.000
β-blocker	291	74.6	34	69.4	0.489	291	74.4	25	73.5	9	64.3	0.676
CCB	65	16.7	7	14.3	0.838	65	16.6	5	14.7	2	14.3	1.000
ACE-I/ARB	234	60.0	23	47.0	0.091	235	60.1	17	50.0	5	35.7	0.121
Statin	259	66.4	34	69.4	0.749	260	66.5	24	70.6	9	64.3	0.872
Influenza vaccination	205	52.6	16	32.7	0.010	206	52.7	11	32.4	4	28.6	0.020

DM, diabetes mellitus; HT, hypertension; COPD, chronic obstructive pulmonary disease; MI, myocardial infarction; CKD, chronic kidney disease; SCr, serum creatinine; HF, heart failure; ACS, acute coronary syndrome; STEMI, ST-segment elevation myocardial infarction; NSTEMI, non-ST-elevation myocardial infarction; UA, unstable angina; LVEF, left ventricular ejection fraction; CCB, calcium channel blocker; ACE-I, angiotensin-converting enzyme inhibitor; ARB, angiotensin II receptor blocker; Composite hospitalization, composite hospitalization due to ACS, HF, or stroke; event-free (B), free events from composite hospitalization due to ACS, HF, or stroke; event-free (C), free events from hospitalization due to ACS or HF.

hazard ratios (Tables 3 and 4). Age above 65 years was indicated as a significant prognostic indicator for death in the nonvaccination group (HR = 10.78, 95% CI = 1.39–83.62, $P = 0.023$) but not in the vaccination group (HR = 2.28, 95% CI = 0.42–12.48, $P = 0.341$). However, the effect size of age did not significantly vary between vaccination groups ($P = 0.252$) (Table 4). Differently, the CKD variable was a promising poor prognostic indicator in both groups, (HR = 5.12, 95% CI = 1.27–20.65, $P = 0.022$) and (HR = 24.01, 95% CI = 1.34–417.20, $P = 0.029$). However, the effect size of CKD hazard ratio seemed to diverge with a wide range of confidence intervals; a significant difference was not demonstrated ($P = 0.340$) (Table 4).

Receiving beta-blockers was shown as a nonprotective indicator as well as demonstrating no prognostic value in the nonvaccination group, but it was shown as a potential

The Modification Effect of Influenza Vaccine on Prognostic Indicators for Cardiovascular Events after...

95

TABLE 3: Multivariable hazard ratios stratified by influenza vaccination for each cardiovascular event, which was analyzed by multivariable stratified Cox's regression analysis.

Prognostic indicators	No vaccination		Influenza vaccination	
	HR (95% CI)	P value	HR (95% CI)	P value
MACEs				
LVEF (%)				
≤40	2.07 (1.12–3.82)	0.021	2.37 (1.01–5.59)	0.048
Medication				
ACE-I/ARB	0.44 (0.23–0.83)	0.012	1.12 (0.45–2.78)	0.806
Death				
Age (year)				
>65	10.78 (1.39–83.62)	0.023	2.28 (0.42–12.48)	0.341
Medication				
ACE-I/ARB	0.26 (0.07–0.94)	0.041	1.15 (0.21–6.30)	0.870
Composite hospitalization due to ACS, HF, or stroke				
LVEF (%)				
≤40	2.25 (1.14–4.45)	0.020	2.16 (0.81–5.76)	0.124
Medication				
ACE-I/ARB	0.48 (0.24–0.99)	0.046	1.23 (0.43–3.54)	0.701
Hospitalization due to ACS				
No indicator was found				
Hospitalization due to HF				
CKD	5.12 (1.27–20.65)	0.022	24.01 (1.38–417.20)	0.029
LVEF (%)				
≤40	7.93 (1.63–38.66)	0.010	8.37 (0.72–97.72)	0.090
Medication				
Beta-blocker	1.63 (0.34–7.78)	0.542	0.05 (0.003–0.76)	0.037

MACEs, major adverse cardiovascular events; LVEF, left ventricular ejection fraction; ACE-I, angiotensin-converting enzyme inhibitor; ARB, angiotensin II receptor blocker; ACS, acute coronary syndrome; HF, heart failure; CKD, chronic kidney disease.

protective indicator in the vaccination group (HR = 0.05, 95% CI = 0.003–0.76, P = 0.037) (Table 3). Moreover, the comparison of hazard ratio between vaccination groups indicated a remarkable difference (P = 0.03) (Table 4).

In summary, the influenza vaccination influenced the prognostic value of clinical predictors for each cardiovascular outcome when compared with nonvaccination group, except two predictors of impaired LVEF for MACEs (HR = 2.07, 95% CI = 1.12–3.82, P = 0.021 and HR = 2.37, 95% CI = 1.01–5.59, P = 0.048) and CKD for hospitalization due to HF (HR = 5.12, 95% CI = 1.27–20.65, P = 0.022 and HR = 24.01, 95% CI = 1.34–417.20, P = 0.029). However, no significant difference

was observed of hazard ratios between influenza vaccination groups, but receiving beta-blockers revealed the differences (P = 0.030) (Table 4).

Multivariable Cox's regression (Table 5) demonstrated that influenza vaccination and beta-blockers coadministration indicated a potential protective effect (HR = 0.05, 95% CI = 0.004–0.71, P = 0.027) after adjusting for sex, dyslipidemia, CKD, SCr, and LVEF, but both factors were independent prognostic indicators for hospitalization due to HF.

The interaction of influenza vaccination among patients receiving beta-blockers was described by a significant reduction of the hazard ratio among patients who had vaccination.

TABLE 4: Discrimination of multivariable hazard ratios by the influenza vaccination for each cardiovascular event.

Prognostic indicators	No vaccination HR (95% CI)	Influenza vaccination HR (95% CI)	Z	P value
MACEs				
LVEF (%)				
≤40	2.07 (1.12–3.82)	2.37 (1.01–5.59)	−0.26	0.797
Medication				
ACE-I/ARB	0.44 (0.23–0.83)	1.12 (0.45–2.78)	−1.65	0.098
Death				
Age (year)				
>65	10.78 (1.39–83.62)	2.28 (0.42–12.48)	1.14	0.252
Medication				
ACE-I/ARB	0.26 (0.07–0.94)	1.15 (0.21–6.30)	−1.38	0.169
Composite hospitalization due to ACS, HF, or stroke				
LVEF (%)				
≤40	2.25 (1.14–4.45)	2.16 (0.81–5.76)	0.07	0.948
Medication				
ACE-I/ARB	0.48 (0.24–0.99)	1.23 (0.43–3.54)	−1.43	0.152
Hospitalization due to ACS				
No indicator was found				
Hospitalization due to HF				
CKD	5.12 (1.27–20.65)	24.01 (1.38–417.20)	−0.95	0.340
LVEF (%)				
≤40	7.93 (1.63–38.66)	8.37 (0.72–97.72)	−0.04	0.971
Medication				
Beta-blocker	1.63 (0.34–7.78)	0.05 (0.003–0.76)	2.18	0.030

MACEs, major adverse cardiovascular events; LVEF, left ventricular ejection fraction; ACE-I, angiotensin-converting enzyme inhibitor; ARB, angiotensin II receptor blocker; ACS, acute coronary syndrome; HF, heart failure; CKD, chronic kidney disease.

TABLE 5: Multivariable hazard ratios and 95% confidence intervals of influenza vaccination and beta-blocker for hospitalization due to HF.

Influenza vaccine	Beta-blocker	HR	95% CI	P value
No	No	Reference		
No	Yes	1.29	0.27–6.16	0.750
Yes	No	2.46	0.40–15.22	0.334
Yes	Yes	0.05	0.01–0.71	0.027

Note. All analyses were adjusted for gender, dyslipidemia, SCr, and LVEF, which are independent prognostic indicators for hospitalization due to HF.

This protective interaction showed benefits of receiving influenza vaccination with beta-blocker for hospitalization due to HF among ACS patients.

4. Discussion

This post hoc study demonstrated that the significant prognostic indicators for cardiovascular events in patients with ACS were age, LVEF, CKD, and receiving ACE-I/ARB. Even though the hazard ratio of each individual prognostic factor may differ between the vaccination and nonvaccination groups, the difference was not significant, except for receiving beta-blockers. Receiving beta-blockers presented the prognostic indicator for the reduction of hospitalization due to HF when influenza vaccine was given.

The evidence from seasonal patterns of cardiovascular deaths was similar to patterns of influenza circulation [29]. Clinical findings among patients with influenza presented systemic effects such as myalgia, high fever, and fatigue, as well as frequent myocardial involvement [29]. The influenza virus has extensive effects on the inflammatory and coagulation pathways, leading to destabilization of vulnerable atherosclerotic plaques and coronary occlusion, which are major causes of acute MI [29]. Moreover, host response to acute infections can facilitate ACS by affecting coronary arteries and atherosclerotic lesions, such as increased sympathetic activity [28].

The upregulated sympathetic nervous system shown in heart failure [18] may reduce the influenza vaccine response [31–33] or cause persistence decline of antibody titers [32].

The sympathetic nervous system will increase proinflammatory cytokines and exacerbate influenza infection, as shown in animal models [34]. In the lung of infected animals, the anti-influenza CD8+ T cell response could be limited by sympathetic nervous system [35], while cytotoxic T lymphocytes could effectively respond to different subtypes of influenza A virus with a specific antibody response [36]. Cytotoxic T cells were described as important factors for recovering from influenza infection in humans [36].

Human T and B lymphocytes express beta-2 adrenergic receptors, where the catecholamine effect via beta-2 adrenergic receptors on cytokine regulation decreased responses to vaccines [37]. In contrast, T cell responses were enhanced by the administration of beta-2 adrenergic antagonists [35].

The study in mice showed that acute stress reduced the number of NK cells in the intraparenchymal region of the lungs and this event could be reversed by the administration of beta-adrenergic antagonists [38]. Acute stress can be hypothesized as the cause of lung lymphocyte redistribution through beta-adrenergic stimulation by elevating catecholamine level [38]. Therefore, beta-blockers could reduce the inflammatory response and the degree of lung injury. Some animal models revealed survival benefits, particularly when beta-blockers were administered before the septic insult [39].

Beta-blockers are recommended as a secondary prevention for ACS patients recovering from acute MI and without contraindication [40]. ACS was indicated as an important cause of worsening or new-onset of HF and also a common factor precipitating acute decompensated HF [18]. Consequently, prescribing beta-blockers to chronic HF patients is recommended due to their protective results [18, 41].

The decrease in heart rate, contractility, and blood pressure due to beta-blockers could inhibit the effects of circulating catecholamines and oxygen demand [42]. Beta-blockers can reduce the sympathetic tone by inhibiting an increase in catecholamine circulation [43], as a cause of proinflammatory cytokines [34, 43] and disrupt the immune response [43].

Moreover, the administration of influenza vaccine can prevent influenza infection and also reduce acute infection effects by promoting inflammation, the progression of atherosclerosis, and triggering acute MI [9–15, 17].

In this study, solely administration of beta-blockers or influenza vaccination was not shown to be the protective evidence for hospitalization due to HF among ACS patients. However, the combination of the two showed very synergistic effect during a year of follow-up time.

4.1. Limitation. Incomplete data was a limitation of this study. Only 2 incomplete variables were found from 20 variables. The variables of SCr and LVEF had 6.83% and 54.67% of missing values, respectively. However, multiple imputations were conducted and imputed data were categorized for appropriate data management.

5. Conclusion

The study showed that influenza vaccination influenced the prognostic abilities of clinical predictors for cardiovascular outcomes when compared between patients who received vaccination and the nonvaccination group. However, two predictors of impaired LVEF for MACEs and CKD for hospitalization due to HF were not affected. Moreover, different prognostic ability between influenza vaccination groups was not significantly observed, but receiving beta-blockers was acknowledged.

This study presented the strong modification effect of influenza vaccine among ACS patients who received beta-blockers to reduce hospitalization due to HF. This benefit of influenza vaccination should be noteworthily considered in clinical practice for ACS patients. However, further studies of influenza vaccine and beta-blocker synergy should be established in a larger population involving clinical trials.

Although, this study disclosed a new benefit of influenza vaccine and beta-blockers coadministration in preventing HF hospitalization, a further study involving influenza vaccine among HF patients is strongly recommended.

Competing Interests

The authors declare no competing interests in this work.

References

[1] B. C. G. Voordouw, P. D. van der Linden, S. Simonian, J. van der Lei, M. C. J. M. Sturkenboom, and B. H. C. Stricker, "Influenza vaccination in community-dwelling elderly," *Archives of Internal Medicine*, vol. 163, no. 9, pp. 1089–1094, 2003.

[2] R. Praditsuwan, P. Assantachai, C. Wasi, P. Puthavatana, and U. Kositanont, "The efficacy and effectiveness of influenza vaccination among Thai elderly persons living in the community," *Journal of the Medical Association of Thailand*, vol. 88, no. 2, pp. 256–264, 2005.

[3] T. Jefferson, D. Rivetti, A. Rivetti, M. Rudin, C. Di Pietrantonj, and V. Demicheli, "Efficacy and effectiveness of influenza vaccines in elderly people: a systematic review," *The Lancet*, vol. 366, no. 9492, pp. 1165–1174, 2005.

[4] J. Nordin, J. Mullooly, S. Poblete et al., "Influenza vaccine effectiveness in preventing hospitalizations and deaths in persons 65 years or older in Minnesota, New York, and Oregon: data from 3 health plans," *Journal of Infectious Diseases*, vol. 184, no. 6, pp. 665–670, 2001.

[5] T. Jefferson, C. Di Pietrantonj, L. A. Al-Ansary, E. Ferroni, S. Thorning, and R. E. Thomas, "Vaccines for preventing influenza in the elderly," *Cochrane Database of Systematic Reviews*, no. 2, Article ID CD004876, 2010.

[6] K. L. Nichol, J. D. Nordin, D. B. Nelson, J. P. Mullooly, and E. Hak, "Effectiveness of influenza vaccine in the community-dwelling elderly," *The New England Journal of Medicine*, vol. 357, no. 14, pp. 1373–1381, 2007.

[7] K. L. Nichol, J. Nordin, J. Mullooly, R. Lask, K. Fillbrandt, and M. Iwane, "Influenza vaccination and reduction in hospitalizations for cardiac disease and stroke among the elderly," *The New England Journal of Medicine*, vol. 348, no. 14, pp. 1322–1332, 2003.

[8] A. Vila-Córcoles, T. Rodriguez, C. de Diego et al., "Effect of influenza vaccine status on winter mortality in Spanish community-dwelling elderly people during 2002–2005 influenza periods," *Vaccine*, vol. 25, no. 37-38, pp. 6699–6707, 2007.

[9] A. Phrommintikul, S. Kuanprasert, W. Wongcharoen, R. Kanjanavanit, R. Chaiwarith, and A. Sukonthasarn, "Influenza vaccination reduces cardiovascular events in patients with acute coronary syndrome," *European Heart Journal*, vol. 32, no. 14, pp. 1730–1735, 2011.

[10] J. A. Udell, R. Zawi, D. L. Bhatt et al., "Association between influenza vaccination and cardiovascular outcomes in high-risk patients: a meta-analysis," *The Journal of the American Medical Association*, vol. 310, no. 16, pp. 1711–1720, 2013.

[11] E. P. Gurfinkel, R. L. De La Fuente, O. Mendiz, and B. Mautner, "Influenza vaccine pilot study in acute coronary syndromes and planned percutaneous coronary interventions: the FLU Vaccination Acute Coronary Syndromes (FLUVACS) study," *Circulation*, vol. 105, no. 18, pp. 2143–2147, 2002.

[12] E. Gurfinkel, "Flu vaccination in acute coronary syndromes and planned percutaneous coronary interventions (FLUVACS) Study One-year follow-up," *European Heart Journal*, vol. 25, no. 1, pp. 25–31, 2004.

[13] A. Ciszewski, Z. T. Bilinska, L. B. Brydak et al., "Influenza vaccination in secondary prevention from coronary ischaemic events in coronary artery disease: FLUCAD study," *European Heart Journal*, vol. 29, no. 11, pp. 1350–1358, 2008.

[14] M. M. Davis, K. Taubert, A. L. Benin et al., "Influenza vaccination as secondary prevention for cardiovascular disease: a science advisory from the American Heart Association/American College of Cardiology," *Journal of the American College of Cardiology*, vol. 48, no. 7, pp. 1498–1502, 2006.

[15] S. C. Smith, E. J. Benjamin, R. O. Bonow et al., "AHA/ACCF secondary prevention and risk reduction therapy for patients with coronary and other atherosclerotic vascular disease: 2011 update: a guideline from the American Heart Association and American College of Cardiology Foundation," *Circulation*, vol. 124, no. 22, pp. 2458–2473, 2011.

[16] P. T. O'Gara, F. G. Kushner, D. D. Ascheim et al., "2013 ACCF/AHA guideline for the management of ST-elevation myocardial infarction: a report of the American College of Cardiology Foundation/American Heart Association Task Force on Practice Guidelines," *Journal of the American College of Cardiology*, vol. 61, no. 4, pp. e78–e140, 2013.

[17] R. S. Wright, J. L. Anderson, C. D. Adams et al., "2012 ACCF/AHA focused update incorporated into the ACC/AHA 2007 guidelines for the management of patients with unstable Angina/Non–ST-elevation myocardial infarction," *Journal of the American College of Cardiology*, vol. 61, no. 23, pp. e179–e347, 2013.

[18] C. W. Yancy, M. Jessup, B. Bozkurt et al., "2013 ACCF/AHA guideline for the management of heart failure: a report of the american college of cardiology foundation/american heart association task force on practice guidelines," *Journal of the American College of Cardiology*, vol. 62, no. 16, pp. e147–e239, 2013.

[19] J. Scharpé, W. E. Peetermans, J. Vanwalleghem et al., "Immunogenicity of a standard trivalent influenza vaccine in patients on long-term hemodialysis: an open-label trial," *American Journal of Kidney Diseases*, vol. 54, no. 1, pp. 77–85, 2009.

[20] K. A. Birdwell, M. R. Ikizler, E. C. Sannella et al., "Decreased antibody response to influenza vaccination in kidney transplant recipients: a prospective cohort study," *American Journal of Kidney Diseases*, vol. 54, no. 1, pp. 112–121, 2009.

[21] M. J. C. Salles, Y. A. S. Sens, L. S. V. Boas, and C. M. Machado, "Influenza virus vaccination in kidney transplant recipients: serum antibody response to different immunosuppressive drugs," *Clinical Transplantation*, vol. 24, no. 1, pp. E17–E23, 2010.

[22] C. Cavdar, M. Sayan, A. Sifil et al., "The comparison of antibody response to influenza vaccination in continuous ambulatory peritoneal dialysis, hemodialysis and renal transplantation patients," *Scandinavian Journal of Urology and Nephrology*, vol. 37, no. 1, pp. 71–76, 2003.

[23] A. Dvorakova and R. Poledne, "Influenza—a trigger for acute myocardial infarction," *Atherosclerosis*, vol. 172, no. 2, p. 391, 2004.

[24] M. Madjid, M. Naghavi, S. Litovsky, and S. W. Casscells, "Influenza and cardiovascular disease: a new opportunity for prevention and the need for further studies," *Circulation*, vol. 108, no. 22, pp. 2730–2736, 2003.

[25] M. Naghavi, P. Wyde, S. Litovsky et al., "Influenza infection exerts prominent inflammatory and thrombotic effects on the atherosclerotic plaques of apolipoprotein E-deficient mice," *Circulation*, vol. 107, no. 5, pp. 762–768, 2003.

[26] S. E. Epstein, J. Zhu, A. H. Najafi, and M. S. Burnett, "Insights into the role of infection in atherogenesis and in plaque rupture," *Circulation*, vol. 119, no. 24, pp. 3133–3141, 2009.

[27] M. Haidari, P. R. Wyde, S. Litovsky et al., "Influenza virus directly infects, inflames, and resides in the arteries of atherosclerotic and normal mice," *Atherosclerosis*, vol. 208, no. 1, pp. 90–96, 2010.

[28] V. F. Corrales-Medina, M. Madjid, and D. M. Musher, "Role of acute infection in triggering acute coronary syndromes," *The Lancet Infectious Diseases*, vol. 10, no. 2, pp. 83–92, 2010.

[29] C. Warren-Gash, L. Smeeth, and A. C. Hayward, "Influenza as a trigger for acute myocardial infarction or death from cardiovascular disease: a systematic review," *The Lancet Infectious Diseases*, vol. 9, no. 10, pp. 601–610, 2009.

[30] R. Brame, P. Mazerolle, and A. Piquero, "Using the correct statistical test for the equality of regression coefficients," *Criminology*, vol. 36, no. 4, pp. 859–866, 1998.

[31] O. Vardeny, J. J. M. Moran, N. K. Sweitzer, M. R. Johnson, and M. S. Hayney, "Decreased T-cell responses to influenza vaccination in patients with heart failure," *Pharmacotherapy*, vol. 30, no. 1, pp. 10–16, 2010.

[32] C. M. Albrecht, N. K. Sweitzer, M. R. Johnson, and O. Vardeny, "Lack of persistence of influenza vaccine antibody titers in patients with heart failure," *Journal of Cardiac Failure*, vol. 20, no. 2, pp. 105–109, 2014.

[33] O. Vardeny, N. K. Sweitzer, M. A. Detry, J. M. Moran, M. R. Johnson, and M. S. Hayney, "Decreased immune responses to influenza vaccination in patients with heart failure," *Journal of Cardiac Failure*, vol. 15, no. 4, pp. 368–373, 2009.

[34] K. M. K. Grebe, K. Takeda, H. D. Hickman et al., "Cutting edge: sympathetic nervous system increases proinflammatory cytokines and exacerbates influenza A virus pathogenesis," *Journal of Immunology*, vol. 184, no. 2, pp. 540–544, 2010.

[35] K. M. Grebe, H. D. Hickman, K. R. Irvine, K. Takeda, J. R. Bennink, and J. W. Yewdell, "Sympathetic nervous system control of anti-influenza CD8$^+$ T cell responses," *Proceedings of the National Academy of Sciences of the United States of America*, vol. 106, no. 13, pp. 5300–5305, 2009.

[36] A. J. McMichael, F. M. Gotch, G. R. Noble, and P. A. S. Beare, "Cytotoxic T-cell immunity to influenza," *The New England Journal of Medicine*, vol. 309, no. 1, pp. 13–17, 1983.

[37] M. Montminy, "Transcriptional regulation by cyclic AMP," *Annual Review of Biochemistry*, vol. 66, pp. 807–822, 1997.

[38] O. Kanemi, X. Zhang, Y. Sakamoto, M. Ebina, and R. Nagatomi, "Acute stress reduces intraparenchymal lung natural killer cells via beta-adrenergic stimulation," *Clinical and Experimental Immunology*, vol. 139, no. 1, pp. 25–34, 2005.

[39] A. Rudiger, "Beta-block the septic heart," *Critical Care Medicine*, vol. 38, no. 10, pp. S608–S612, 2010.

[40] J. López-Sendón, K. Swedberg, and J. McMurray, "Expert consensus document on beta-adrenergic receptor blockers," *European Heart Journal*, vol. 25, no. 15, pp. 1341–1362, 2004.

[41] J. J. V. McMurray, S. Adamopoulos, S. D. Anker et al., "ESC Guidelines for the diagnosis and treatment of acute and chronic heart failure 2012: the Task Force for the Diagnosis and Treatment of Acute and Chronic Heart Failure 2012 of the European Society of Cardiology. Developed in collaboration with the Heart Failure Association (HFA) of the ESC," *European Heart Journal*, vol. 33, no. 14, pp. 1787–1847, 2012.

[42] C. W. Hamm, J.-P. Bassand, S. Agewall et al., "ESC Guidelines for the management of acute coronary syndromes in patients presenting without persistent ST-segment elevation: the Task Force for the management of Acute Coronary Syndromes (ACS) in patients presenting without persistent ST-segment elevatio," *European Heart Journal*, vol. 32, no. 23, pp. 2999–3054, 2011.

[43] I. J. Elenkov, R. L. Wilder, G. P. Chrousos, and E. S. Vizi, "The sympathetic nerve—an integrative interface between two super-systems: the brain and the immune system," *Pharmacological Reviews*, vol. 52, no. 4, pp. 595–638, 2000.

14

RyR2 QQ2958 Genotype and Risk of Malignant Ventricular Arrhythmias

Francesca Galati,[1] **Antonio Galati,**[2] **and Serafina Massari**[1]

[1]*Department of Biological and Environmental Sciences and Technologies, University of Salento, 73100 Lecce, Italy*
[2]*Department of Cardiology, "Card. G. Panico" Hospital, Tricase, 73039 Lecce, Italy*

Correspondence should be addressed to Francesca Galati; francesca.galati.82@gmail.com

Academic Editor: Kai Hu

Ventricular arrhythmias are one of the most common causes of death in developed countries. The use of implantable cardiac defibrillators is the most effective treatment to prevent sudden cardiac death. To date, the ejection fraction is the only approved clinical variable used to determine suitability for defibrillator placement in subjects with heart failure. The purpose of this study was to assess whether genetic polymorphisms found in the ryanodine receptor type 2 (Q2958R) and histidine-rich calcium-binding protein (S96A) might serve as markers for arrhythmias. Genotyping was performed in 235 patients treated with defibrillator for primary and secondary prevention of arrhythmias. No significant association was found between the S96A polymorphism and arrhythmia onset, whereas the QQ2958 genotype in the ryanodine receptor gene was correlated with an increased risk of life-threatening arrhythmias. Concurrent stressor conditions, such as hypertension, seem to increase this effect. Our findings might help to better identify patients who could benefit from defibrillator implantation.

1. Introduction

Sudden cardiac death (SCD) is one of the most frequent causes of death in industrialized countries. SCD is commonly the result of ventricular tachycardia (VT) and/or ventricular fibrillation (VF) that occur secondary to a complex interplay between a susceptible myocardial substrate typically affected by cardiomyopathy and a transient trigger. The use of implantable cardioverter-defibrillator (ICD) is the most effective treatment to prevent this disease, because it may terminate the arrhythmia by low-voltage antitachycardia pacing or high-energy cardioversion. However, only a minority of patients benefit from these devices, because the majority of patients with an ICD have never received a shock appropriate for VT or VF. Furthermore, a substantial number of patients, who die suddenly, are not identified as high risk prior to death and do not receive an ICD implantation [1]. Although numerous clinical and serum biomarkers have been investigated for use in the risk stratification of SCD [2], the ejection fraction (EF) remains the only approved clinical variable that is used to determine suitability for ICD placement in subjects

with heart failure (HF). As a result, there is a substantial interest in identifying more reliable predictors that could help to discriminate which patients are most likely to benefit from an ICD implant. The identification of genetic alterations responsible for rare hereditary arrhythmic diseases, such as Brugada syndrome, long QT, and catecholaminergic polymorphic ventricular tachycardia (CPVT), has focused the attention on the molecular basis of arrhythmias, particularly on the role of the calcium channels and associated proteins. The ryanodine receptor type 2 (RyR2), which is expressed primarily in cardiac muscle [3], is one of the three isoforms of the family of ryanodine receptors that regulate the duration and amplitude of the Ca^{2+} flow from the sarcoplasmic reticulum (SR). It is well known that aberrant diastolic Ca^{2+} release via RyR2 leads to contractile dysfunction by reducing the SR Ca^{2+} content. This provides a substrate for delayed after depolarisation (DAD), which ultimately leads to lethal arrhythmias [4]. Recently, Ran et al. [5] found that the G1886S variant (rs3766871) of the *RyR2* gene was associated with an increased risk of ventricular arrhythmias and sudden cardiac death. The histidine-rich Ca-binding protein (HRC), expressed predominantly in striated muscle, is another SR component involved in the regulation of the Ca^{2+} uptake [6, 7], accumulation [8], and release from the sarcoplasmic reticulum [7, 9]. As reported in previous studies [10–12], ion channels polymorphisms have the potential to modify the clinical phenotype. These findings suggested the idea that also polymorphisms in RyR2 and HRC genes might have the same potential, thus representing an important factor in determining the risk of arrhythmia in HF patients who could benefit from an ICD implantation. The most common RyR2 polymorphism is RyR2-Q2958R (rs34967813, A/G), described for the first time by Tiso et al. [13], with a heterozygous prevalence of 34% in Caucasians and 10% in African Americans. It is localized within the area of interaction with the RyR2 modulator [14] and has remained highly conserved during the evolution of the ryanodine receptors [14–17]. Therefore, it will be of interest to study the functional consequences of this variation. HRC is known as an effective regulator of RyR2 activity and SR Ca^{2+} release. A genetic variant of HRC, Ser96Ala (rs3745297, G/T), disrupts the Ca^{2+} microdomain around the RyR2, as it alters the Ca^{2+} dependent association of RyR2 and HRC [18] and may enhance RyR2 activity from the SR luminal side, increasing uncontrolled Ca^{2+} release and induced Ca^{2+} instability. Arvanitis et al. [19] identified an association between HRC-S96A and malignant ventricular arrhythmias in patients with idiopathic dilated cardiomyopathy. In this study, we investigated whether these two polymorphisms (RyR2-Q2958R and HRC-S96A) are associated with the occurrence of spontaneous ventricular arrhythmias in patients receiving an ICD for primary and secondary prevention of SCD.

2. Materials and Methods

2.1. Patients and Procedures. We enrolled 235 unrelated Caucasian patients, from Salento (Southern Italy), who were consecutively admitted between January 2009 and September 2012 at the Department of Cardiology of Hospital "Card. G. Panico," and treated with an ICD, according to class I or class II indications of ACC/AHA/HRS guidelines [20, 21]. Patients with long QT syndrome, Brugada syndrome, or CPVT were excluded from the study. 157 subjects (66.8%) had an ICD implantation for primary prevention and 78 patients (33.2%) for secondary prevention. Reversible causes of ventricular arrhythmias, such as acute ischemia, electrolyte abnormalities, and QT prolonging medication use, were ruled out. During a mean follow-up time of 44 ± 13 months, 23 patients of the 157 experienced at least one episode of ventricular arrhythmia and they formed group I with the 78 patients of the secondary prevention. The remaining 134 patients of the 157, who did not develop ventricular arrhythmias, formed group II. Ventricular tachycardia was defined by the following characteristics: (i) a regular wide QRS complex (>120 milliseconds) tachycardia at a rate of more than 100 beats per minute and with a uniform and stable QRS morphology of the consecutive beats and (ii) the arrhythmia lasting ≥30 seconds or causing hemodynamic collapse in <30 seconds.

Demographic, clinical, and routine laboratory data were collected from all patients using a structured data form. Before implantation, a transthoracic echocardiogram and a coronary angiography were performed for all patients.

The presence of ischemic heart disease was defined as prior myocardial infarction and/or angina with hospitalization and/or an infarct and/or major ischemia patterns on electrocardiogram or angiographically documented coronary artery disease (>50% stenosis in ≥1 coronary artery). Dilated cardiomyopathy was defined as enlargement of the heart cavity and systolic dysfunction of one or both ventricles in the absence of congenital, coronary, hypertensive, valvular, or pericardial heart disease. The diagnostic criteria included the identification of an ejection fraction (EF) ≤35% and/or a fractional shortening <25%, in association with a left ventricular (LV) end-diastolic dimension >112% of the predicted value corrected for age and body surface area. LV ejection fraction was categorized as ≤35% or >35% according to the ACC/AHA/HRS guidelines [20] for ICD implantation. Patients were divided into the four NYHA (New York Heart Association) classes, based on how much they were limited during physical activity.

Hypertension was defined as a systolic blood pressure ≥140 mmHg or a diastolic blood pressure ≥90 mmHg or the use of antihypertensive medications. Diabetes was defined as a fasting plasma glucose level >7.0 mmol/L or a nonfasting plasma glucose level >11.1 mmol/L or the use of antidiabetic medications. Dyslipidemia was defined as elevated total (>240 mg/dL) or low-density lipoprotein (LDL >130 mg/dL) cholesterol levels or low levels of high-density lipoprotein cholesterol (HDL <40 mg/dL) or elevated triglycerides levels (>150 mg/dL). Smoking was categorized as nonsmoking or current smoking (currently smoking or stopped <1 year ago).

All patients had an ICD with a VT and VF programming which allowed the analysis of stored intracardiac electrograms and/or RR-intervals of ventricular tachyarrhythmias with a cycle length (CL) ≤330 ms. ICDs employed a stepwise analysis of morphology, rate, stability, atrioventricular association, and onset (ventricular acceleration, atrial acceleration or nonacceleration). All patients were followed up in our outpatient clinic at six-month intervals.

100 healthy subjects from the same population were also enrolled. We ruled out any disease by studying patients' medical history, by performing a physical examination, or by performing an echocardiogram and a chest radiograph.

The study was approved by the local ethics committee and conducted in accordance with the guidelines of the declaration of Helsinki. Informed consent was obtained from all subjects prior to participation.

2.2. DNA Analysis. DNA extraction was carried out on total blood using Archive Pure DNA Blood Kit (5-PRIME, Hamburg, Germany) according to the manufacturer's recommended protocol.

We genotyped our patients for the following two variants:

(i) *RyR2* Q2958R (rs34967813, A/G), involving a substitution of adenine with guanine within exon 61, which results in the substitution of arginine for glutamine;

TABLE 1: Primers sequences, annealing temperatures, and fragment size.

Gene	SNP	Allele	Primer sequence $5' \rightarrow 3'$	Fragment size (bp)	T_a
RyR2	Q2958R (A>G)	A	_Upper:_ GGAGAACATTTCCCTTATGA<u>C</u>CA _Lower:_ GCAGGACTAAGGTCCCACAA	476	60°C
		G	_Upper:_ GAGAACATTTCCCTTATGA<u>C</u>CG _Lower:_ GCAGGACTAAGGTCCCACAA	476	60°C
HRC	S96A (G>T)	G	_Upper:_ AAGGAGGATGAAGATG<u>C</u>CG _Lower:_ TCCTCTTCCTCCTCCTCCTC	347	62°C
		T	_Upper:_ AAAAGGAGGATGAAGATG<u>C</u>CT _Lower:_ TCCTCTTCCTCCTCCTCCTC	347	62°C

Bold letters in primer sequences highlight the allele-specific nucleotide, while underlined letters highlight mismatch nucleotide.

(ii) _HRC_ S96A (rs3745297, G/T), involving a substitution of guanine with thymine within exon 1, which results in the substitution of alanine for serine.

The DNA polymorphism analyses were performed using AS-PCR. The primers were designed with the Primer3 software [22]. Primer sequences, annealing temperature, and amplification product sizes are shown in Table 1. PCR amplifications were carried out in a total reaction volume of 25 μL, with each reaction containing 100 ng of gDNA, 5 pmol of each primer, 10 mM dNTPs, 2.5 U Taq 5-Prime Eppendorf (5-PRIME, Hamburg, Germany), and 1x reaction buffer. The reaction cycle conditions consisted of an initial denaturation step at 94°C for 5 min, followed by 35 cycles of 30 s denaturation at 94°C, 30 s annealing at varying temperatures (see Table 1 for specific annealing temperatures), and 30 s extension at 68°C, with a final extension at 68°C for 5 min.

Allele-specific primers were constructed by introducing a one-base mismatch sequence before the SNP site. After agarose-gel electrophoresis, the PCR product was visualized with ethidium bromide, photographed, and genotyped.

Due to deviation from Hardy-Weinberg equilibrium (HWE), to exclude genotyping errors, all genomic DNAs genotyped for _RyR2_ Q2958R were subjected to direct sequencing. Primers used for direct sequencing were CTACA-GATGGTGGCAGCAGA (upper primer) and GCAGGAC-TAAGGTCCCACAA (lower primer).

2.3. Statistical Analysis. Continuous data are expressed as the mean ± standard deviation; categorical data are expressed as a percentage. A goodness of fit test for normality and a Brown-Forsythe or Levene test for homogeneity of variances were used to assess the applicability of parametric tests. Differences between mean data were compared by Student's t-test for the normally distributed continuous variables or by the Mann-Whitney test for nonnormally distributed variables. Differences in genotype frequencies and other categorical data between cases and controls were compared with Fisher's exact test (mid-p exact p value) and, in Hardy-Weinberg disequilibrium (HWD), with Armitage trend test. The consistency of the genotype frequencies with the HWE was tested using a chi-squared goodness-of-fit test on a contingency table of observed versus expected genotypic frequencies in cases and controls. Post hoc evaluations, where necessary, were performed by means of the Bonferroni correction. The MedCalc Statistical Software version 13.3 (MedCalc Software bvba,

Ostend, Belgium; http://www.medcalc.org; 2014) was used for the multivariate logistic regression analysis. A two-sided p value <0.05 was considered significant for all tests.

3. Results

Table 2 provides a summary of the characteristics of our study population. Overall, 83 (35.3%) patients had idiopathic dilated cardiomyopathy (IDCM), 108 (46.0%) patients had dilated ischemic heart disease (IHD), 29 (12.3%) patients exhibited nondilated IHD, and 15 (6.4%) patients had other heart diseases (HDs). Of the total patients in our study, simultaneous cardiac resynchronization therapy was used in 64 (27.2%) patients, 18 (17.8%) in group I and 46 (34.3%) in group II.

Although more male patients were included in group I than in group II, no other significant differences were observed between the two groups with regard to demographic data. With respect to HF aetiology, the difference in the distribution of cardiac pathologies was due to the different ACC/AHA/HRS guidelines indications (in nondilated IHD, an ICD is implanted only for secondary prevention, while in dilated cardiomyopathy, it is indicated in primary prevention). Comparable values for the clinical (NYHA classification) and echocardiographic (EF and ventricular size) prognostic markers were obtained in both groups. Over 45.5% of the total population was hypertensive, 38.3% was diabetic and 40.8% was dyslipidemic; however, hypertension, diabetes, and dyslipidemia were distributed in a uniform manner between the two groups (49.5% versus 42.5%, 39.6% versus 37.3%, and 41.6% versus 40.3%, resp.). Atrial fibrillation was present in 19.1% of our patients and was equally distributed between the two groups (14.9% versus 22.4%; $p = 0.1807$). No significant difference in pharmacological treatment was observed between the groups, with the exception of the antiarrhythmic drug amiodarone, which was taken by 60.4% of patients with VT/VF versus 25.4% of patients in the other group, because it was always given after the first episode of VT/VF documented by the ICD to prevent further arrhythmic episodes and ICD discharge.

No patient was lost to follow-up, during which 2 patients (2.0%) in group I and 2 patients (1.5%) in group II died, all for refractory heart failure. 11 patients (10.9%) in group I and 26 patients (19.4%) in group II were hospitalized for heart failure ($p = 0.1028$).

TABLE 2: Demographic data and clinical features of the study population according to arrhythmias occurrence.

	Total $n = 235$	Group I $n = 101$	Group II $n = 134$	p value
Demographic				
Male sex, n (%)	182 (77.4%)	86 (85.1%)	96 (71.6%)	0.0177
Age (years)	73 ± 8	73 ± 8	73 ± 8	1.0000
BMI (kg/m^2)	27 ± 5	28 ± 5	27 ± 4	0.0887
Current smoking, n (%)	122 (51.5%)	53 (52.5%)	69 (50.7%)	0.5958
HF etiology				
IDCM, n (%)	83 (35.3%)	19 (18.8%)	64 (47.8%)	0.0001
Dilated IHD, n (%)	108 (46.0%)	42 (41.6%)	66 (49.2%)	
Nondilated IHD, n (%)	29 (12.3%)	29 (28.7%)	0 (0%)	
Other HD, n (%)	15 (6.4%)	11 (10.9%)	4 (3.0%)	
CRT, n (%)	64 (27.2%)	18 (17.8%)	46 (34.3%)	0.0051
NYHA class, n (%)				
I	34 (14.5%)	16 (15.8%)	18 (13.4%)	0.4548
II	106 (45.1%)	50 (49.5%)	56 (41.8%)	
III	92 (39.1%)	34 (33.7%)	58 (43.3%)	
IV	3 (1.3%)	1 (1%)	2 (1.5%)	
Comorbidities				
Hypertension, n (%)	107 (45.5%)	50 (49.5%)	57 (42.5%)	0.2936
Diabetes, n (%)	90 (38.3%)	40 (39.6%)	50 (37.3%)	0.7866
Dyslipidemia, n (%)	96 (40.8%)	42 (41.6%)	54 (40.3%)	0.8937
Atrial fibrillation, n (%)	45 (19.1%)	15 (14.9%)	30 (22.4%)	0.1807
Echo				
LVEDD, (mm)	59 ± 10	60 ± 12	57 ± 13	0.0716
LVESD, (mm)	47 ± 9	48 ± 8	46 ± 10	0.1002
LVEF, (%)	33 ± 10	32 ± 9	34 ± 11	0.1377
Drug therapy				
Beta-blockers, n (%)	200 (85.1%)	86 (85.1%)	114 (85.1%)	1.0000
ACE-inhibitors or ARB, n (%)	184 (78.3%)	82 (81.2%)	102 (76.1%)	0.4247
Antialdosterone, n (%)	150 (63.8%)	61 (60.3%)	89 (66.4%)	0.4107
Diuretics, n (%)	210 (89.4%)	85 (84.1%)	123 (93.3%)	0.0971
Amiodarone, n (%)	95 (40.4%)	61 (60.4%)	34 (25.4%)	0.0001

ARB: angiotensin receptor blockers; BMI: body mass index; HD: heart disease; HF: heart failure; IDCM: idiopathic dilated cardiomyopathy; IHD: ischemic heart disease; CRT: cardiac resynchronization therapy; LVEDD: left ventricular end-diastolic diameter; LVEF: left ventricular ejection fraction; LVESD: left ventricular end-systolic diameter.

The genotypic distribution of the two polymorphisms in the overall cohort and with respect to arrhythmia occurrence is reported in Table 3.

The genotype distribution of the HRC S96A polymorphism is in HWE in the total population as in the two study groups. Conversely, the genotype distribution of the RyR2 Q2958R variant showed deviation from HWE with a high percentage of heterozygotes in the total population and in the two groups.

However, the RyR2 polymorphism genotypic distribution was not significantly different than that of a control population of 100 healthy subjects recruited within the same medical centre (4% QQ, 94% QR, and RR 2%).

When we compared our group of 101 subjects with ventricular arrhythmias (group I) to 134 patients without documented arrhythmias (group II), we found no significant difference in the distribution of the HRC S96A genotypes between them. Conversely, the distribution of RyR2 Q2958R genotypes was significantly different between the two groups ($p = 0.0040$ with Fisher's exact test and $p = 0.0086$ using Armitage trend test), with a higher percentage of the QQ genotype in group I (13.9%) compared to group II (3.0%). A post hoc analysis with Bonferroni's correction for pairwise comparisons confirmed the significant difference. According to these data, the subjects with the QQ genotype seem to be more susceptible to VT/VF development (RR 1.95; IC 95% 1.45–2.62; $p = 0.0018$).

Multiple logistic regression analysis revealed that the correlation between the QQ genotype and the risk of VT/VF (OR 2.5559; 1.1394 to 5.7334; $p = 0.0228$) is independent from other clinical characteristics such as age, smoking, BMI, hypertension, diabetes, dyslipidemia, and HRC S96A polymorphism (Table 4).

TABLE 3: Genotypic frequency of the two analyzed polymorphisms in the study population and according to arrhythmias occurrence.

	Total	Group I	Group II	p value
RyR2 Q2958R (A>G) (*n* = 235)				
QQ	18 (7.7%)	14 (13.9%)	4 (3.0%)	
QR	213 (90.6%)	85 (84.2%)	128 (95.5%)	0.0040*
RR	4 (1.7%)	2 (1.9%)	2 (1.5%)	
HRC S96A (G>T) (*n* = 235)				
SS	38 (16.2%)	12 (11.9%)	26 (19.4%)	
SA	145 (61.7%)	69 (68.3%)	76 (56.7%)	0.1750
AA	52 (22.1%)	20 (19.8%)	32 (23.9%)	

* with Fisher's exact test, while $p = 0.0086$ using Armitage trend test.

TABLE 4: Multiple logistic regression analysis.

	Odds ratio	95% CI	p value
Age	0.9983	0.9643 to 1.0335	0.9235
BMI	0.9926	0.5558 to 1.7724	0.9799
Diabetes	0.9320	0.5275 to 1.6468	0.8085
Dyslipidemia	0.8714	0.4977 to 1.5257	0.6300
Hypertension	0.7225	0.4106 to 1.2715	0.2597
Smoking	0.9118	0.5100 to 1.6302	0.7554
HRC	0.6929	0.4720 to 1.0173	0.0612
RyR2	2.5559	1.1394 to 5.7334	0.0228

BMI: body mass index.

TABLE 5: Genotypic frequency of *RyR2* Q2958R in the study population subgroups according to arrhythmias occurrence.

	Group I	Group II	p value
Hypertensive patients (*n* = 107)			
QQ	12 (24.0%)	0 (0%)	
QR	37 (74.0%)	56 (98.2%)	0.0001*
RR	1 (2.0%)	1 (1.8%)	
Not hypertensive patients (*n* = 118)			
QQ	2 (4.3%)	3 (4.2%)	
QR	43 (93.5%)	68 (94.4%)	1
RR	1 (2.2%)	1 (1.4%)	
Dyslipidemic patients (*n* = 96)			
QQ	5 (11.9%)	6 (11.1%)	
QR	36 (85.7%)	47 (87.0%)	1
RR	1 (2.4%)	1 (1.9%)	
Not dyslipidemic patients (*n* = 129)			
QQ	4 (7.4%)	3 (4.0%)	
QR	49 (90.8%)	71 (94.7%)	0.6777
RR	1 (1.8%)	1 (1.3%)	
Diabetic patients (*n* = 90)			
QQ	6 (15.0%)	2 (4.0%)	
QR	33 (82.5%)	48 (96.0%)	0.0696
RR	1 (2.5%)	0 (0%)	
Not diabetic patients (*n* = 137)			
QQ	8 (14.3%)	2 (2.5%)	
QR	47 (83.9%)	77 (95.0%)	0.0204
RR	1 (1.8%)	2 (2.5%)	

* with Fisher's exact test, while $p = 0.0004$ using Armitage trend test.

Given the large percentage of hypertensive, dyslipidemic, and diabetic subjects in our cohort, we conducted a stratified association analysis of the genetic variants in the presence or absence of these comorbidities.

Also in the subgroups, Hardy-Weinberg equilibrium was not reached for the *RyR2* Q2958R variant.

The distribution of *RyR2* Q2958R genotypes was not significantly different in dyslipidemic and nondyslipidemic patients between the two groups (Table 5). The same is true in diabetic and nondiabetic individuals, as we believe that the difference apparently emerging is exclusively linked to the low number of patients with diabetes. On the contrary, in hypertensive subjects we found a higher, statistically significant frequency of *RyR2* QQ genotype among VT/VF patients ($p = 0.0001$ with Fisher's exact test and $p = 0.004$ using Armitage trend test), which was associated with an increased risk of malignant ventricular arrhythmias (RR 2.51; IC 95% 1.96–3.23; $p = 0.0001$), whereas in hypertension-free patients the genotypic percentages were the same in the two groups ($p = 1$).

Additionally, in these subgroups, no significant association was observed between the *HRC* S96A genotypes and ventricular arrhythmias (data not shown).

When analyzed by allele status (Table 6), there were no significant differences in baseline clinical characteristics between *RyR2*QQ patients and QR or RR individuals; however, we observed an increase in the percentage of hypertensive subjects in the QQ genotype (66.7%) compared to the other genotypes (43.8%). This analysis indicates that the correlation between the 2958QQ genotype and the history

of sustained VT/VF in our patients is independent of other clinical characteristics.

4. Discussion

In the present study we found that the *RyR2*QQ genotype seems to be associated with a strong trend towards increased

TABLE 6: Clinical characteristics and events stratified according to *RyR2* allele status.

	RyR2 QQ $n = 18$	RyR2 QR + RR $n = 217$	p value
Demographic			
Male sex, n (%)	13 (72.2%)	170 (78.3%)	0.5581
Age (years)	74 ± 7	72 ± 6	0.1811
BMI (kg/m^2)	28 ± 6	28 ± 3	1.0000
Current smoking, n (%)	7 (38.9%)	98 (45.2%)	0.6330
HF etiology			0.6598
IDCM, n (%)	5 (27.8%)	76 (35.0%)	
Dilated IHD, n (%)	8 (44.5%)	100 (46.1%)	
Nondilated IHD, n (%)	3 (16.6%)	28 (12.9%)	
Other HD, n (%)	2 (11.1%)	13 (6.0%)	
NYHA class, n (%)			0.8741
I	3 (16.7%)	30 (13.8%)	
II	9 (50.0%)	98 (45.2%)	
III	6 (33.3%)	86 (39.6%)	
IV	0	3 (1.4%)	
VT/VF, n (%)	14 (77.8%)	87 (40.1%)	0.0025
Comorbidities			
Hypertension, n (%)	12 (66.7%)	95 (43.8%)	0.0837
Diabetes, n (%)	8 (44.4%)	82 (37.8%)	0.6187
Dyslipidemia, n (%)	11 (61.1%)	85 (39.2%)	0.0827
Echo			
LVEDD, (mm)	58 ± 10	61 ± 8	0.1354
LVESD, (mm)	47 ± 8	48 ± 6	0.5093
LVEF (%)	35 ± 10	32 ± 11	0.2643

BMI: body mass index; HD: heart disease; HF: heart failure; IDCM: idiopathic dilated cardiomyopathy; IHD: ischemic heart disease; LVEDD: left ventricular end-diastolic diameter; LVEF: left ventricular ejection fraction; LVESD: left ventricular end-systolic diameter.

susceptibility to life-threatening arrhythmias in patients receiving ICD therapy for primary and secondary prevention. The association was significant in the general population ($p = 0.004$) and was more evident in hypertensive patients ($p = 0.0001$). A marked HWD in the genotypic distribution of Q2958R polymorphism for *RyR2* gene was observed. Moreover, this SNP seems to be an independent risk factor for an increased risk of ventricular arrhythmias, as evidenced by multivariate analysis. Tiso et al. [13] described for the first time the Q2958R polymorphism in *RyR2* gene. As reported in dbSNP (http://www.ncbi.nlm.nih.gov/SNP/), the Q2958 allele frequency was estimated to be 72.1% in the European population (573 subjects) and 64% in the population of North America (120 subjects). In our cohort (335 subjects), the frequency is lowered to 53% with a heterozygous prevalence of 90.6%. Deviation from HWE may be due to biologic or nonbiologic reasons. Genotyping errors are one of the possible sources of HWD, but they are generally small and do not generate sufficient deviations from HWE to be detected. However, to rule out genotyping errors, we reanalyzed this polymorphism by the use of direct sequencing and in all cases sequencing data were consistent with AS-PCR results. To exclude a selection bias (population stratification) due to our inclusion and exclusion criteria, we enrolled and genotyped 100 healthy subjects, obtaining the same genotype distribution.

Another possible cause of deviation from HWE could be a differential survival of subjects with different genotypes: while the newborns of a population may be in HWE, the elderly individuals deviate from HWE. So we think that the prevalence of heterozygosity could be explained by a relatively benign effect of the QR condition on RyR2 channel function. However, this advantage is lacking in the homozygous QQ, becoming risk-conferring in the setting of imposed stress load due to hypertension.

In recent reports, it has been shown that defective interdomain interaction between the IP-domain (putative partner domain of I-domain, which remains to be identified) and the I-domain (amino acids 3722–4610) causes various proarrhythmic states, such as increased frequency of spontaneous Ca^{2+} sparks and the appearance of DAD [23]. We hypothesize that the presence of glutamic acid in position 2958 could weaken the IP-domain/I-domain interaction, keeping RyR2 in a slightly less closed form, resulting in greater Ca^{2+} release. In this context, stress factors such as hypertension can amplify the phenotypic effects of the Q2958 allele [24]. Furthermore, the Q2958R polymorphism lies within the proposed modulator region (MR1, residues 2618–3015) that has been highly conserved during ryanodine receptor evolution [14]. Three potential calmodulin-binding sites, from residues 2774–2806, 2876–2897, and 2997–3015, have been found in this region [25]. The presence of glutamic acid in this region could weaken the interaction of RyR2 with modulators especially in hypertensive patients.

Alternatively, this variant might be in linkage disequilibrium with a gene that contributes to disease susceptibility or affects survival, or with a gene that is associated with the choice of mates, justifying the Hardy-Weinberg disequilibrium.

Different from Arvanitis et al. [19] in our cohort, we did not find any association with the S96A polymorphism in the HRC gene and an increased risk of arrhythmias. The discordant results may be due to the different method of patient recruitment. Only patients with idiopathic dilated cardiomyopathy were analyzed in the work of Arvanitis et al. [19].

5. Conclusions

To date, our study is the first one to analyze the possible role of *RyR2* Q2958R polymorphism in SCD, showing that it might contribute to the onset of malignant cardiac arrhythmias. Stress load due to hypertension seems to modulate this effect. The association that we found may help to determine the arrhythmic risk in HF patients, who could benefit from an ICD implantation according to the ACC/AHA guidelines. The limit of our study is that the genotype distribution of the *RyR2* Q2958R variant showed deviation from HWE. This implies a selected rather than a random sample, invalidating direct comparisons with other populations.

However, we must keep in mind that single-nucleotide polymorphisms are only partial contributors to an individual's risk for developing a disease.

Therefore, our results should be regarded with caution and our findings regarding RyR2 polymorphism should be confirmed in future prospective larger-scale clinical trials specifically designed, comparing similar study groups in primary prevention with the same phenotype (i.e., underlying disease) and adequately powered to detect genotype-specific differences.

Acknowledgments

The financial support of the MIUR (PON 254/Ric. Potenziamento del Centro di Ricerche per la Salute dell' Uomo e dell'Ambiente Cod. PONa3_00334) is gratefully acknowledged.

References

[1] H. V. Huikuri, A. Castellanos, and R. J. Myerburg, "Sudden death due to cardiac arrhythmias," *The New England Journal of Medicine*, vol. 345, no. 20, pp. 1473–1482, 2001.

[2] R. Havmöller and S. S. Chugh, "Plasma biomarkers for prediction of sudden cardiac death: another piece of the risk stratification puzzle?" *Circulation: Arrhythmia and Electrophysiology*, vol. 5, no. 1, pp. 237–243, 2012.

[3] J. Nakai, T. Imagawa, Y. Hakamata, M. Shigekawa, H. Takeshima, and S. Numa, "Primary structure and functional expression from cDN A of the cardiac ryanodine receptor/calcium release channel," *FEBS Letters*, vol. 271, no. 1-2, pp. 169–177, 1990.

[4] M. Yano, T. Yamamoto, N. Ikemoto, and M. Matsuzaki, "Abnormal ryanodine receptor function in heart failure," *Pharmacology and Therapeutics*, vol. 107, no. 3, pp. 377–391, 2005.

[5] Y. Ran, J. Chen, N. Li et al., "Common RyR2 variants associate with ventricular arrhythmias and sudden cardiac death in chronic heart failure," *Clinical Science*, vol. 119, no. 5, pp. 215–223, 2010.

[6] K. N. Gregory, K. S. Ginsburg, I. Bodi et al., "Histidine-rich Ca binding protein: a regulator of sarcoplasmic reticulum calcium sequestration and cardiac function," *Journal of Molecular and Cellular Cardiology*, vol. 40, no. 5, pp. 653–665, 2006.

[7] D. A. Arvanitis, E. Vafiadaki, G.-C. Fan et al., "Histidine-rich Ca-binding protein interacts with sarcoplasmic reticulum Ca-ATPase," *American Journal of Physiology—Heart and Circulatory Physiology*, vol. 293, no. 3, pp. H1581–H1589, 2007.

[8] E. Kim, D. W. Shin, C. S. Hong, D. Jeong, D. H. Kim, and W. J. Park, "Increased Ca^{2+} storage capacity in the sarcoplasmic reticulum by overexpression of HRC (histidine-rich Ca^{2+} binding protein)," *Biochemical and Biophysical Research Communications*, vol. 300, no. 1, pp. 192–196, 2003.

[9] H. G. Lee, H. Kang, D. H. Kim, and W. J. Park, "Interaction of HRC (histidine-rich Ca^{2+}-binding protein) and triadin in the lumen of sarcoplasmic reticulum," *The Journal of Biological Chemistry*, vol. 276, no. 43, pp. 39533–39538, 2001.

[10] S. Poelzing, C. Forleo, M. Samodell et al., "SCN5A polymorphism restores trafficking of a Brugada syndrome mutation on a separate gene," *Circulation*, vol. 114, no. 5, pp. 368–376, 2006.

[11] J. C. Makielski, B. Ye, C. R. Valdivia et al., "A ubiquitous splice variant and a common polymorphism affect heterologous expression of recombinant human SCN5A heart sodium channels," *Circulation Research*, vol. 93, no. 9, pp. 821–828, 2003.

[12] A. M. Lahtinen, P. A. Noseworthy, A. S. Havulinna et al., "Common genetic variants associated with Sudden cardiac death: the FinSCDgen Study," *PLoS ONE*, vol. 7, no. 7, Article ID e41675, 2012.

[13] N. Tiso, D. A. Stephan, A. Nava et al., "Identification of mutations in the cardiac ryanodine receptor gene in families affected with arrhythmogenic right ventricular cardiomyopathy type 2 (ARVD2)," *Human Molecular Genetics*, vol. 10, no. 3, pp. 189–194, 2001.

[14] R. E. A. Tunwell, C. Wickenden, B. M. A. Bertrand et al., "The human cardiac muscle ryanodine receptor-calcium release channel: identification, primary structure and topological analysis," *Biochemical Journal*, vol. 318, no. 2, pp. 477–487, 1996.

[15] Y. Nakashima, S. Nishimura, A. Maeda et al., "Molecular cloning and characterization of a human brain ryanodine receptor," *FEBS Letters*, vol. 417, no. 1, pp. 157–162, 1997.

[16] K. Otsu, H. F. Willard, V. K. Khanna, F. Zorzato, N. M. Green, and D. H. MacLennan, "Molecular cloning of cDNA encoding the Ca^{2+} release channel (Ryanodine receptor) of rabbit cardiac muscle sarcoplasmic reticulum," *The Journal of Biological Chemistry*, vol. 265, no. 23, pp. 13472–13483, 1990.

[17] J. Fujii, K. Otsu, F. Zorzato et al., "Identification of a mutation in porcine ryanodine receptor associated with malignant hyperthermia," *Science*, vol. 253, no. 5018, pp. 448–451, 1991.

[18] J. Z. Zhang, J. C. McLay, and P. P. Jones, "The arrhythmogenic human HRC point mutation S96A leads to spontaneous Ca^{2+} release due to an impaired ability to buffer store Ca^{2+}," *Journal of Molecular and Cellular Cardiology*, vol. 74, pp. 22–31, 2014.

[19] D. A. Arvanitis, D. Sanoudou, F. Kolokathis et al., "The Ser96Ala variant in histidine-rich calcium-binding protein is associated with life-threatening ventricular arrhythmias in idiopathic dilated cardiomyopathy," *European Heart Journal*, vol. 29, no. 20, pp. 2514–2525, 2008.

[20] A. E. Epstein, J. P. Di Marco, K. A. Ellenbogen et al., "ACC/AHA/HRS 2008 Guidelines for device-based therapy of cardiac rhythm abnormalities: a report of the American College of Cardiology/American Heart Association Task Force on Practice Guidelines (writing committee to revise the ACC/AHA/NASPE 2002 guideline update for implantation of cardiac pacemakers and antiarrhythmia devices) developed in collaboration with the American Association for Thoracic Surgery and Society of Thoracic Surgeons," *Journal of the American College of Cardiology*, vol. 51, no. 21, pp. e1–e62, 2008.

[21] C. M. Tracy, A. E. Epstein, D. Darbar et al., "2012 ACCF/AHA/HRS focused update incorporated into the ACCF/AHA/HRS 2008 guidelines for device-based therapy of cardiac rhythm abnormalities: a report of the American college of cardiology foundation/American heart association task force on practice guidelines and the heart rhythm society," *Journal of the American College of Cardiology*, vol. 61, no. 3, pp. e6–e75, 2013.

[22] S. Rozen and H. Skaletsky, "Primer3 on the WWW for general users and for biologist programmers," *Methods in Molecular Biology*, vol. 132, pp. 365–386, 2000.

[23] H. Tateishi, M. Yano, M. Mochizuki et al., "Defective domain-domain interactions within the ryanodine receptor as a critical

cause of diastolic Ca^{2+} leak in failing hearts," *Cardiovascular Research*, vol. 81, no. 3, pp. 536–545, 2009.

[24] R. J. Van Oort, I. L. Respress, N. Li et al., "Accelerated development of pressure overload-induced cardiac hypertrophy and dysfunction in an RyR2-R176Q knockin mouse model," *Hypertension*, vol. 55, no. 4, pp. 932–938, 2010.

[25] D. B. Witcher, R. J. Kovacs, H. Schulman, D. C. Cefali, and L. R. Jones, "Unique phosphorylation site on the cardiac ryanodine receptor regulates calcium channel activity," *The Journal of Biological Chemistry*, vol. 266, no. 17, pp. 11144–11152, 1991.

15

Impact of Rosuvastatin Treatment on HDL-Induced PKC-βII and eNOS Phosphorylation in Endothelial Cells and Its Relation to Flow-Mediated Dilatation in Patients with Chronic Heart Failure

Ephraim B. Winzer,[1] **Pauline Gaida,**[2] **Robert Höllriegel,**[1] **Tina Fischer,**[1] **Axel Linke,**[1] **Gerhard Schuler,**[1] **Volker Adams,**[1] **and Sandra Erbs**[1]

[1]*Leipzig Heart Center, Department of Cardiology, Leipzig University, 04289 Leipzig, Germany*
[2]*Saechsisches Krankenhaus Altscherbitz, 04435 Leipzig, Germany*

Correspondence should be addressed to Ephraim B. Winzer; bece@medizin.uni-leipzig.de

Academic Editor: Robert Chen

Background. Endothelial function is impaired in chronic heart failure (CHF). Statins upregulate endothelial NO synthase (eNOS) and improve endothelial function. Recent studies demonstrated that HDL stimulates NO production due to eNOS phosphorylation at Ser^{1177}, dephosphorylation at Thr^{495}, and diminished phosphorylation of PKC-βII at Ser^{660}. The aim of this study was to elucidate the impact of rosuvastatin on HDL mediated eNOS and PKC-βII phosphorylation and its relation to endothelial function. *Methods.* 18 CHF patients were randomized to 12 weeks of rosuvastatin or placebo. At baseline, 12 weeks, and 4 weeks after treatment cessation we determined lipid levels and isolated HDL. Human aortic endothelial cells (HAEC) were incubated with isolated HDL and phosphorylation of eNOS and PKC-βII was evaluated. Flow-mediated dilatation (FMD) was measured at the radial artery. *Results.* Rosuvastatin improved FMD significantly. This effect was blunted after treatment cessation. LDL plasma levels were reduced after rosuvastatin treatment whereas drug withdrawal resulted in significant increase. HDL levels remained unaffected. Incubation of HAEC with HDL had no impact on phosphorylation of eNOS or PKC-βII. *Conclusion.* HDL mediated eNOS and PKC-βII phosphorylation levels in endothelial cells do not change with rosuvastatin in CHF patients and do not mediate the marked improvement in endothelial function.

1. Introduction

Patients with chronic heart failure (CHF) are characterized by endothelial dysfunction which is associated with worse prognosis [1]. Different mechanisms have been shown to contribute to endothelial dysfunction. A hallmark is an imbalance of nitric oxide (NO) production via the endothelial NO synthase (eNOS) and NO degradation via oxidant radicals resulting in a diminished NO bioavailability [2, 3].

High-density lipoprotein (HDL) plasma levels are of prognostic relevance for cardiovascular diseases. Nevertheless, several pharmacological approaches to increase HDL quantity failed to reduce cardiovascular events [4]. Therefore, functional properties of HDL are of increasing interest [5]. HDL from healthy subjects has been shown to activate NO

synthesis in endothelial cells [6, 7]. In vitro experiments demonstrated that the incubation of murine aortic rings with human HDL induces NO dependent vasorelaxation [6]. The role of HDL in endothelial function is underscored by in vivo studies showing that intravenous infusion of reconstituted HDL in hypercholesterolemic men rapidly restores endothelial function by increasing NO bioavailability [8]. Furthermore, endothelial function in children was found to be correlated to the ability of isolated HDL to induce eNOS activating phosphorylation in cultured endothelial cells [9].

In CHF, functional properties of HDL are altered. With increasing disease severity, more malondialdehyde is bound to HDL particles and subsequent activation of protein kinase-βII (PKC-βII) results in pronounced phosphorylation of eNOS at its inhibitory site Thr^{495} whereas the eNOS activating phosphorylation at Ser[1177], mediated by PI3K and Akt, is reduced. Thereby, the stimulating effect of isolated HDL on NO production in endothelial cells is blunted. However, this process seems partially reversible with exercise training [7].

Numerous studies have shown that statins improve endothelial function mediated by increased eNOS expression, reduced oxidant stress, and restored endothelial repair mechanisms via circulating endothelial progenitor cells [10–12].

Recently, Chang et al. found that HDL isolated from patients with valvular heart disease in comparison to healthy controls inhibited phosphorylation of eNOS at Ser[1177] and increased phosphorylation at Thr[495] in cultured endothelial cells. This was associated with reduced eNOS-dependent NO production and increased superoxide generation and resulted in impaired vasodilation of murine aortic rings in response to acetylcholine. Interestingly, a short time treatment with simvastatin partially corrected these dysfunctional properties of HDL [13].

These findings indicate that the statin related improvement in endothelial function in humans might be partially mediated by functional properties of HDL.

Previously, we reported the effects of a high-dose rosuvastatin therapy for 12 weeks in patients with CHF on flow-mediated dilatation (FMD) of the radial artery and endothelial repair mechanisms [11]. To further elucidate the role of HDL in this context, the aim of the present study was to analyse the effect of isolated HDL on the phosphorylation of PKC-βII and eNOS at Ser[1177] and Thr[495] in cultured endothelial cells. Furthermore, we report for the first time the effect of statin withdrawal on blood lipids and endothelial function in CHF patients.

2. Methods

The main clinical trial is registered at https://clinicaltrials.gov/ with the following number: NCT00176332.

2.1. Patient Selection and Study Protocol. The study protocol was approved by the ethics committee of the University of Leipzig and written informed consent was obtained from all patients.

In a subgroup of 18 patients from the main study cohort, further evaluation of HDL function was performed (rosuvastatin group $n = 9$, placebo group $n = 9$). Patients with CHF as a result of either ischemic heart disease or dilated cardiomyopathy, clinically stable at New York Heart Association class II or class III for at least one month, left ventricular-ejection fraction <40%, end diastolic left ventricular diameter >55 mm, and peak oxygen uptake <20 mL/min/kg body weight were included. Significant valvular disease and ongoing nicotine abuse served as exclusion criterions. Patients were randomly assigned in a double blind manner to an intervention group receiving 40 mg rosuvastatin daily or a placebo group. At the beginning of the study (bsl), after 12 weeks of active treatment (12 wk), and 4 weeks after discontinuation of the study drug (16 wk), blood samples were taken from all patients to determine blood lipid levels and isolate HDL particles.

2.2. Endothelial Function Measurement. Flow-mediated dilatation (FMD) of the radial artery was measured using a high-resolution ultrasound scanning echo-tracking angiometer (NIUS 02, Asulab Research Laboratory, Neuchatel, Switzerland) as described previously [11].

2.3. Isolation of HDL. HDL was isolated from serum by sequential density ultracentrifugation ($d = 1.006$–1.21 g/mL) as recently described in detail [7].

2.4. Cell Culture and Incubation with Isolated HDL. Human aortic ECs (HAEC; Cell Systems Biotechnology, Troisdorf, Germany) were cultured in EGM-2 cell culture medium (Lonza, Walkersville, MD): Cells were incubated for 0, 5, 10, 15, 30, or 60 minutes with 50 μg/mL isolated HDL in EGM-2 medium (containing growth factors and 10% fetal calf serum) as recently described [7, 14, 15]. Thereafter, cells were harvested with ice-cold lysis buffer (50 mmol/L Tris-HCl; pH 7.4; 1% NP-40; 0,25% Na-deoxycholate; 150 mmol/L NaCl; 1 mmol/L EDTA; 0.1% Triton X-100; 0.2% SDS) containing protease inhibitor mix M (Serva, Heidelberg, Germany) as well as phosphatase inhibitor mix II (Serva). Protein concentration was determined using BSA as standard (BCA method; Pierce, Rockford, IL).

2.5. Western Blot Analysis. Ten micrograms of total protein was separated on a denaturing polyacrylamide gel and transferred to a PVDF membrane. To detect specific proteins, the following antibodies were applied: anti-eNOS (Santa Cruz), antiphospho-eNOS-Ser[1177] and antiphospho-eNOS-Thr[495] (both BD Biosciences, Heidelberg, Germany), and anti-PKC-βII and antiphospho-PKC-βII-Ser[660] (both Santa Cruz). For the evaluation of HDL-induced phosphorylation of the respective protein, the maximal stimulation was used as recently described [7]. All samples were analysed in triplicate.

2.6. Statistical Analysis. Data were analysed using SPSS version 22 (IBM Corp.). For the descriptive statistics of clinical parameters, median and interquartile range were calculated. Mean values ± standard error (SEM) was calculated for all other variables. Repeated measures ANOVA were used to test for change over time. Comparisons from baseline were performed using an analysis of covariance. Categorical variables were tested applying Fisher's exact test. Correlation between selected variables was estimated by Spearman's rank correlation coefficient. A p value of less than 0.05 was considered statistically significant.

3. Results

3.1. Study Patients. The characteristics of the study patients are depicted in Table 1. The randomly assigned patients for HDL function analysis represent well the whole study group of the main study (data not shown) [11]. Clinical characteristics of the patients and cardiac medication did not differ between groups.

TABLE 1: Clinical characteristics.

	Rosuvastatin $n = 9$	Placebo $n = 9$	p value
Clinical profile			
Age [years]	67 (57–72)	60 (55–73)	0.65
Male gender [n]	7 (78%)	5 (56%)	0.62
Characterization of CHF			
Ischemic heart disease [n]	3 (33%)	4 (44%)	1.00
LV ejection fraction [%]	34 (24–36)	30 (30–37)	0.37
LV end diastolic diameter [mm]	64 (58–71)	59 (58–65)	0.19
VO_2 max [mL/min/kg]	13.7 (11.5–17.0)	16.7 (13.8–19.1)	0.18
NYHA class II/III [n/n]	4/5 (44/56%)	6/3 (67/33%)	0.64
Cardiac medication			
Beta blocker [n]	9 (100%)	9 (100%)	n.a.
ACE inhibitor or AT II blocker [n]	9 (100%)	9 (100%)	n.a.
Aldosterone antagonist [n]	7 (78%)	6 (67%)	1.00
Other diuretics [n]	8 (89%)	8 (89%)	1.00
Digitalis [n]	1 (11%)	3 (33%)	0.24

n.a.: not applicable, median (IQR).

TABLE 2: Flow-mediated dilatation and blood lipids.

	Baseline	12 weeks	16 weeks
FMD [%]			
Rosuvastatin	7.56 ± 1.61	21.36 ± 3.49*	6.23 ± 1.16**
Placebo	4.73 ± 0.88	4.74 ± 1.01	5.14 ± 0.68
LDL [mmol/L]			
Rosuvastatin	3.30 ± 0.17	1.53 ± 0.09*	3.49 ± 0.19**
Placebo	3.91 ± 0.27	3.12 ± 0.36	3.31 ± 0.45
HDL [mmol/L]			
Rosuvastatin	1.17 ± 0.10	1.26 ± 0.08	1.16 ± 0.09
Placebo	1.21 ± 0.12	1.19 ± 0.10	1.28 ± 0.14

*Repeated measures ANOVA $p < 0.01$ for baseline versus 12 weeks.
**Repeated measures ANOVA $p < 0.01$ for 12 weeks versus 16 weeks.

3.2. Blood Lipid Levels. LDL plasma levels were reduced after 12 weeks of rosuvastatin treatment, whereas drug withdrawal resulted in a significant LDL increase (bsl 3.30 ± 0.17 mmol/L, 12 wk 1.53 ± 0.09 mmol/L, and 16 wk 3.49 ± 0.19 mmol/L; $p < 0.001$ for bsl versus 12 wk and 12 wk versus 16 wk). However, HDL levels remained unaffected (bsl 1.17 ± 0.10 mmol/L, 12 wk 1.26 ± 0.08 mmol/L, and 16 wk 1.16 ± 0.09 mmol/L; $p =$ n.s.) (Table 2).

3.3. Endothelial Function. As already shown in an earlier publication, the flow-mediated dilatation of the radial artery significantly improved by 183% with rosuvastatin treatment without any change in the placebo group [11]. The FMD data of the presented subgroup here are depicted in Table 2. The treatment effect did not persist four weeks after drug withdrawal.

3.4. Phosphorylation of Endothelial NO Synthase and Protein Kinase C-βII. Incubation of HAEC with HDL from rosuvastatin treated patients had no impact on phosphorylation of eNOS at Ser[1177] (bsl 2.91 ± 0.86-fold, 12 wk 3.45 ± 1.0-fold, and 16 wk 4.35 ± 1.47-fold versus unstimulated cells; $p =$ n.s.) or Thr[495] (bsl 2.03 ± 0.41-fold, 12 wk 1.98 ± 0.39-fold, and 16 wk 2.30 ± 0.62-fold versus unstimulated cells; $p =$ n.s.) and does not influence phosphorylation of PKC-βII at Ser[660] (bsl 2.23 ± 0.27-fold, 12 wk 2.66 ± 0.71-fold, and 16 wk 2.43 ± 0.53-fold versus unstimulated cells; $p =$ n.s.). In the placebo group, no change in these parameters was evident (Figure 1).

3.5. Correlation between Endothelial Function and Phosphorylation of eNOS. In the rosuvastatin group, we found no correlation between flow-mediated dilatation and phosphorylation of eNOS neither at Ser[1177] at any time point (bsl $r = -0.65$, $p = 0.06$; 12 wk $r = 0.15$, $p = 0.70$; 16 wk $r = 0.15$, $p = 0.70$) nor at Thr[495] (bsl $r = 0.20$, $p = 0.61$; 12 wk $r = -0.13$, $p = 0.73$; 16 wk $r = 0.63$, $p = 0.07$) or PKC-βII at Ser[660] (bsl $r = -0.18$, $p = 0.64$; 12 wk $r = -0.17$, $p = 0.67$; 16 wk $r = -0.40$, $p = 0.29$).

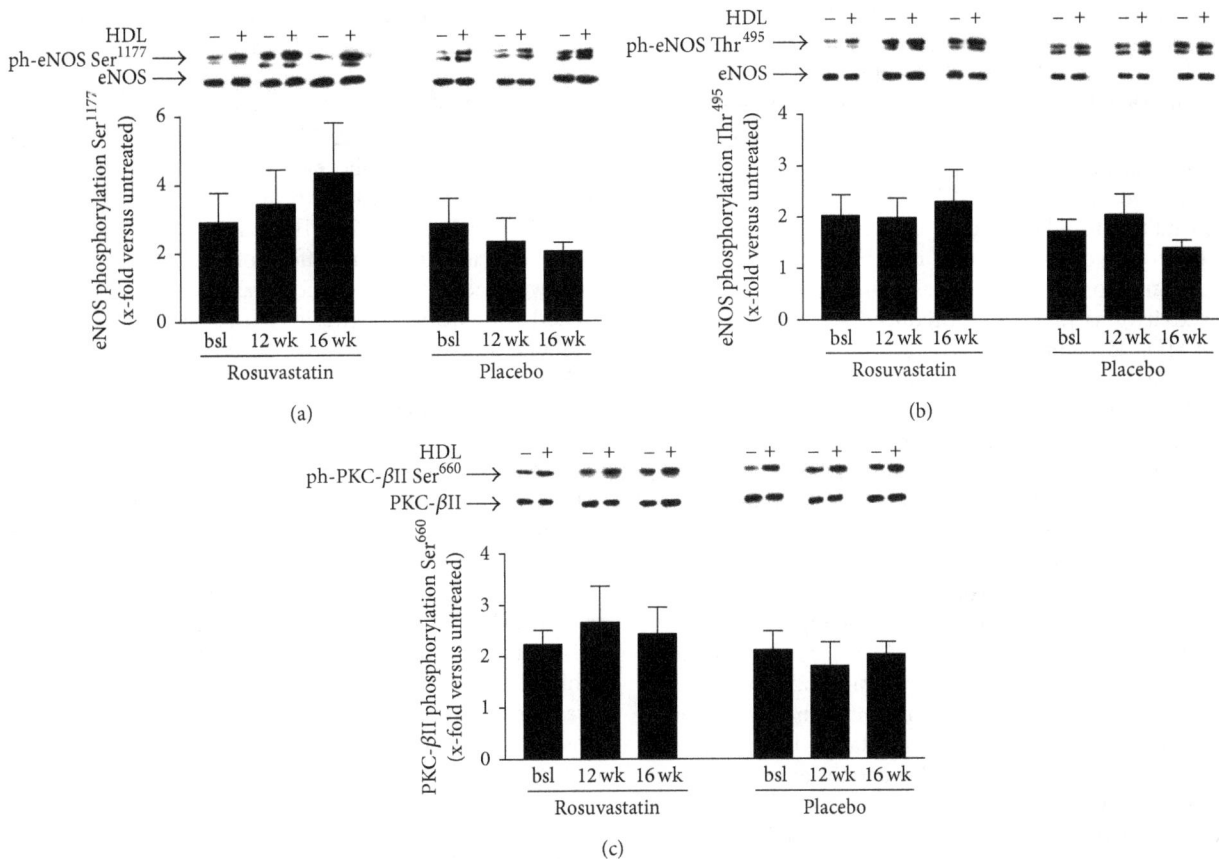

FIGURE 1: (a) X-fold increase in eNOS phosphorylation at Ser^{1177} of human aortic endothelial cells stimulated with HDL from patients treated with rosuvastatin or placebo versus unstimulated cells. (b) X-fold increase in eNOS phosphorylation at Thr^{495} of human aortic endothelial cells stimulated with HDL from patients treated with rosuvastatin or placebo versus unstimulated cells. (c) X-fold increase in PKC-βII phosphorylation at Ser^{660} of human aortic endothelial cells stimulated with HDL from patients treated with rosuvastatin or placebo versus unstimulated cells.

4. Discussion

The following findings emerge from this study: (i) Treatment with rosuvastatin 40 mg for 12 weeks in patients with chronic heart failure does not affect the ability of isolated HDL to change the phosphorylation of PKC-βII at Ser^{660} and the phosphorylation of eNOS at its activity regulating sites Ser^{1177} and Thr^{495} in cultured endothelial cells. (ii) Four weeks after rosuvastatin withdrawal, the treatment effect on LDL cholesterol level and endothelial function is completely abolished.

Our data are in contrast to findings by Chang et al. who demonstrated that low-dose simvastatin treatment with 20 mg per day even for the short period of 5–7 days in patients with valvular heart disease was sufficient to induce HDL-mediated phosphorylation of Akt and eNOS at Ser^{1177} and to inhibit eNOS phosphorylation at the Thr^{495} site in cultured human umbilical vein endothelial cells, resulting in enhanced NO production. Vasodilation of murine aortic rings significantly increased when incubated with HDL from simvastatin treated patients compared to HDL from untreated patients in this study [13].

Beside different statins used with different dosages and treatment periods, the patient groups studied differ significantly. We selected heart failure patients with reduced left ventricular-ejection fraction (mean LV-EF 30% compared to 62% in the study by Chang et al.) and excluded those with more than mild-to-moderate valvular disease. Additionally, more than one-third of patients in our group suffered from ischemic heart disease due to coronary artery disease whereas Chang et al. excluded patients with coronary artery disease. A previous study from our group indicated that HDL dysfunction in patients with reduced LV-EF is related to disease severity with lower HDL-induced NO production in patients according to New York Heart Association Classification class IIIb compared to those in class II [7]. Interestingly, Chang et al. did not find a relation between heart failure symptoms caused by valvular disease and HDL function with a higher proinflammation index in patients in NYHA class II than those in class III. This raises the question whether different mechanisms result in HDL dysfunction in patients with ischemic or dilative cardiomyopathy compared to those with valvular heart disease with subsequently different responsiveness to statin treatment.

The amount of malondialdehyde (MDA) bound to HDL particles has been shown to be crucial for HDL-mediated activation of PKC-βII and downstream eNOS phosphorylation at Thr^{495} resulting in diminished NO production and endothelial dysfunction [7, 16]. Paraoxonase (Pon), an enzyme associated with HDL, protects lipoproteins from oxidative modifications. In CHF, Pon activity of HDL is significantly reduced when compared to healthy controls and might thereby contribute to reduced HDL function in CHF [7]. Also in coronary artery disease patients, HDL associated Pon activity was found to be reduced and associated with higher MDA levels bound to HDL and the inability of isolated HDL to induce NO production in cultured endothelial cells [17]. It has been shown that simvastatin as well as atorvastatin significantly increases serum Pon activity in association with reduced lipid peroxide concentration and serum levels of MDA in hypercholesterolemia [18, 19]. In the present study, PKC-βII phosphorylation remained totally unchanged in response to rosuvastatin even though serum markers of oxidant stress including oxidized LDL and lipid peroxide concentration were reduced as already reported [11]. We therefore assume that rosuvastatin does not reduce the level of MDA bound to HDL particles significantly in CHF. We speculate that the previously demonstrated changes in serum Pon activity and MDA level with statin therapy do not necessarily reflect the activity of Pon and the amount of MDA associated with HDL particles. Nevertheless, differences in patient population as well as type of statin and dosage might contribute to these conflicting results.

However, results from cell culture experiments indicate that statin treatment might improve HDL-mediated eNOS activity via changes on the receptor site: Apolipoprotein A1, a key lipoprotein in HDL particles, binds to the scavenger receptor-BI on endothelial cells [6]. The stimulation of human umbilical vein endothelial cells with HDL resulted in an SR-BI dependent upregulation and activation of eNOS. Prior treatment of these cells with simvastatin increased SR-BI expression through a RhoA and PPAR-α dependent mechanism and thereby enhanced downstream effects on eNOS [20].

Additionally, another signalling pathway evolved in HDL-mediated eNOS activation was found to be modified by statins: sphingosine 1-phosphate (S1P), which is enriched in HDL fractions, binds to G-protein-coupled S1P receptors on endothelial cells and regulates eNOS activation [21]. The incubation of bovine aortic endothelial cells with pitavastatin or atorvastatin led to a dose-dependent increase in S1P1-receptor expression and enhanced eNOS activation in response to HDL [22]. Both of these signalling pathways regulate eNOS activity via phosphorylation at Ser^{1177} in a PI3K/Akt-dependent manner [16, 23, 24].

To demonstrate such treatment effects in humans, endothelial cells would have to be harvested before and after oral statin treatment. This has not been performed in the present study.

Recent analysis of the West of Scotland Coronary Prevention Study identified a long-term legacy benefit from five years of cholesterol lowering therapy with pravastatin in middle aged men at increased risk for atherosclerosis

through decreased cardiovascular event rates and death from cardiovascular causes even 15 years after the active treatment period [25]. However, in our trial, LDL cholesterol level as well as FMD reached baseline levels four weeks after rosuvastatin withdrawal. This is in line with findings in patients with metabolic syndrome showing that the discontinuation of fluvastatin results in deterioration of FMD already after 24 hours [26]. This might be of clinical relevance since an early rebound effect of endothelial dysfunction following acute statin withdrawal is discussed to be associated with worse prognosis at least in patients with acute vascular stress such as stroke or acute coronary syndrome [27].

There are some limitations: First, the sample size for the analysis of HDL function is quite low. However, we found not even a trend towards altered eNOS phosphorylation levels after rosuvastatin therapy, whereas lipid levels and endothelial function clearly changed with therapy and drug withdrawal. Second, we did not evaluate the effect of rosuvastatin on SR-BI or S1P receptor expression and Pon activity and MDA. Nevertheless, primary goal of the study was to investigate the influence of rosuvastatin on eNOS activity. Third, NO generation in endothelial cells in response to HDL was not quantified, and we cannot rule out the possibility that rosuvastatin ameliorates NO generation independent of the evaluated phosphorylation levels.

5. Conclusion

Rosuvastatin treatment in CHF patients does not alter the ability of isolated HDL on the phosphorylation levels of PKC-βII and eNOS at Ser^{1177} and Thr^{495} in cultured endothelial cells. We did not find any relation between FMD and HDL-induced PKC-βII and eNOS phosphorylation with or without rosuvastatin treatment. This indicates that HDL function, at least its effect on eNOS phosphorylation, does not mediate the marked improvement in endothelial function with rosuvastatin treatment in CHF patients.

Abbreviations

Akt:	Protein kinase B
CHF:	Chronic heart failure
eNOS:	Endothelial nitric oxide synthase
FMD:	flow-mediated dilatation
HAEC:	Human aortic endothelial cell
HDL:	High-density lipoprotein
LDL:	Low-density lipoprotein
LV-EF:	Left ventricular-ejection fraction
MDA:	Malondialdehyde
NO:	Nitric oxide
PI3K:	Phosphatidyl inositol 3 phosphate kinase
PKC:	Protein kinase C
Pon:	Paraoxonase
S1P:	Sphingosine 1 phosphate
ser:	Serine
SR-BI:	Scavenger receptor-BI
thr:	Threonine.

Competing Interests

The authors declare that there is no conflict of interests regarding the publication of this paper.

Acknowledgments

This work was supported by an unrestricted grant from AstraZeneca. AstraZeneca provided the study medication (rosuvastatin and placebo).

References

[1] D. Fischer, S. Rossa, U. Landmesser et al., "Endothelial dysfunction in patients with chronic heart failure is independently associated with increased incidence of hospitalization, cardiac transplantation, or death," *European Heart Journal*, vol. 26, no. 1, pp. 65–69, 2005.

[2] A. Linke, S. Erbs, and R. Hambrecht, "Effects of exercise training upon endothelial function in patients with cardiovascular disease," *Frontiers in Bioscience*, vol. 13, no. 2, pp. 424–432, 2008.

[3] E. B. Winzer and A. Linke, "Exercise training improves endothelial function in human cardiovascular disease—role of oxidative stress," in *Systems Biology of Free Radicals and Antioxidants*, I. Laher, Ed., pp. 3831–3853, 2014.

[4] D. Keene, C. Price, M. J. Shun-Shin, and D. P. Francis, "Effect on cardiovascular risk of high density lipoprotein targeted drug treatments niacin, fibrates, and CETP inhibitors: meta-analysis of randomised controlled trials including 117,411 patients," *The British Medical Journal*, vol. 349, Article ID g4379, 2014.

[5] S. Gielen and U. Landmesser, "A new look at HDL in coronary disease: can we escape natural history?" *Heart*, vol. 97, no. 23, pp. 1899–1901, 2011.

[6] I. S. Yuhanna, Y. Zhu, B. E. Cox et al., "High-density lipoprotein binding to scavenger receptor-BI activates endothelial nitric oxide synthase," *Nature Medicine*, vol. 7, no. 7, pp. 853–857, 2001.

[7] V. Adams, C. Besler, T. Fischer et al., "Exercise training in patients with chronic heart failure promotes restoration of high-density lipoprotein functional properties," *Circulation Research*, vol. 113, no. 12, pp. 1345–1355, 2013.

[8] L. E. Spieker, I. Sudano, D. Hürlimann et al., "High-density lipoprotein restores endothelial function in hypercholesterolemic men," *Circulation*, vol. 105, no. 12, pp. 1399–1402, 2002.

[9] U. Müller, Y. Matsuo, M. Lauber et al., "Correlation between endothelial function measured by finger plethysmography in children and HDL-mediated eNOS activation—a preliminary study," *Metabolism: Clinical and Experimental*, vol. 62, no. 5, pp. 634–637, 2013.

[10] U. Landmesser, F. Bahlmann, M. Mueller et al., "Simvastatin versus ezetimibe: pleiotropic and lipid-lowering effects on endothelial function in humans," *Circulation*, vol. 111, no. 18, pp. 2356–2363, 2005.

[11] S. Erbs, E. B. Beck, A. Linke et al., "High-dose rosuvastatin in chronic heart failure promotes vasculogenesis, corrects endothelial function, and improves cardiac remodeling—results from a randomized, double-blind, and placebo-controlled study," *International Journal of Cardiology*, vol. 146, no. 1, pp. 56–63, 2011.

[12] S. Dimmeler, A. Aicher, M. Vasa et al., "HMG-CoA reductase inhibitors (statins) increase endothelial progenitor cells via the PI 3-kinase/Akt pathway," *The Journal of Clinical Investigation*, vol. 108, no. 3, pp. 391–397, 2001.

[13] F.-J. Chang, H.-Y. Yuan, X.-X. Hu et al., "High density lipoprotein from patients with valvular heart disease uncouples endothelial nitric oxide synthase," *Journal of Molecular and Cellular Cardiology*, vol. 74, pp. 209–219, 2014.

[14] A. Oberbach, V. Adams, N. Schlichting et al., "Proteome profiles of HDL particles of patients with chronic heart failure are associated with immune response and also include bacteria proteins," *Clinica Chimica Acta*, vol. 453, pp. 114–122, 2016.

[15] S. Riedel, S. Radzanowski, T. S. Bowen et al., "Exercise training improves high-density lipoprotein-mediated transcription of proangiogenic microRNA in endothelial cells," *European Journal of Preventive Cardiology*, vol. 22, no. 7, pp. 899–903, 2015.

[16] A. Javaheri and D. J. Rader, "High-density lipoprotein: NO failure in heart failure," *Circulation Research*, vol. 113, no. 12, pp. 1275–1277, 2013.

[17] C. Besler, K. Heinrich, L. Rohrer et al., "Mechanisms underlying adverse effects of HDL on eNOS-activating pathways in patients with coronary artery disease," *The Journal of Clinical Investigation*, vol. 121, no. 7, pp. 2693–2708, 2011.

[18] M. Tomás, M. Sentí, F. García-Faria et al., "Effect of simvastatin therapy on paraoxonase activity and related lipoproteins in familial hypercholesterolemic patients," *Arteriosclerosis, Thrombosis, and Vascular Biology*, vol. 20, no. 9, pp. 2113–2119, 2000.

[19] A. Nagila, T. Permpongpaiboon, S. Tantrarongroj et al., "Effect of atorvastatin on paraoxonase1 (PON1) and oxidative status," *Pharmacological Reports*, vol. 61, no. 5, pp. 892–898, 2009.

[20] T. Kimura, C. Mogi, H. Tomura et al., "Induction of scavenger receptor class B type I is critical for simvastatin enhancement of high-density lipoprotein-induced anti-inflammatory actions in endothelial cells," *The Journal of Immunology*, vol. 181, no. 10, pp. 7332–7340, 2008.

[21] T. Kimura, K. Sato, H. Tomura, and F. Okajima, "Cross-talk between exogenous statins and endogenous high-density lipoprotein in anti-inflammatory and anti-atherogenic actions," *Endocrine, Metabolic and Immune Disorders—Drug Targets*, vol. 10, no. 1, pp. 8–15, 2010.

[22] Y. Higashi, H. Matsuoka, H. Umei et al., "Endothelial function in subjects with isolated low HDL cholesterol: role of nitric oxide and circulating progenitor cells," *American Journal of Physiology—Endocrinology and Metabolism*, vol. 298, no. 2, pp. E202–E209, 2010.

[23] C. Mineo, I. S. Yuhanna, M. J. Quon, and P. W. Shaul, "High density lipoprotein-induced endothelial nitric-oxide synthase activation is mediated by Akt and MAP kinases," *The Journal of Biological Chemistry*, vol. 278, no. 11, pp. 9142–9149, 2003.

[24] J.-R. Nofer, M. van der Giet, M. Tölle et al., "HDL induces NO-dependent vasorelaxation via the lysophospholipid receptor S1P3," *The Journal of Clinical Investigation*, vol. 113, no. 4, pp. 569–581, 2004.

[25] I. Ford, H. Murray, C. McCowan, and C. J. Packard, "Long term safety and efficacy of lowering LDL cholesterol with statin therapy: 20-Year Follow-Up of West of Scotland Coronary Prevention study," *Circulation*, vol. 133, no. 11, pp. 1073–1080, 2016.

[26] S. Westphal, C. Abletshauser, and C. Luley, "Fluvastatin treatment and withdrawal: effects on endothelial function," *Angiology*, vol. 59, no. 5, pp. 613–618, 2008.

[27] A. Pineda and L. X. Cubeddu, "Statin rebound or withdrawal syndrome: does it exist?" *Current Atherosclerosis Reports*, vol. 13, no. 1, pp. 23–30, 2011.

16

Human Induced Pluripotent Stem Cell-Derived Cardiomyocytes Afford New Opportunities in Inherited Cardiovascular Disease Modeling

Daniel R. Bayzigitov,[1,2,3] Sergey P. Medvedev,[1,2,3,4]
Elena V. Dementyeva,[1,2,3] Sevda A. Bayramova,[3] Evgeny A. Pokushalov,[3]
Alexander M. Karaskov,[3] and Suren M. Zakian[1,2,3,4]

[1]Federal Research Center, Institute of Cytology and Genetics, Siberian Branch of the Russian Academy of Sciences, Academy Lavrentyev Avenue 10, Novosibirsk 630090, Russia
[2]Institute of Chemical Biology and Fundamental Medicine, Siberian Branch of the Russian Academy of Sciences, Academy Lavrentyev Avenue 8, Novosibirsk 630090, Russia
[3]State Research Institute of Circulation Pathology, Rechkunovskaya Street 15, Novosibirsk 630055, Russia
[4]Novosibirsk State University, Pirogova Street 2, Novosibirsk 630090, Russia

Correspondence should be addressed to Suren M. Zakian; zakian@bionet.nsc.ru

Academic Editor: Vicky A. Cameron

Fundamental studies of molecular and cellular mechanisms of cardiovascular disease pathogenesis are required to create more effective and safer methods of their therapy. The studies can be carried out only when model systems that fully recapitulate pathological phenotype seen in patients are used. Application of laboratory animals for cardiovascular disease modeling is limited because of physiological differences with humans. Since discovery of induced pluripotency generating induced pluripotent stem cells has become a breakthrough technology in human disease modeling. In this review, we discuss a progress that has been made in modeling inherited arrhythmias and cardiomyopathies, studying molecular mechanisms of the diseases, and searching for and testing drug compounds using patient-specific induced pluripotent stem cell-derived cardiomyocytes.

1. Introduction

Cardiovascular diseases (CVDs) include a wide range of diseases which greatly differ in their manifestations and underlying causes. Among CVDs there are acute conditions such as myocardial infarction, congenital heart diseases, and inherited diseases induced by genetic mutations. To search for new drugs and approaches to CVD treatment, the modern experimental medicine applies several types of model systems. First of all, these are animal models, mainly rodents: laboratory mice and rats. To date rodents are actively used to create models of acute myocardial infarction, different types of arrhythmia, and vessel diseases. Besides, there are lines of laboratory animals that carry mutations causing inherited

CVDs [1, 2]. Despite the great amount of data on CVD pathogenesis and ways of their treatment obtained using laboratory animals, these model systems have some restrictions that are due to differences in the cardiovascular physiology (heart rate, peculiarities of the repolarization phase of action potential, etc.) between animals and humans (Table 1). This is particularly important in modeling of diseases caused by malfunctioning of potassium channels, as different types of potassium channels play a key role in cardiomyocyte repolarization in different species [1]. This problem can be solved by using human cardiomyocytes. However, myocardial tissue biopsy is an invasive procedure and requires a special surgical interference (e.g., abdominal operation), which cannot be carried out for the whole CVD range. In addition, the biopsy

TABLE 1: Electrophysiological characteristics of heart that differ in humans and laboratory animals (modified from [91]).

	Mouse	Rat	Guinea pig	Rabbit	Dog	Human
Heart rate (bpm)	500	300	230	200	70	75
Coronary collaterals	Variable	Low	High	None	Middle	Low
Ventricular AP duration (ms)	25–40	50	140	120–140	250	250
Primary repolarizing current	I_{Kto}	I_{Kto}	$I_{Kr,s}$	$I_{Kr,s}$	$I_{Kr,s}$	$I_{Kr,s}$
Q wave in ECG	No	No	Yes	Yes	Yes	Yes
ST segment in ECG	No	No	Yes	Yes	Yes	Yes

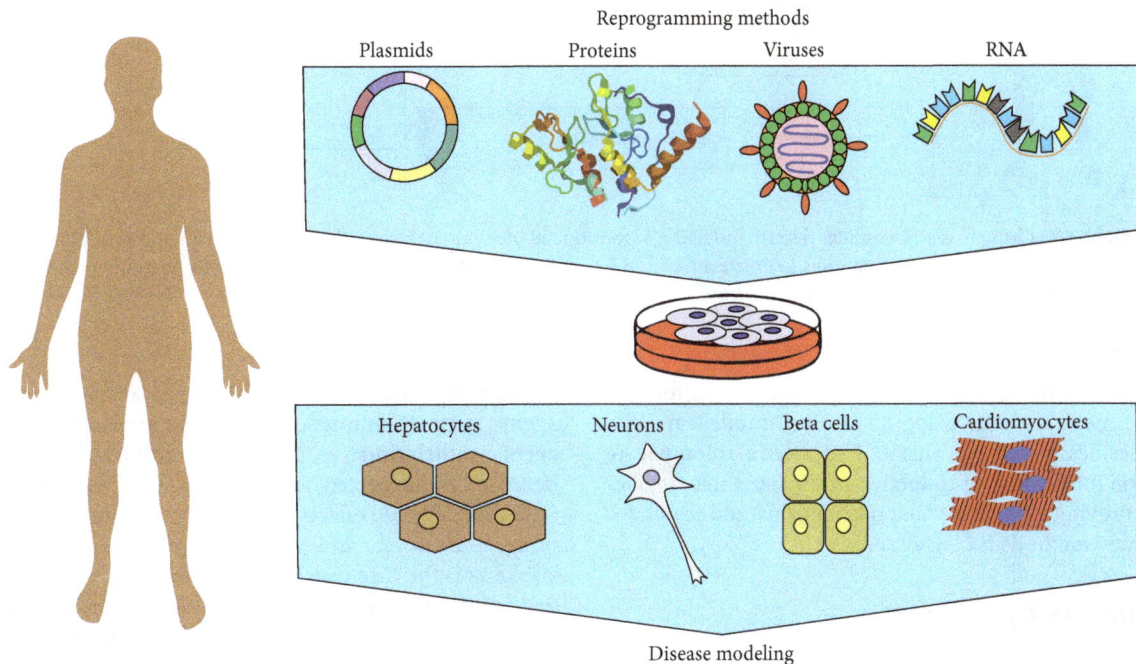

FIGURE 1: Induced pluripotent stem cell-based approach for human disease modeling. hiPSCs can be generated from human somatic cells using viruses, plasmids, modified RNA, and recombinant proteins. iPSCs are differentiated into various cell types for disease modeling, drug screening, and cell therapy.

size is very small and differentiated cardiac cells have low survival and proliferation potentials. The obstacles can be overcome by techniques of generation and directed differentiation of human pluripotent cells. In 2006, Takahashi and Yamanaka reported a pioneering work on reprogramming of adult somatic cells into induced pluripotent stem cells (iPSCs) by overexpression of four transcription factors—Oct3/4, Sox2, Klf4, and c-Myc [3]. These factors are able to turn back terminally differentiated cells to a pluripotent state. iPSCs have been generated from various donor cell types—keratinocytes [4, 5], neuronal cells [6, 7], T-lymphocytes [8, 9], and adipose stromal cells [10]. Like human embryonic stem cells (hESCs), iPSCs can be differentiated into any cell type of human organism (Figure 1). Since then, iPSCs have developed into impetuous, spectacular, and groundbreaking research field promising a great and powerful approach for personalized medicine in the future. However, large-scale and safe application of iPSCs and their derivatives in substitutive cell therapy, including cardiovascular disease treatment, still requires experiments on animal models. At the same time, creation of cell models of inherited cardiovascular diseases

using patient-specific iPSCs-derived cardiomyocytes is being developed.

One of the advantages of the iPSC-based approach is that iPSCs can be generated in any period of patient's life from any type of differentiated cells. Cardiomyocytes obtained during iPSC differentiation are very similar to native cardiomyocytes in morphology, gene expression pattern, electrophysiological rates, and sensitivity to chemical substances. Reliable and efficient methods of iPSC differentiation into various types of cardiomyocytes (atrial, ventricular, and nodal cardiomyocytes) are being currently established. Generating patient-specific iPSCs with subsequent differentiation into cardiomyocytes was already applied to model such CVDs as long QT syndrome, arrhythmogenic cardiomyopathy/right ventricular dysplasia, heart failure, hereditary supravalvular stenosis, catecholaminergic polymorphic ventricular tachycardia, and others. The cell models provide a good opportunity to study CVD pathogenesis at the cellular and molecular levels, search for new drugs, make toxicological researches, and examine possibilities of CVD cell and gene therapy (see Table 6) (Figure 2).

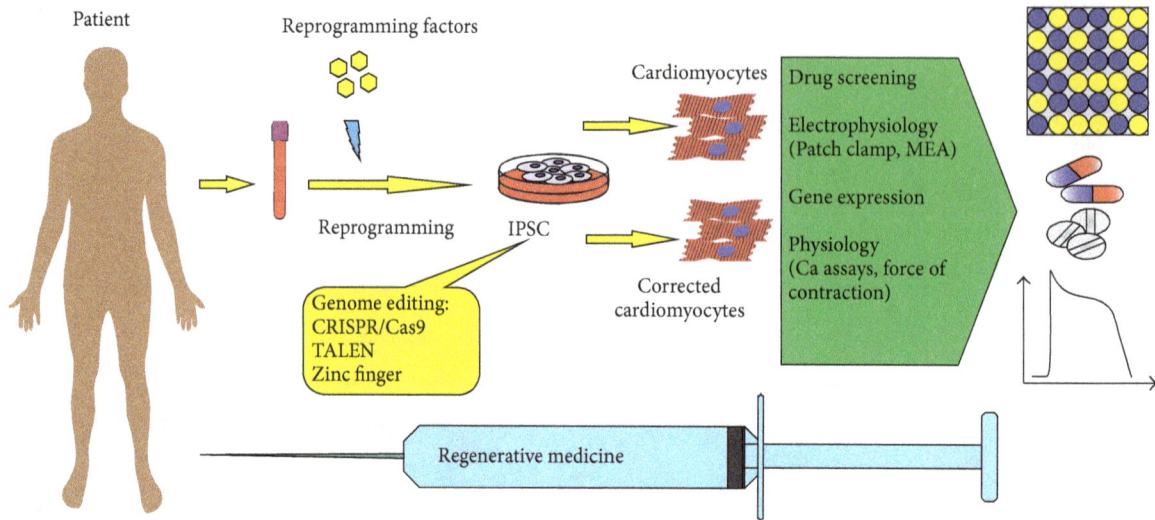

FIGURE 2: Genome editing in cardiovascular disease modeling with induced pluripotent stem cells. Patient-specific induced pluripotent stem cells are corrected using genome editing tools to create a panel of isogenic iPSC lines that are differentiated into cardiomyocytes for disease modeling, drug discovery and screening, and cell therapy.

In this review, the problems concerning search for and testing of medical drugs using disease cell models are discussed. Besides, patient-specific iPSC-derived cardiomyocyte application for *in vitro* reproduction of CVD pathologic phenotype, studying CVD molecular mechanisms, and search for new therapy methods is considered.

2. Cardiotoxicity of Drugs

The Caucasian population is the most studied population, although risk alleles and their frequencies may vary between populations. There are approximately 150 FDA-approved drugs containing pharmacogenomic information in their labeling, describing polymorphic drug targets, genotype-specific dosing, risk of adverse dosing, or clinical response variability. However, individual genetic and epigenetic variations are usually not taken into consideration, making the drugs less effective, ineffective, or even harmful for some patients. The personalized medicine may help physicians to treat patients effectively and without risk of adverse drug reactions. The latter is one of the leading causes of hospitalization in the USA and accounts for more than 110000 deaths annually and more than 700000 serious outcomes (e.g., death, hospitalization, life-threatening disability, and congenital anomaly) [11]. According to FAERS (FDA Adverse Events Reporting System), the number of adverse drug reactions is steadily growing, which may be potentially prevented by an individualized approach to treatment. The median cost of drug developing from discovery to shelf in pharmacy is 1–5 billion US dollars. Nevertheless, while pharmaceutical companies spend money to develop new drugs that pass preclinical and clinical studies, the drugs may be further removed from market. Cardiovascular events or disorders were the main reasons for drug withdrawal in the last 10 years. About thirty drugs belonging to various drug categories (histamine antagonists, antipsoriatic agent, peripheral vasodilator, anorectic and hypolipidaemic agent, sympathomimetics, cough suppressant, antiobesity agents, anthelmintic, etc.) have been withdrawn from market because of unexpected side effects on cardiovascular system (see Table 2). Side effects can damage structure and survival of cardiomyocytes and promote myocardial infarction and stroke as is the case with the anti-inflammatory drug, Vioxx, and many anticancer drugs, such as doxorubicin [12, 13].

Heart rate and QT duration (prolongation or shortening) can also be affected, which can lead to polymorphic ventricular tachyarrhythmia, seizures, and even sudden death. Indeed, in 2010 this was the reason for the US FDA's request for withdrawal of propoxyphene, an opioid analgesic marketed by Xanodyne Pharmaceuticals, and sibutramine, an appetite depressant marketed by Abbott Laboratories. The serotonin agonist, cisapride, had caused about a hundred deaths before its use was ceased. Unexpected side effects are damaging both for companies that spend much money on drug development and promotion and for patients taking the medication.

As discussed earlier, there are significant differences in gene expression pattern and physiology of heart between species, which can hamper efficient extrapolating toxicology studies from laboratory animals to humans. According to the MHRA report in 2006, concordance between toxicities in humans and laboratory animals was concluded to be 71% when using both rodents (mice and rats) and nonrodents (dogs and monkeys). When using rodents only, the concordance was just 43% [14]. Remarkably, humans are more sensitive to drugs than rats, dogs, and mice. The latter tolerates 6–400-fold higher concentration of various antineoplastic agents compared to humans (e.g., Amethopterin, Nitromin, Cytoxan, ThioTEPA, Myleran, Pactamycin, Carboplatin, Amsacrine, Thalicarpine, Chlorozotocin, and Fludarabine) [15]. Conversely, potentially valuable drugs may

TABLE 2: List of drugs withdrawn from the market for safety reasons because of severe cardiovascular effects.

Drug name	Drug class or use	Year of withdrawal	Adverse reaction or safety concern
Astemizole	Histamine antagonists	1999	Fatal arrhythmia
Azaribine	Antipsoriasis	1976	Thromboembolism
Buflomedil	Peripheral vasodilator	2011	Neurological and cardiac disorders
Benfluorex	Anorectic and hypolipidemic	2009	Risk of heart valve disease
Chlorphentermine	Sympathomimetics	1969	Cardiovascular toxicity
Cisapride monohydrate	Serotonin receptor agonists	2000	Fatal arrhythmia
Cloforex	Sympathomimetic	1969	Cardiovascular toxicity
Clobutinol	Cough suppressant	2007	QT prolongation
Dexfenfluramine	Serotonin uptake inhibitors, antiobesity agents	1997	Cardiac valvular disease
Dithiazanine iodide	Anthelmintic	1964	Cardiovascular and metabolic reaction
Dofetilide	Antiarrhythmia agents, potassium channel blockers	2004	Prolonged QT
Encainide HCl	Antiarrhythmic, sodium channel blockers	1991	Cardiotoxicity, ventricular arrhythmias
Fenfluramine	Sympathomimetic, serotonin uptake inhibitors	1997	Cardiac valvular disease
Grepafloxacin	Antimicrobial	1999	QT prolongation
Levomethadyl acetate HCl	Analgesics, opioid	2003	Cardiac arrhythmias and cardiac arrest
Mibefradil dihydrochloride	Calcium channel blockers	1998	Fatal arrhythmia
Orciprenaline	Sympathomimetic, bronchodilator, tocolytic	2010	Cardiac side effects, mainly palpitations and tachycardia
Pergolide mesylate	Dopamine agonists, antidyskinetics	2007	Risk for heart valve damage
Prenylamine	Vasodilator, calcium channel blockers	1988	Polymorphic ventricular tachycardia and death
Propoxyphene	Analgesics, opioid	2010	Increased risk of heart attacks and stroke
Rofecoxib	COX-2 selective NSAID	2004	Risk for heart attack and stroke
Rosiglitazone	Antidiabetic treatment	2011	Risk of heart failure
Sertindole	Antipsychotic	1998	Arrhythmias and sudden cardiac death
Sibutramine	Appetite depressants	2010	Cardiovascular disorders
Sparfloxacin	Fluoroquinolone antibiotic	2001	QT prolongation
Tegaserod maleate	Serotonin receptor agonists	2007	Risk for heart attack and stroke and Unstable angina
Terfenadine	Histamine antagonists	1998	Cardiovascular toxicity, prolonged QT interval
Terodiline	Antispasmodic	1991	Ventricular tachycardia and arrhythmia
Thioridazine	Antipsychotic, dopamine antagonists	2005	cardiac disorders
Valdecoxib	Nonsteroidal anti-inflammatory	2005	Risk for heart attack and stroke

be removed from the pipeline because of toxicity in animals whereas they might be completely nontoxic in humans.

To address this, the FDA proposed a new paradigm labeled the "Comprehensive *In Vitro* Proarrhythmia Assay" to assess the cardiac safety of new or existing drugs in phase 1 studies. Essential to the new paradigm is a focus on understanding mechanisms by in silico reconstruction of human cellular ventricular electrophysiology and confirmation of the electrophysiological effects on human iPSC-derived cardiomyocyte assays [16].

The reason why drugs with lethal side effects are not removed from the pipeline before they reach the clinic is the use of inadequate drug screening and safety assessment platforms. Drugs are tested for ion channel targets on immortalized cell lines (e.g., Chinese hamster ovary (CHO) or human embryonic kidney (HEK) cells) engineered to overexpress appropriate ion channels [17]. However, these cell lines do not reproduce exactly ion channel functioning under normal and pathological conditions (e.g., in case of long QT syndrome). Therefore, human cardiomyocytes are an ideal object to study CVDs. In turn, pluripotent cells, in particular iPSCs, can be an unlimited source of human cardiomyocytes. The examples of iPSC use in inherited CVD modeling are given below.

3. Long QT Syndrome

Long QT (LQT) syndrome is a cardiovascular disease which is diagnosed by QT interval prolongation on the ECG. QT duration depends on sex, age, and heart rate. Therefore, corrected QT interval is used. It is calculated taking into account both QT duration and heart rate. The QT interval is thought to be prolonged when duration of the corrected QT interval is more than 460 ms. According to different estimates, the prevalence of this disease is $1:2000-1:3000$. QT interval prolongation is caused by extension of repolarization during action potential in ventricular cardiomyocytes. This increases the risk of early afterdepolarization, which, in turn, can cause polymorphic ventricular tachycardia. The most frequent ventricular tachycardia in LQT syndrome is torsade de pointes which leads to syncope and may transform into ventricular fibrillation causing the cardiac arrest and sudden death [18].

There are two forms of LQT syndrome, which are acquired and congenital [19]. Acquired form can be caused by a wide range of reasons like other CVDs, disorders of electrolyte exchange, central nervous system diseases, endocrine abnormalities, stress, abstinence from food, diets, poisoning by chemical compounds, and side effects of some drugs. The list of drugs which can prolong the QT interval is being expanded. It includes antiarrhythmic, antihistamine, antibiotic, anaesthetic, and antidepressant drugs and many others. Congenital form is due to mutations in genes encoding proteins involved in potassium, sodium, and calcium channel structure and functioning in cardiomyocytes. The majority of the mutations is autosomal-dominant. To date 13 genes have been identified, mutations in which induce LQT syndrome. According to the genes, there are 13 types of congenital syndrome (LQT1–LQT13) (see Table 3). It is worth mentioning that the first three types are most common; they account for more than 90% of all affected by congenital LQTS [19].

Nowadays, beta blockers as well as implantable cardioverter-defibrillators or cardiostimulators are used to treat LQT syndrome. However their efficiency is insufficient which requires developing new approaches to LQTs treatment. The problem is that the disease is very heterogeneous. There are hundreds of LQT syndrome causing mutations that are located in different parts of the genes and lead to different severity of disease manifestations. Moreover, carriers of the same mutation (even within one family) may demonstrate different disease severity—from early onset of cardiac events to absence of any symptoms. The factors defining LQT syndrome severity need to be clarified. Nevertheless, sex and age (level of sex hormones), other diseases, and administration of some drugs are believed to influence the QT interval duration [20, 21]. Additionally, amount of data on correlations between some single nucleotide polymorphisms (SNPs), QT duration, and disease severity is currently increasing [20, 22, 23]. This heterogeneity requires personalized approaches to LQT syndrome therapy, which can not be provided by existing animal models and heterogeneous systems. iPSC-based technology opened new perspectives in creating more advanced personalized models of LQT syndrome. Several groups have already generated patient-specific iPSC lines carrying mutations causing LQT syndrome types 1, 2, 3, and 8 (see Table 3), that is, for four types of congenital syndrome out of thirteen. The patient-specific iPSC lines were differentiated into cardiomyocytes that showed increase in action potential duration and disturbances in functioning of ion channels involved in appropriate type of LQT syndrome.

iPSC-derived cardiomyocytes to model LQT syndrome were firstly obtained in 2010. Two patients, representatives of one family, carrying the missense mutation c.569G>A (p.R190Q) in KCNQ1 encoding alpha-subunit of slow delayed rectifier potassium current (I_{Ks}) channels were used. The R190Q mutation was found to disrupt KCNQ1 trafficking to cell membrane, which resulted in reduced number of I_{Ks} channels in the patients. As a result, I_{Ks} decreased by 70–80% in the patient-specific cardiomyocytes as compared to control ones. Patient-specific cardiomyocytes were also prone to catecholamine-induced tachycardia that could be managed by beta blockers [24]. In another study, patient-specific iPSCs having the 1893delC mutation in KCNQ1 were generated [25]. The electrophysiological analysis of contracting areas of embryoid bodies (EBs) showed significant increase in the field potential duration. The blocker of fast delayed rectifier potassium current (I_{Kr}) channels, E4031, greatly increased the field potential duration in both control and patient-specific EBs. However, E4031 induced arrhythmia only in patient-specific EBs. At the same time, I_{Ks} channel blocker, chromanol 293B, increased the field potential duration in control EBs, but not in patient-specific EBs. This fact suggests that LQT syndrome was due to disorders in I_{Ks} channel functioning. Studying individual patient's cardiomyocytes by patch-clamp and immunocytochemistry showed that the 1893delC mutation also interfered with mutant protein trafficking from cytoplasm to cell membrane [25]. These studies confirm that cardiomyocytes obtained in the course of patient-specific iPSC differentiation adequately reproduce the main features of the pathological phenotype of LQT syndrome type 1.

iPSC-based models were also created for LQT syndrome type 2. Patient-specific iPSCs carrying different mutations in KCNH2 that encodes alpha-subunit of I_{Kr} channels have been generated. Electrophysiological studies of the iPSC-derived cardiomyocytes revealed a number of pathological manifestations. For example, cardiomyocytes obtained from the patient having the missense A614V mutation in KCNH2 showed a

TABLE 3: Human IPSC-derived patient-specific LQT syndrome cell models.

Syndrome type	Gene	Protein	Mutation	Donor cell types	Reprogramming method	References
LQT1	KCNQ1	Potassium voltage-gated channel subfamily KQT member 1	p.R190Q	Fibroblasts	RV[a], OSKM[b]	[24]
			1893delC (P631fs/33)	Fibroblasts	LV[c], OSKM	[25]
LQT2	KCNH2	Potassium voltage-gated channel subfamily H member 2	p.A614V	Fibroblasts	RV, OSK[b]	[26]
			p.A561T	Fibroblasts	LV, ONSL[b]	[27]
			p.R176W	Fibroblasts	RV, OSKM	[29]
			p.G603D	T-lymphocytes	SV[d], OSKM	[92]
			p.N996I	Fibroblasts	RV, OSKM	[35]
LQT3	SCN5A	Sodium channel protein type 5 subunit alpha	p.F1473C	Fibroblasts	RV, OSKM	[30]
			p.V1763M	Fibroblasts	mRNA, OSKM	[31]
LQT4	ANK2	Ankyrin-2				
LQT5	KCNE1	Potassium voltage-gated channel subfamily E member 1				
LQT6	KCNE2	Potassium voltage-gated channel subfamily E member 2				
LQT7	KCNJ2	Inward rectifier potassium channel 2				
LQT8	CACNA1	Voltage-dependent P-type/Q-type calcium channel subunit alpha-1A	p.G406R	Fibroblasts	RV, OSKM	[5]
LQT9	CAV3	Caveolin-3				
LQT10	SCN4B	Sodium channel subunit beta-4 precursor				
LQT11	AKAP9	A-kinase anchor protein 9				
LQT12	SNTA1	Alpha-1-syntrophin				
LQT13	KCNJ5	G protein-activated inward rectifier potassium channel 4				

RV[a]: retroviruses, LV[c]: lentiviruses, SV[d]: sendai virus , and OCT4 (O), SOX2 (S), KLF4 (K), c-MYC (M), NANOG (N), and LIN28 (L)[b]. Ion channels: I_{Ks}: slow delayed rectifier K+ current; I_{Kr}: rapid delayed rectifier K+ current; I_{Na}: sodium channel current; I_{K1}: inwardly rectifying K+ current; $I_{Ca,L}$: L-type calcium current; and I_{KAch}: acetylcholine activated potassium current.

decrease in I_{Kr} (by about 60%) and increase in duration of action and field potentials as compared to control cells [26]. In addition, the cardiomyocytes demonstrated signs of early afterdepolarization (about 66% of cells) and premature contractions (about 36% of cells). The interesting fact is that action potential prolongation and early afterdepolarization were greatly inhibited while using nifedipine, a blocker of calcium channels, and pinacidil that stimulates opening of ATP-dependent potassium channels.

Patient-specific iPSC-derived cardiomyocytes can be used for search for and study of new drug combinations as was successfully demonstrated in the study by Matsa et al. [27]. iPSCs were obtained from a fifteen-year-old female that showed symptoms of LQT syndrome and carried the missense c.1681G>A (p.A561T) mutation in KCNH2 and her mother who was an asymptomatic carrier of the mutation. Cardiomyocytes obtained from both daughter's and mother's iPSCs showed prolonged field/action potential duration as compared to control cells. However, the daughter's cardiomyocytes had a more pronounced elongation of the action potential. Adding of isoprenaline shortened the action potential duration but caused early afterdepolarization in a great number of cardiomyocytes. Effect of isoprenaline was reversed by beta blockers (nadolol and propranolol). Use of potassium channel activators, nicorandil and/or PD-118057, also led to decrease in the action potential duration; however, no arrhythmogenic early afterdepolarization was observed [27]. Another study showed that roscovitine was able to deactivate L-type calcium current ($I_{Ca,L}$) channels and restore normal calcium currents and electrophysiological properties of cardiomyocytes derived from iPSCs of Timothy syndrome patients [5]. This syndrome is associated with autosomal-dominant mutations in CACNA1C encoding alpha-subunit of $I_{Ca,L}$ channels and is accompanied not only by QT prolongation and arrhythmias (LQT syndrome type 8) but also by a wide range of disorders, congenital heart disorders and syndactyly and autism and backwardness and high risk of sudden death at an early age [28].

Thus, iPSC-derived cardiomyocytes of particular patients can be used for selection of individual drug combinations, which may help to avoid complications during drug therapy. This approach is strongly supported by the fact that patients' iPSC-derived cardiomyocytes are able to adequately reproduce individual peculiarities of disease manifestation. For example, cardiomyocytes of a patient having the R176W mutation in *KCNH2* demonstrate a significant increase in action and field potentials but do not show any signs of early afterdepolarization, which agrees with the absence of arrhythmic events in this patient [29]. The relationships between genotype and clinical symptoms seen in patients were fully reproduced in iPSC-based models for LQT syndrome types 3 and 8 [5, 30, 31].

Cardiomyocytes obtained from iPSCs of LQT syndrome patients can be also a tool for development and testing new therapy methods. In one study, allele-specific RNA interference was used to correct a mutant phenotype in patient-specific cardiomyocytes [32]. Using short interfering RNA, the authors managed to decrease the RNA level of a mutant *KCNH2* (*hERG*) allele (c.G1681A) by 61.8%, thereby increasing probability of formation of functional hERG tetramer by 4.5 times. It was enough to normalize the action potential duration, to restore I_{Kr}, and to reduce the frequency of spontaneous and induced arrhythmias (early afterdepolarization) [32]. This fact suggests that the allele-specific RNA interference can be an efficient method to correct LQT syndrome type 2 and other diseases with autosomal-dominant inheritance. However, to apply this method in clinic, a number of difficult issues need to be solved. One of them is targeted siRNA delivery in specific cell types of affected organ, for example, in cardiomyocytes. Experiments on mouse LQT syndrome models may be required to find a solution of this issue [33, 34].

In addition, cardiomyocytes obtained from patient-specific iPSCs can be used to test newly detected mutations, to clarify relationships between the mutations and disease phenotype, and to study molecular mechanisms of disease pathogenesis. For example, Bellin et al. obtained iPSCs of a female LQT syndrome patient who was asymptomatic and diagnosed only based on electrocardiogram results [35]. The genetic screening showed that the patient had the c.A2987T (p.N996I) mutation in *KCNH2*. In order to verify the role of this mutation in LQT syndrome development, two pairs of isogenic pluripotent cell lines that had the same genetic background and differed only by one point mutation were used. One pair was two patient-specific iPSC lines. One carried the N996I mutation whereas in the other the mutation was corrected by homologous recombination. The second pair was two ESC lines that differed in presence/absence of the N996I mutation. Electrophysiological analysis of the iPSC- and ESC-derived cardiomyocytes showed that only the presence of the N996I mutation increased the action potential duration and damaged I_{Kr}. Correction of the mutation improved these parameters. Further studies demonstrated that this mutation disrupted hERG trafficking to cell membrane, which seemed to underlie pathology development [35].

Thus, iPSC-derived cardiomyocytes of LQT syndrome patients are being used to study molecular mechanisms of disease development, to examine new disease causing mutations, to search for new therapy methods, and to test existing drugs for QT interval prolongation and proarrhythmic activity.

4. Catecholaminergic Polymorphic Ventricular Tachycardia

Catecholaminergic polymorphic ventricular tachycardia (CPVT) is a severe inherited cardiovascular disease. Its prevalence is about 1 : 10000. CPVT is defined by absence of structural heart damage and severe tachycardia induced by physical or emotional stress [36]. CPVT causes syncope and is a frequent reason of sudden death among young people [37]. About 30% of CPVT patients show the symptoms under the age of 10, and the death rate under the age of 35 is 30–35%. The only methods of CPVT therapy are beta blockers and automatic cardioverter-defibrillator implantation [38]. Mutations in two genes are known to cause CPVT. One of the genes *(RyR2)* encodes a ryanodine receptor. This protein is involved in calcium ions release from sarcoplasmic reticulum and plays a key role in cardiomyocyte contractions. There are over 150 mutations in *RyR2* which have autosomal-dominant inheritance, cause CPVT type I, and are responsible for up to 55% of CPVT cases. Mutations in another gene *(CASQ2)*, which encodes the calcium binding protein (calsequestrin), are much rarer and cause about 3–5% of CPVT cases. 15 mutations were identified in *CASQ2*. The mutations have autosomal-recessive inheritance and cause CPVT type II [39].

To model CPVT *in vivo*, mice that had mutations in *RyR2* or were *CASQ2* knockouts were used. To study the disease *in vitro*, myocytes were transduced with recombinant adenoviruses expressing mutant CASQ2 forms. Both model types were found to reproduce the CPVT clinical pattern including delayed afterdepolarization in response to adrenergic stimulation [40–44]. However, the method of inducing the pluripotent state in somatic cells has opened new perspectives in studying mechanisms of this severe disease and searching for new ways of its treatment.

A research group generated iPSCs of patients from a Bedouin tribe living in the northern part of Israel and having rare homozygous missense p.D307H mutation in *CASQ2* [39]. Beta-adrenergic agonist (isoproterenol) stimulation of the patient-specific iPSC-derived cardiomyocytes caused delayed afterdepolarization, arrhythmogenic oscillating prepotentials, and postcontractions. The effects were not detected in control cardiomyocytes [39]. Analysis by electronic microscopy showed that the patient-specific cardiomyocytes had immature phenotype, less organized myofibrils, enlarged cisterns of sarcoplasmic reticulum, and reduced number of caveolae [39]. The patients' cardiomyocytes were also defined by decreased contraction frequency. This agreed with clinical data, according to which CPVT type II patients had bradycardia at rest.

Using patient-specific iPSCs, CPVT type I models were also obtained [45–47]. Fatima et al. generated iPSCs of a

TABLE 4: Human IPSC-derived patient-specific CPVT syndrome cell models.

Gene	Protein	Mutation	Donor cell types	Reprogramming method	References
CASQ2	Calsequestrin 2	p.D307H	Fibroblasts	LV[a], OSKM[b]	[39]
RyR2	Ryanodine receptor 2	p.P2328S	Fibroblasts	RV[c], OSKM	[47]
RyR2	Ryanodine receptor 2	p.F2483I	Fibroblasts	RV, OSKM	[45]
RyR2	Ryanodine receptor 2	p.S406L	Fibroblasts	RV, OSKM	[46]

LV[a]: lentiviruses, RV[c]: retroviruses, and OCT4 (O), SOX2 (S), KLF4 (K), and c-MYC (M)[b].

46-year-old woman having the dominant missense p.F2483I mutation in *RyR2* which was within FKBP12.6-binding domain of ryanodine receptor [45]. Unlike control cardiomyocytes, isoproterenol treatment of the patient-specific cardiomyocytes resulted in a negative chronotropic effect, delayed afterdepolarization, and arrhythmia. Visualization of calcium ion currents in the patient's cardiomyocytes showed a high amplitude and duration of calcium ion release, even without adrenergic stimulation. Similar results were obtained upon studying cardiomyocytes of a 25-year-old male patient having the missense p.P2328S mutation in *RyR2* [47]. As was shown by patch-clamp, the patient-specific cardiomyocytes had the signs of delayed afterdepolarization in case of spontaneous contractions and in presence of adrenaline as well as early afterdepolarization in case of spontaneous contractions. Besides, the patient's cardiomyocytes had a lower content of calcium ions in the sarcoplasmic reticulum, which suggested its possible abnormal leakage [47].

iPSC-based model of CPVT type I was also created for a female patient carrying the p.S406L mutation in the RyR2 N-terminal domain [46]. Cardiomyocytes of a healthy donor and the patient showed that they had similar levels of calcium ions in systole and diastole and equal content of calcium ions in the sarcoplasmic reticulum. However, during isoproterenol stimulation the level of calcium ions in diastole sharply increased in the patient's cells as compared to control ones, while the level of calcium ions in systole did not change. The calcium ion content in sarcoplasmic reticulum did not increase in the patient's cardiomyocytes in response to isoproterenol. Under the intact condition in the patient-specific cardiomyocytes, abnormal sparks of calcium ion release and more extended plateau phase and decay phase were observed. In response to isoproterenol the frequency of such sparks increased and they acquired longer decay phases. The use of dantrolen (the drug effectively used for treatment of the malignant hyperthermia) was shown to normalize parameters of calcium ion release sparks and prevent cells from arrhythmia [46].

Thus, as in the case of LQT syndrome, patient-specific iPSC-derived cardiomyocytes adequately reproduce the disease *in vitro* and are a good tool for studying CPVT molecular mechanisms and drug searching (see Table 4).

5. Inherited Cardiomyopathies

Cardiomyopathies (CMPs) are a group of cardiovascular diseases that are defined by structural and functional changes of the cardiac muscle forming even in the absence of coronary artery pathologies, increased arterial pressure, or cardiac valvulopathy. There are several types of primary cardiomyopathies: arrhythmogenic right ventricular dysplasia, dilated (congestive) CMP, hypertrophic CMP, specific CMP (metabolic, inflammatory, ischemic, cirrhotic, etc.), and unclassified CMP (fibroelastosis, noncompaction cardiomyopathy (spongiform cardiomyopathy), mitochondriopathies, etc.). Primary CMPs can be caused by viruses, bacteria, autoimmune disorders, toxic action of the alcohol, and medical drugs and also by genetic mutations. In most cases, the only way of CMP therapy is cardiac transplantation. In 2012-2013, several research groups obtained cell models of inherited arrhythmogenic right ventricular dysplasia (ARVD) and dilated (DCMP) and hypertrophic (HCMP) cardiomyopathies using patient-specific iPSCs (see Table 5) [31, 48–52].

6. Arrhythmogenic Right Ventricular Dysplasia (ARVD)

ARVD is defined by progressive replacement of healthy tissue of cardiac muscle, mainly in the right ventricle, with fibroadipose tissue and enhanced apoptosis of cardiomyocytes. These changes lead to ventricular tachycardia and increased risk of sudden death. Despite the disease severity and high incidence, there are still few data on the mechanisms of its onset and development. This mainly is due to low availability of the material (myocardial biopsy) for research, especially at the early stages of disease development. Nearly 50% of patients suffering from ARVD have mutations in genes which encode desmosomes components—desmoplakin, plakoglobin, plakophilin-2, desmoglein-2, and desmocollin-2 [53]. Mutations in *PKP2* encoding plakophilin-2 are the most frequent. In three studies, iPSC-derived cardiomyocytes of patients with diagnosed ARVD have been obtained [48, 49, 54]. In one case, a patient was homozygous for the c.2484C>T mutation in *PKP2* [49]. This mutation interrupts transcript splicing and induces 7-nucleotide deletion in the *PKP2* exon 12. Main pathological hallmarks of ARVD are progressive fibrofatty replacement of cardiomyocytes with increased cardiomyocyte apoptosis. However, changes in plakoglobin localization in patient iPSC-derived cardiomyocytes did not influence lipogenesis and apoptosis in mutant cardiomyocytes as compared to the control ones. The fact is that iPSC-derived cardiomyocytes were immature and corresponded to embryonic cardiomyocytes. To produce energy embryonic cardiomyocytes use glycolysis while adult cardiomyocytes do fatty acid oxidation. In order to reproduce ARVD pathogenesis *in vitro*, energy metabolism of adult cardiomyocytes was activated with insulin, dexamethasone, and

TABLE 5: Human IPSC-derived patient-specific cardiomyopathy cell models.

Disease	Gene	Protein	Mutation	Donor cell types	Reprogramming method	References
Arrhythmogenic right ventricular dysplasia (ARVD)	PKP2	Plakophilin 2	c.2484C>T	Fibroblasts	PB[a], OSKM[b]	[49]
	PKP2	Plakophilin 2	c.2013delC	Fibroblasts	Epi[c], OSKM	
Arrhythmogenic right ventricular dysplasia (ARVD)	PKP2	Plakophilin 2	c.972InsT/N	Fibroblasts	RV[d], OSK[b]	[48]
Arrhythmogenic right ventricular dysplasia (ARVD)	PKP2	Plakophilin 2	c.1841T>C (p.L614P)	Fibroblasts	RV, OSKM	[54]
Dilated cardiomyopathy	DES	Desmin	c.940C>T (p.A285V)	Fibroblasts	RV, OSKM	[52]
Barth syndrome (dilated cardiomyopathy)	TAZ1	Tafazzin	c.590G>T, p. G197V c.110-1AG>AC 170G>T, p. R57L	Fibroblasts	LV[f], OSKM	[60]
Dilated cardiomyopathy	TNNT2	Troponin T type 2 (cardiac)	p.R173W	Fibroblasts	LV, OSKM	[51]
Hypertrophic cardiomyopathy	MYH7	Myosin heavy chain beta	p.R663H	Fibroblasts	LV, OSKM	[50]
LEOPAPD syndrome (hypertrophic cardiomyopathy)	PTPN11	Protein tyrosine phosphatase, nonreceptor type 11	p.T468M	Fibroblasts	RV, OSKM	[62]

PB[a]: PiggyBac, RV[d]: retroviruses, LV[f]: lentiviruses, Epi[c]: episomes, and OCT4 (O), SOX2 (S), KLF4 (K), and c-MYC (M)[b].

3-isobutyl-1-methylxanthine. The stimulation activated transcription of the main regulator of fatty acid oxidation, PPAR- (peroxisome proliferator-activated receptor-) alpha, but this did not induce statistically significant changes in the mutant cardiomyocytes properties. Then adipogenic differentiation in combination with rosiglitazone and indomethacin that are activators of the PPAR-gamma receptor was applied. Activation of the PPAR-gamma signaling cascade, which is abnormally active in cardiac muscle of ARVD patients, resulted in enhanced lipogenesis and apoptosis in the iPSC-derived mutant cardiomyocytes. Interestingly, insulin, dexamethasone, and 3-isobutyl-1-methylxanthine used for PPAR-alpha activation adequately reproduced hormone action in adult human body. At the same time, there are no ligands activating the PPAR-gamma and similar to rosiglitazone and indomethacin in their chemical structure. Nevertheless, it was found that rosiglitazone and indomethacin could be replaced with 13-hydroxy-octadecadienoic acid, main component of oxidized low-density lipoproteins, during PPAR-gamma activation. Application of PPAR-gamma antagonists (GW9662 and T0070907) upon reproducing the pathological condition could prevent cardiomyocyte lipogenesis and apoptosis. Finally, pathological features were shown to be inhibited by either PPAR-alpha inactivation or PPAR-gamma activation only. This means that pathological mechanisms involve activation of both PPAR-alpha and PPAR-gamma signaling cascades. The conclusion was confirmed using iPSC-derived cardiomyocytes of a patient heterozygous for

the c.2013delC deletion inducing frameshift mutation and transcription termination in the PKP2 exon 10 [49].

In the other two studies, iPSC-derived cardiomyocytes of patients carrying two different mutations in PKP2 were generated. One mutation was the heterozygous c.972InsT/N insertion leading to frameshift mutation [48] and the other was the missense c.1841T>C (p.L614P) mutation [54]. Increased lipogenesis, damage of desmosome structure, and PPAR-gamma activation were observed in the patient-specific iPSC-derived cardiomyocytes. One of the studies also showed that the adipogenic stimulation intensified changes in the desmosomes structure and lipid accumulation. These effects could be prevented by a specific inhibitor of glycogen synthase kinase 3 beta [48].

7. Dilated Cardiomyopathy (DCM)

Dilated cardiomyopathy is a myocardial disease characterized by ventricular chamber enlargement and systolic dysfunction with no increase in ventricular wall thickness. DCM is one of the most common reasons of cardiac failure after coronary vessels disease and elevated blood pressure [55, 56]. About 30–35% of DCM cases are inherited. Mutations in more than 30 genes encoding proteins of cytoskeleton, sarcomere, and nuclear lamina can cause DCM [57].

iPSC-derived cardiomyocytes have been also obtained for patients with inherited DCM [51, 52]. In one study, a patient demonstrated such cardiological symptoms as palpitation

TABLE 6: Summary of published studies in cardiovascular disease with patient-specific iPSC.

Disease name	Cell type made	Phenotype displayed in iPSC-derived cells	Drug tested	References
Arrhythmogenic right ventricular cardiomyopathy/dysplasia	CMs	Reduced expression of plakophilin-2 and plakoglobin; evidence of myofibril disorganization; elevated lipid content relative to control CMs when they are exposed to adipogenic differentiation media	Nifedipine-inhibited contraction; isoproterenol increased contraction rate	[54]
Barth syndrome	CMs	Impaired cardiolipin biogenesis; ROS production was markedly increased and ATP levels were significantly lower; maximal electron transport chain activity was severely impaired in CMs	Linoleic acid improved sarcomere organization and increased twitch stress to nearly normal levels; mitoTEMPO treatment normalized sarcomere organization and contractility	[93]
Carnitine palmitoyltransferase II (CPT II) deficiency	Myocytes	CPT II-deficient myocytes accumulated more palmitoylcarnitine	Bezafibrate reduced the amount of palmitoylcarnitine	[94]
CPVT	CMs	Immature cardiomyocytes with less organized myofibrils and enlarged sarcoplasmic reticulum cisternae and reduced number of caveolae; DADs; oscillatory arrhythmic prepotentials; after-contractions and diastolic $[Ca^{2+}]_i$ rise	None	[39]
CPVT	CMs	Higher amplitudes and longer durations of spontaneous Ca^{2+} transients; Ca^{2+} release events after repolarization; abnormal Ca^{2+} response to phosphorylation induced by increased cAMP levels	None	[45]
CPVT	CMs	Elevated diastolic Ca^{2+} concentrations, a reduced sarcoplasmic reticulum Ca^{2+} content, and an increased susceptibility to arrhythmias	Dantrolene restored normal Ca^{2+} spark properties and rescued the arrhythmogenic phenotype	[46]
CPVT	CMs	Similar to above, but also evidence of early afterdepolarizations (EADs)	Flecainide and Thapsigargin blocked ads-beta blockers improved Ca^{2+} transient anomalies	[95]
CPVT	CMs	Aberrant Ca^{2+} cycling resulting in DAD and EAD	None	[47]
Familial dilated cardiomyopathy	CMs	Punctate sarcomeric α-actinin distribution; altered Ca^{2+} handling, decreased contractility	Norepinephrine markedly increased the number of CMs with punctate sarcomeric α-actinin distribution from DCM iPSC clones; metoprolol improved myofilament organization and significantly prevented aggravation of the DCM iPSC-CMs that is induced by norepinephrine treatment	[51]

TABLE 6: Continued.

Disease name	Cell type made	Phenotype displayed in iPSC-derived cells	Drug tested	References
LEOPARD syndrome	CMs	CMs are larger and have a higher degree of sarcomeric organization and preferential localization of NFATC4 in the nucleus compared to normal CMs	None	[62]
LQT1	CMs	Longer and slower repolarization velocity; abnormal subcellular distribution of R190Q KCNQ1; reduction of outward K^+ current	Isoproterenol induced EAD was prevented by propranolol, simulating clinical LQT1	[24]
LQT2	CMs	Prolongation of the action potential duration; reduction of potassium current I_{Kr}; EADs	Nifedipine: complete elimination of EADs; pinacidil: abolished EADs; ranolazine: pronounced anti-EAD effect at both cellular and multicellular level	[26]
LQT2	CMs	Same as above	Nicorandil and PD118057: action potential shortening and reduction of EADs; E4031: induced EADs; isoprenaline induced EADs and was blocked by nadolol and propranolol, simulating clinical treatment	[27]
LQT3	CMs	Dysfunction in Na^+ channel gating, increase in I_{NaL}, right-shifted steady-state channel availability, and faster recovery from inactivation	Mexiletine corrects Na^+ channel inactivation	[30]
LQT3	CMs	Significantly prolonged APD and in patient-derived V-like hiPSC-CMs during the spontaneous contraction and during electrical pacing. Tetrodotoxin-sensitive late Na^+ current (dA/dF) was significantly larger in patient-derived hiPSC-CMs	Mexiletine reduced the late Na^+ current, moderate effect of mexiletine in shortening the APD	[31]
LQT8 (Timothy syndrome)	CMs	Irregular contractions; excessive Ca^{2+} influx; prolonged action potentials; irregular electric activity; abnormal Ca^{2+} transients	Roscovitine normalized the Ca^{2+} defects and improved channel inactivation	[5]
Overlap syndrome of cardiac sodium channel disease	CMs	Significant decrease in I_{Na} density and upstroke velocity; a larger persistent I_{Na} leading to an increased persistent I_{Na}	None	[33]
Marfan type 1	Mesenchymal cells	Elevated TGF-β signaling; inhibited osteogenesis and spontaneous chondrogenesis	None	[96]
Pompe disease (infantile onset)	CMs	Glycogen accumulation; ultrastructurally abnormal mitochondria; accumulation of autophagosomes; carnitine deficiency	L-carnitine increased O_2 consumption and suppressed mitochondrial structural phenotype; treatment with rhGAA with autophagy inhibitor 3-MA normalized glycogen content	[97]
SAS	SMCs	Significantly lower level of ELN protein in SMCs and proliferate at a higher rate and migrate significantly faster in response to the chemotactic cytokine platelet-derived growth factor	Recombinant elastin or small GTPase RhoA rescues defective SM α-actin filament bundles	[69]

and precollaptoid states as well as nonsustained ventricular tachycardias were detected by the Holter monitoring. The patient's father and brother suddenly died because of non-defined cardiac disease. Exome sequencing revealed previously unknown heterozygous missense c.940C>T (p.A285V) mutation in *DES* encoding desmin [52]. *DES* mutations were previously shown to induce various forms of DCM [57–59]. iPSC-derived cardiomyocytes of the patient carrying the c.940C>T mutation had a number of structural abnormalities such as presence of diffuse desmin-containing aggregates and weak interaction of desmin with troponin T, alpha-actin, and F-actin. Scanning electron microscopy analysis showed structure damage of sarcomere Z-disks and presence of pleomorphic dense structures near Z-disks or between myofibrils. In comparison with control cardiomyocytes, the patient-specific ones demonstrated a lower contractile rate and inadequate response to adrenergic stress induced by isoproterenol [52].

In another study, genetic screening of 7 family members was performed to identify DCM causing mutation [51]. Four individuals, representatives of three generations, had the missense p.R173W mutation in *TNNT2* which encodes cardiac troponin T. iPSC-derived cardiomyocytes were generated for each mutation carrier. The mutant cardiomyocytes demonstrated changes in regulation of calcium ion currents and elevated contractility and most cells had irregular distribution of sarcomeric alpha-actin. Beta-adrenergic agonists increased intensity of the pathological changes, while beta blockers or ectopic expression of Serca2a (calcium-dependent adenosine triphosphatase of sarcoplasmic reticulum) restored the functions in the mutant cardiomyocytes [51].

DCM may also be a trait of some complex inherited syndromes. For example, DCM is a symptom of the Barth syndrome along with skeletal muscle myopathy, neutropenia, growth retardation, and 3-methylglutaric aciduria. The Barth syndrome is caused by mutations in *TAZ1* located on X-chromosome (Xq28) and encoding mitochondrial protein tafazzin. Cell models based on iPSCs of patients having *TAZ1* mutations have been successfully obtained and used to study effect of the mutations on mitochondria functioning [60].

A recent study showed that cardiomyocyte treatment with antisense oligonucleotides to Ser14450fsX4 mutation in the TTN exon 326 improves DCM phenotype at both structural and functional levels in mice and patient-derived cells. Skipping of the exon with Ser14450fsX4 mutation in patient cardiomyocytes improved myofibril assembly and stability and normalized expression of TTN regulated genes. TTN knock-in in homozygous and heterozygous mice confirmed the effect of exon skipping. This may potentially provide more effective treatment and early prevention of heart failure. However, preclinical research is needed to determine the optimal regimen of treatment with antisense oligonucleotides and to make pharmacokinetic/pharmacodynamic analysis [61].

8. Inherited Hypertrophic Cardiomyopathy

Inherited hypertrophic cardiomyopathy (HCM) is an autosomal-dominant disease which is characterized by structural damage of cardiomyocyte sarcomeres. HCM patients have abnormal increase in left ventricle wall thickness in the absence of enhanced haemodynamic activity and high risk of progressive cardiac failure, arrhythmia, and sudden cardiac death. HCM is one of the most common inherited cardiovascular diseases [55].

In 2013, an iPSC-based model of HCM was created [50]. iPSCs were generated from a family consisting of ten individuals. In the family, mother and four children had missense p.R663H mutation in *MYH7* encoding beta-myosin heavy chain. iPSC-derived mutant cardiomyocytes demonstrated HCM features—enlarged cell size and arrhythmia. The cardiomyocytes had irregular circulation of calcium ions and their content in the cells was highly increased, which was the main mechanism of disease pathogenesis. Furthermore, several drugs that had prevented hypertrophy and electrophysiological disorders were identified [50].

Hypertrophic cardiomyopathy is the main manifestation of a rare inherited syndrome—the LEOPARD syndrome. This name is the acronym of the words denoting its manifestations: lentigines, electrocardiographic abnormalities, ocular hypertelorism, pulmonary valve stenosis, abnormal genitalia, retardation of growth, and deafness. Nearly 90% of the LEOPARD syndrome cases and 45% of Noonan's syndrome cases are caused by missense mutations in *PTPN11* encoding the SHP2 tyrosine phosphatase. In 2010, iPSC-derived cardiomyocytes of two patients having missense p.T468M mutation in *PTPN11* were generated. The patients' cardiomyocytes had a larger size and irregular sarcomere organization and most cells had nuclear localization of NFATC4 which belongs to transcriptional factors involved in hypertrophy development [62].

9. Supravalvular Aortic Stenosis

Supravalvular aortic stenosis (SAS) is a serious disease accompanied by increased proliferation of vascular smooth muscle cells. This results in stenosis and blocking of ascending artery and other major arteries. Patients suffering from the disease are under high risk of sudden cardiac death. Its therapy includes surgical vessel correction, vessel prosthesis, and cardiac transplantation [63]. SAS is caused by heterozygous mutations in *ELN* or deletions in the q-arm of chromosome 7 (7q11.23, Williams-Beuren syndrome) which also involve *ELN*. As deletions in 7q11.23 usually involve up to 28 genes, Williams-Beuren syndrome patients have a more complex phenotype including craniofacial defects and neurobehavioral disorders. Although the Williams-Beuren syndrome is a rare disease with prevalence of 1 : 10000, it is one of the most common vessel diseases having proven inherited nature [63, 64].

ELN encodes the monomeric precursor protein (tropoelastin) which is secreted by arterial smooth muscle cells. Tropoelastin polymerizes and forms elastin which is the main component of extracellular matrix of smooth muscle cells defining vessel elasticity and resistance to constant dynamic action. At present, there are SAS models obtained using laboratory animals [65, 66]. However, application of the models is limited because of functional differences between animal and human smooth muscle cells. Studying SAS is also complicated by insufficient biopsy material of patients and low viability of smooth muscle cells in culture [67, 68]. Thus, using patient-specific iPSCs as well as their directed differentiation into smooth muscle cells seems to be a very prospective tool for generating SAS models.

Such iPSCs have been obtained from a patient having 4-nucleotide insertion in *ELN* causing a frameshift mutation and premature transcription termination in exon 10 and from Williams-Beuren syndrome patients [4, 69]. As compared to the control cells, the patient-specific iPSC-derived smooth muscle cells were found to have abnormal organization of alpha-actin filaments, high rate of proliferation and migration, low sensitivity to vasoactive drugs (carbachol and endothelin-1), and decreased capacity of vessel-like structure formation [4, 69]. Application of recombinant elastin and small GTPase RhoA activation by tropomyosin allowed correcting the process of actin filament formation [69]. Furthermore, a specific kinase inhibitor ERK1/2 or rapamycin (mTOR signaling cascade inhibitor) significantly reduced abnormal rate of mutant cells proliferation [4, 69].

10. Problems and Prospects of Creating and Application of Inherited Cardiovascular Disease Cell Models

Protocols allowing highly efficient iPSC differentiation into cardiomyocytes have been developed. In some protocols, treatment of embryoid bodies (EBs) with different combinations of growth factors was used [70–72]. Later, protocols based on monolayer differentiation and TGF-beta subfamily receptor stimulation with activin A and bone morphogenetic protein 4 (BMP4) were developed [73, 74]. Another approach to cardiac monolayer differentiation is WNT signaling pathway activation with GSK3 protein kinase inhibitor, CHIR99021, followed by WNT repression with IWP2 [75]. An optimized inexpensive and simple cardiac differentiation protocol using metabolic selection for cardiomyocyte enrichment was also developed [76].

Although protocols of directed cardiac differentiation are being improved, most iPSC-CMs are known to have immature phenotype. Although iPSC-CMs express relevant ion channel genes (SCN5A, KCNJ2, CACNA1C, KCNQ1, and KCNH2), structural genes (MYH6, MYLPF, MYBPC3, DES, TNNT2, and TNNI3), and transcription factors (NKX2.5, GATA4, and GATA6) [77], they differ from adult ventricular cardiomyocytes in a number of properties. iPSC-CMs have smaller cell size, exhibit reduced inward rectifier K currents and the presence of prominent pacemaker currents, and manifest spontaneous membrane depolarizations. In addition, lack of t-tubules and disorganized sarcomeres are observed in iPSC-CMs. The relative immaturity of iPSC-CMs limits their usage in disease modeling, drug screening, and regenerative medicine [78]. Attempts to circumvent this limitation have shown that long-term cultivation of iPSC-CMs improves sarcomere organization [79]. In addition, external signals, such as electrical stimulation and mechanical cyclic stretching, were reported to promote functional iPSC-CM maturation [80, 81].

To date a great number of experimental evidences confirm that cell models can reproduce *in vitro* various aspects of disease pathologic phenotype. In addition, there are successful attempts to create systems to test drugs for their ability to treat disease symptoms at the cell level and their potential cardiotoxicity [82]. However, the number of iPSC lines with a certain genotype obtained for each disease is limited. Therefore, researches have to use cells carrying a limited spectrum of mutations whereas the real number of disease causing mutations can be tens or even hundreds of times higher. For example, more than 1400 mutations in more than 20 genes are known for inherited hypertrophic cardiomyopathy [83]. Such genetic diversity can cause variability in disease manifestations, which may require different approaches to disease therapy [84, 85]. This problem can be solved by creating biobanks of patient-specific iPSCs which would cover a wide range of genotypes including the rare ones (reviewed in [86, 87]). In the biobanks patient-specific iPSC lines are fully characterized, stored under common conditions, and licensed for use in research. The cell lines from the biobanks can be available to a wide range of researchers from academic institutions and pharmaceutical companies.

Another problem is selection of control cells for modeling and studying inherited cardiovascular diseases. Control cells are usually obtained from healthy people so they have another genetic background (SNPs set). Moreover, pluripotent cell lines can differ from each other in their differentiation potentials, proliferation rates, and other features, even if they were generated by one method and in one laboratory. The peculiarities may have effect on accuracy of research results. The problem can be solved by using new methods of genome engineering such as homologous recombination mediated by TALENs (Transcription Activator-Like Effector Nucleases) and CRISPR (Clustered Regularly Interspaced Short Palindromic Repeats)/Cas9. The method allows correcting existing mutations in genomes of pluripotent cells and creating so-called isogenic pluripotent cell lines that differ from each other in only one mutation. TALENs and CRISPR/Cas9 can also be used to introduce new mutations in pluripotent cell genomes. This is especially important in the case of rare mutations because the problem of availability of patients carrying the rare mutations is still acute. Genetic constructions that express dominant-negative forms of proteins and are placed in safe harbor loci, such as *AAVS1*, can be applied as well [35, 88]. Besides, the CRISPR/Cas9 system allows studying gene functions and their interaction during formation of a complex pathological phenotype. Moreover, analysis of gene influence on manifestation of phenotypic features can be carried out on genome-wide scale [89, 90]. This is essential for inherited diseases with incomplete penetrance, and this makes it possible to detect modifying genes. Knowledge of existing gene networks, modifying genes, and individual SNPs can give additional possibilities for genetic testing of patients, prediction of disease state pattern, and personalized development of optimal treatment strategy.

Thus, creation of more modern collection, storage, and distribution systems of patient-specific cell lines, as well as new genome editing technologies, can significantly promote application of cardiovascular disease cell models in translational biomedical testing.

11. Conclusion

Search for safer and more effective methods of cardiovascular disease therapy is one of the most important trends in modern pharmacology. Among all cardiovascular diseases, inherited ones are of special interest. Most of them have Mendel inheritance pattern. Several hundreds of disease causing mutations have been described. However, disease pathogenesis at the molecular and cellular levels is still poorly understood in most cases. Studying patient-specific iPSC-derived cardiomyocytes has shown that they are able to reproduce most peculiarities of pathological phenotype, such as electrophysiological abnormalities, sensitivity to some drugs, and other factors. iPSC-derived cardiomyocytes can be also used as platforms for drug testing that may become a basis for large-scale screening of small-molecular compound libraries. Additionally, the models can be successfully applied to study new methods of genome engineering, for example, TALENs and CRISPR/Cas9. To date obtaining a collection of iPSC lines that correspond to maximum genetic diversity (mutation variants and disease modifying SNPs), creating biobanks of cell models, improving methods of directed iPSC differentiation into cardiomyocytes, and scaling of the technology are current tasks of regenerative medicine.

Competing Interests

The authors declare that they have no competing interests.

Acknowledgments

This work was supported by the Federal Research Center Institute of Cytology and Genetics SB RAS budget Project VI.60.1.2 and the Russian Foundation for Basic Research (Grants nos. 14-04-00082 and 14-04-31906).

References

[1] G. Salama and B. London, "Mouse models of long QT syndrome," *The Journal of Physiology*, vol. 578, no. 1, pp. 43–53, 2007.

[2] J. Egido, C. Zaragoza, C. Gomez-Guerrero et al., "Animal models of cardiovascular diseases," *Journal of Biomedicine and Biotechnology*, vol. 2011, Article ID 497841, 13 pages, 2011.

[3] K. Takahashi and S. Yamanaka, "Induction of pluripotent stem cells from mouse embryonic and adult fibroblast cultures by defined factors," *Cell*, vol. 126, no. 4, pp. 663–676, 2006.

[4] C. Kinnear, W. Y. Chang, S. Khattak et al., "Modeling and rescue of the vascular phenotype of Williams-Beuren syndrome in patient induced pluripotent stem cells," *Stem Cells Translational Medicine*, vol. 2, no. 1, pp. 2–15, 2013.

[5] M. Yazawa, B. Hsueh, X. Jia et al., "Using induced pluripotent stem cells to investigate cardiac phenotypes in Timothy syndrome," *Nature*, vol. 471, no. 7337, pp. 230–236, 2011.

[6] S. P. Paşca, T. Portmann, I. Voineagu et al., "Using iPSC-derived neurons to uncover cellular phenotypes associated with Timothy syndrome," *Nature Medicine*, vol. 17, no. 12, pp. 1657–1662, 2011.

[7] D. Prè, M. W. Nestor, A. A. Sproul et al., "A time course analysis of the electrophysiological properties of neurons differentiated from human induced pluripotent stem cells (iPSCs)," *PLoS ONE*, vol. 9, no. 7, Article ID e103418, 2014.

[8] M. E. Brown, E. Rondon, D. Rajesh et al., "Derivation of induced pluripotent stem cells from human peripheral blood T lymphocytes," *PLoS ONE*, vol. 5, no. 6, Article ID e11373, 2010.

[9] T. Seki, S. Yuasa, and K. Fukuda, "Derivation of induced pluripotent stem cells from human peripheral circulating T cells," in *Current Protocols in Stem Cell Biology*, John Wiley & Sons, 2007.

[10] N. Sun, N. J. Panetta, D. M. Gupta et al., "Feeder-free derivation of induced pluripotent stem cells from adult human adipose stem cells," *Proceedings of the National Academy of Sciences of the United States of America*, vol. 106, no. 37, pp. 15720–15725, 2009.

[11] M. Lee, A. J. Flammer, L. O. Lerman, and A. Lerman, "Personalized medicine in cardiovascular diseases," *Korean Circulation Journal*, vol. 42, no. 9, pp. 583–591, 2012.

[12] T. Shinozawa, H. Furukawa, E. Sato, and K. Takami, "A novel purification method of murine embryonic stem cell- and human-induced pluripotent stem cell-derived cardiomyocytes by simple manual dissociation," *Journal of Biomolecular Screening*, vol. 17, no. 5, pp. 683–691, 2012.

[13] T. Grosser, S. Fries, and G. A. FitzGerald, "Biological basis for the cardiovascular consequences of COX-2 inhibition: therapeutic challenges and opportunities," *The Journal of Clinical Investigation*, vol. 116, no. 1, pp. 4–15, 2006.

[14] J. E. May, J. Xu, H. R. Morse, N. D. Avent, and C. Donaldson, "Toxicity testing: the search for an in vitro alternative to animal testing," *British Journal of Biomedical Science*, vol. 66, no. 3, pp. 160–165, 2009.

[15] P. S. Price, R. E. Keenan, and J. C. Swartout, "Characterizing interspecies uncertainty using data from studies of antineoplastic agents in animals and humans," *Toxicology and Applied Pharmacology*, vol. 233, no. 1, pp. 64–70, 2008.

[16] P. T. Sager, G. Gintant, J. R. Turner, S. Pettit, and N. Stockbridge, "Rechanneling the cardiac proarrhythmia safety paradigm: a meeting report from the Cardiac Safety Research Consortium," *American Heart Journal*, vol. 167, no. 3, pp. 292–300, 2014.

[17] D. Rajamohan, E. Matsa, S. Kalra et al., "Current status of drug screening and disease modelling in human pluripotent stem cells," *BioEssays*, vol. 35, no. 3, pp. 281–298, 2013.

[18] L. Crotti, G. Celano, F. Dagradi, and P. J. Schwartz, "Congenital long QT syndrome," *Orphanet Journal of Rare Diseases*, vol. 3, no. 1, article 18, 2008.

[19] P. L. Hedley, P. Jørgensen, S. Schlamowitz et al., "The genetic basis of long QT and short QT syndromes: a mutation update," *Human Mutation*, vol. 30, no. 11, pp. 1486–1511, 2009.

[20] A. S. Amin, Y. M. Pinto, and A. A. M. Wilde, "Long QT syndrome: beyond the causal mutation," *The Journal of Physiology*, vol. 591, no. 17, pp. 4125–4139, 2013.

[21] C. Sims, S. Reisenweber, P. C. Viswanathan, B.-R. Choi, W. H. Walker, and G. Salama, "Sex, age, and regional differences in L-type calcium current are important determinants of arrhythmia phenotype in rabbit hearts with drug-induced long QT type 2," *Circulation Research*, vol. 102, no. 9, pp. e86–e100, 2008.

[22] J. R. Giudicessi and M. J. Ackerman, "Arrhythmia risk in long QT syndrome: beyond the disease-causative mutation,"

Circulation: Cardiovascular Genetics, vol. 6, no. 4, pp. 313–316, 2013.

[23] I. C. R. M. Kolder, M. W. T. Tanck, P. G. Postema et al., "Analysis for genetic modifiers of disease severity in patients with long-QT syndrome type 2," *Circulation: Cardiovascular Genetics*, vol. 8, no. 3, pp. 447–456, 2015.

[24] A. Moretti, M. Bellin, A. Welling et al., "Patient-specific induced pluripotent stem-cell models for long-QT syndrome," *New England Journal of Medicine*, vol. 363, no. 15, pp. 1397–1409, 2010.

[25] T. Egashira, S. Yuasa, T. Suzuki et al., "Disease characterization using LQTS-specific induced pluripotent stem cells," *Cardiovascular Research*, vol. 95, no. 4, pp. 419–429, 2012.

[26] I. Itzhaki, L. Maizels, I. Huber et al., "Modelling the long QT syndrome with induced pluripotent stem cells," *Nature*, vol. 471, no. 7337, pp. 225–230, 2011.

[27] E. Matsa, D. Rajamohan, E. Dick et al., "Drug evaluation in cardiomyocytes derived from human induced pluripotent stem cells carrying a long QT syndrome type 2 mutation," *European Heart Journal*, vol. 32, no. 8, pp. 952–962, 2011.

[28] U. Krause, V. Gravenhorst, T. Kriebel, W. Ruschewski, and T. Paul, "A rare association of long QT syndrome and syndactyly: Timothy Syndrome (LQT 8)," *Clinical Research in Cardiology*, vol. 100, no. 12, pp. 1123–1127, 2011.

[29] A. L. Lahti, V. J. Kujala, H. Chapman et al., "Model for long QT syndrome type 2 using human iPS cells demonstrates arrhythmogenic characteristics in cell culture," *DMM Disease Models and Mechanisms*, vol. 5, no. 2, pp. 220–230, 2012.

[30] C. Terrenoire, K. Wang, K. W. Chan Tung et al., "Induced pluripotent stem cells used to reveal drug actions in a long QT syndrome family with complex genetics," *Journal of General Physiology*, vol. 141, no. 1, pp. 61–72, 2013.

[31] D. Ma, H. Wei, Y. Zhao et al., "Modeling type 3 long QT syndrome with cardiomyocytes derived from patient-specific induced pluripotent stem cells," *International Journal of Cardiology*, vol. 168, no. 6, pp. 5277–5286, 2013.

[32] E. Matsa, J. E. Dixon, C. Medway et al., "Allele-specific RNA interference rescues the long-QT syndrome phenotype in human-induced pluripotency stem cell cardiomyocytes," *European Heart Journal*, vol. 35, no. 16, pp. 1078–1087, 2014.

[33] R. P. Davis, S. Casini, C. W. van den Berg et al., "Cardiomyocytes derived from pluripotent stem cells recapitulate electrophysiological characteristics of an overlap syndrome of cardiac sodium channel disease," *Circulation*, vol. 125, no. 25, pp. 3079–3091, 2012.

[34] D. Malan, S. Friedrichs, B. K. Fleischmann, and P. Sasse, "Cardiomyocytes obtained from induced pluripotent stem cells with Long-QT syndrome 3 recapitulate typical disease-specific features in vitro," *Circulation Research*, vol. 109, no. 8, pp. 841–847, 2011.

[35] M. Bellin, S. Casini, R. P. Davis et al., "Isogenic human pluripotent stem cell pairs reveal the role of a KCNH2 mutation in long-QT syndrome," *The EMBO Journal*, vol. 32, no. 24, pp. 3161–3175, 2013.

[36] N. Liu, Y. Ruan, and S. G. Priori, "Catecholaminergic polymorphic ventricular tachycardia," *Progress in Cardiovascular Diseases*, vol. 51, no. 1, pp. 23–30, 2008.

[37] M. M. Scheinman and J. Lam, "Exercise-induced ventricular arrhythmias in patients with no structural cardiac disease," *Annual Review of Medicine*, vol. 57, pp. 473–484, 2006.

[38] E. S. Kaufman, "Mechanisms and clinical management of inherited channelopathies: long QT syndrome, Brugada syndrome, catecholaminergic polymorphic ventricular tachycardia, and short QT syndrome," *Heart Rhythm*, vol. 6, no. 8, supplement, pp. S51–S55, 2009.

[39] A. Novak, A. Lorber, J. Itskovitz-Eldor, and O. Binah, "Modeling catecholaminergic polymorphic ventricular tachycardia using induced pluripotent stem cell-derived cardiomyocytes," *Rambam Maimonides Medical Journal*, vol. 3, no. 3, Article ID e0015, 2012.

[40] M. Cerrone, B. Colombi, M. Santoro et al., "Bidirectional ventricular tachycardia and fibrillation elicited in a knock-in mouse model carrier of a mutation in the cardiac ryanodine receptor," *Circulation Research*, vol. 96, no. 10, pp. e77–e82, 2005.

[41] M. R. di Barletta, S. Viatchenko-Karpinski, A. Nori et al., "Clinical phenotype and functional characterization of CASQ2 mutations associated with catecholaminergic polymorphic ventricular tachycardia," *Circulation*, vol. 114, no. 10, pp. 1012–1019, 2006.

[42] P. J. Kannankeril, B. M. Mitchell, S. A. Goonasekera et al., "Mice with the R176Q cardiac ryanodine receptor mutation exhibit catecholamine-induced ventricular tachycardia and cardiomyopathy," *Proceedings of the National Academy of Sciences of the United States of America*, vol. 103, no. 32, pp. 12179–12184, 2006.

[43] N. Liu, B. Colombi, M. Memmi et al., "Arrhythmogenesis in catecholaminergic polymorphic ventricular tachycardia: insights from a RyR2 R4496C knock-in mouse model," *Circulation Research*, vol. 99, no. 3, pp. 292–298, 2006.

[44] D. Terentyev, A. Nori, M. Santoro et al., "Abnormal interactions of calsequestrin with the ryanodine receptor calcium release channel complex linked to exercise-induced sudden cardiac death," *Circulation Research*, vol. 98, no. 9, pp. 1151–1158, 2006.

[45] A. Fatima, G. Xu, K. Shao et al., "In vitro modeling of ryanodine receptor 2 dysfunction using human induced pluripotent stem cells," *Cellular Physiology and Biochemistry*, vol. 28, no. 4, pp. 579–592, 2011.

[46] C. B. Jung, A. Moretti, M. Mederos y Schnitzler et al., "Dantrolene rescues arrhythmogenic RYR2 defect in a patient-specific stem cell model of catecholaminergic polymorphic ventricular tachycardia," *EMBO Molecular Medicine*, vol. 4, no. 3, pp. 180–191, 2012.

[47] K. Kujala, J. Paavola, A. Lahti et al., "Cell model of catecholaminergic polymorphic ventricular tachycardia reveals early and delayed after depolarizations," *PLoS ONE*, vol. 7, no. 9, Article ID e44660, 2012.

[48] O. Caspi, I. Huber, A. Gepstein et al., "Modeling of arrhythmogenic right ventricular cardiomyopathy with human induced pluripotent stem cells," *Circulation: Cardiovascular Genetics*, vol. 6, no. 6, pp. 557–568, 2013.

[49] C. Kim, J. Wong, J. Wen et al., "Studying arrhythmogenic right ventricular dysplasia with patient-specific iPSCs," *Nature*, vol. 494, no. 7435, pp. 105–110, 2013.

[50] F. Lan, A. S. Lee, P. Liang et al., "Abnormal calcium handling properties underlie familial hypertrophic cardiomyopathy pathology in patient-specific induced pluripotent stem cells," *Cell Stem Cell*, vol. 12, no. 1, pp. 101–113, 2013.

[51] N. Sun, M. Yazawa, J. Liu et al., "Patient-specific induced pluripotent stem cells as a model for familial dilated cardiomyopathy," *Science Translational Medicine*, vol. 4, no. 130, Article ID 130ra47, 2012.

[52] H.-F. Tse, J. C. Y. Ho, S.-W. Choi et al., "Patient-specific induced-pluripotent stem cells-derived cardiomyocytes recapitulate the pathogenic phenotypes of dilated cardiomyopathy due to a

novel DES mutation identified by whole exome sequencing," *Human Molecular Genetics*, vol. 22, no. 7, pp. 1395–1403, 2013.

[53] M. M. Awad, H. Calkins, and D. P. Judge, "Mechanisms of disease: molecular genetics of arrhythmogenic right ventricular dysplasia/cardiomyopathy," *Nature Clinical Practice Cardiovascular Medicine*, vol. 5, no. 5, pp. 258–267, 2008.

[54] D. Ma, H. Wei, J. Lu et al., "Generation of patient-specific induced pluripotent stem cell-derived cardiomyocytes as a cellular model of arrhythmogenic right ventricular cardiomyopathy," *European Heart Journal*, vol. 34, no. 15, pp. 1122–1133, 2013.

[55] B. J. Maron, J. A. Towbin, G. Thiene et al., "Contemporary definitions and classification of the cardiomyopathies: an American Heart Association Scientific Statement from the Council on Clinical Cardiology, Heart Failure and Transplantation Committee; Quality of Care and Outcomes Research and Functional Genomics and Translational Biology Interdisciplinary Working Groups; and Council on Epidemiology and Prevention," *Circulation*, vol. 113, no. 14, pp. 1807–1816, 2006.

[56] S. Roura and A. Bayes-Genis, "Vascular dysfunction in idiopathic dilated cardiomyopathy," *Nature Reviews Cardiology*, vol. 6, no. 9, pp. 590–598, 2009.

[57] R. E. Hershberger and J. D. Siegfried, "Update 2011: clinical and genetic issues in familial dilated cardiomyopathy," *Journal of the American College of Cardiology*, vol. 57, no. 16, pp. 1641–1649, 2011.

[58] C. Hedberg, A. Melberg, A. Kuhl, D. Jenne, and A. Oldfors, "Autosomal dominant myofibrillar myopathy with arrhythmogenic right ventricular cardiomyopathy 7 is caused by a des mutation," *European Journal of Human Genetics*, vol. 20, no. 9, pp. 984–985, 2012.

[59] K. Wahbi, A. Béhin, P. Charron et al., "High cardiovascular morbidity and mortality in myofibrillar myopathies due to DES gene mutations: a 10-year longitudinal study," *Neuromuscular Disorders*, vol. 22, no. 3, pp. 211–218, 2012.

[60] J. Dudek, I.-F. Cheng, M. Balleininger et al., "Cardiolipin deficiency affects respiratory chain function and organization in an induced pluripotent stem cell model of Barth syndrome," *Stem Cell Research*, vol. 11, no. 2, pp. 806–819, 2013.

[61] M. Gramlich, L. S. Pane, Q. Zhou et al., "Antisense-mediated exon skipping: a therapeutic strategy for titin-based dilated cardiomyopathy," *EMBO Molecular Medicine*, vol. 7, no. 5, pp. 562–576, 2015.

[62] X. Carvajal-Vergara, A. Sevilla, S. L. Dsouza et al., "Patient-specific induced pluripotent stem-cell-derived models of LEOPARD syndrome," *Nature*, vol. 465, no. 7299, pp. 808–812, 2010.

[63] B. R. Pober, M. Johnson, and Z. Urban, "Mechanisms and treatment of cardiovascular disease in Williams-Beuren syndrome," *The Journal of Clinical Investigation*, vol. 118, no. 5, pp. 1606–1615, 2008.

[64] Z. Urbán, S. Riazi, T. L. Seidl et al., "Connection between elastin haploinsufficiency and increased cell proliferation in patients with supravalvular aortic stenosis and Williams-Beuren syndrome," *American Journal of Human Genetics*, vol. 71, no. 1, pp. 30–44, 2002.

[65] H. C. Dietz and R. P. Mecham, "Mouse models of genetic diseases resulting from mutations in elastic fiber proteins," *Matrix Biology*, vol. 19, no. 6, pp. 481–488, 2000.

[66] S. K. Karnik, J. D. Wythe, L. Sorensen, B. S. Brooke, L. D. Urness, and D. Y. Li, "Elastin induces myofibrillogenesis via a specific domain, VGVAPG," *Matrix Biology*, vol. 22, no. 5, pp. 409–425, 2003.

[67] A. Ruiz-Torres, A. Gimeno, J. Melón, L. Mendez, F. J. Muñoz, and M. Macia, "Age-related loss of proliferative activity of human vascular smooth muscle cells in culture," *Mechanisms of Ageing and Development*, vol. 110, no. 1-2, pp. 49–55, 1999.

[68] J. Thyberg, "Differentiated properties and proliferation of arterial smooth muscle cells in culture," *International Review of Cytology*, vol. 169, pp. 183–265, 1996.

[69] X. Ge, Y. Ren, O. Bartulos et al., "Modeling supravalvular aortic stenosis syndrome with human induced pluripotent stem cells," *Circulation*, vol. 126, no. 14, pp. 1695–1704, 2012.

[70] S. J. Kattman, A. D. Witty, M. Gagliardi et al., "Stage-specific optimization of activin/nodal and BMP signaling promotes cardiac differentiation of mouse and human pluripotent stem cell lines," *Cell Stem Cell*, vol. 8, no. 2, pp. 228–240, 2011.

[71] I. Kehat, D. Kenyagin-Karsenti, M. Snir et al., "Human embryonic stem cells can differentiate into myocytes with structural and functional properties of cardiomyocytes," *Journal of Clinical Investigation*, vol. 108, no. 3, pp. 407–414, 2001.

[72] C. L. Mummery, D. Ward, and R. Passier, "Differentiation of human embryonic stem cells to cardiomyocytes by coculture with endoderm in serum-free medium," *Current Protocols in Stem Cell Biology*, chapter 1, unit 1F.2, 2007.

[73] S. L. Paige, T. Osugi, O. K. Afanasiev, L. Pabon, H. Reinecke, and C. E. Murry, "Endogenous wnt/β-catenin signaling is required for cardiac differentiation in human embryonic stem cells," *PLoS ONE*, vol. 5, no. 6, Article ID e11134, 2010.

[74] J. Zhang, M. Klos, G. F. Wilson et al., "Extracellular matrix promotes highly efficient cardiac differentiation of human pluripotent stem cells: the matrix sandwich method," *Circulation Research*, vol. 111, no. 9, pp. 1125–1136, 2012.

[75] X. Lian, C. Hsiao, G. Wilson et al., "Robust cardiomyocyte differentiation from human pluripotent stem cells via temporal modulation of canonical Wnt signaling," *Proceedings of the National Academy of Sciences of the United States of America*, vol. 109, no. 27, pp. E1848–E1857, 2012.

[76] P. W. Burridge, E. Matsa, P. Shukla et al., "Chemically defined generation of human cardiomyocytes," *Nature Methods*, vol. 11, no. 8, pp. 855–860, 2014.

[77] D. Puppala, L. P. Collis, S. Z. Sun et al., "Comparative gene expression profiling in human-induced pluripotent stem cell—derived cardiocytes and human and cynomolgus heart tissue," *Toxicological Sciences*, vol. 131, no. 1, pp. 292–301, 2013.

[78] I. Karakikes, M. Ameen, V. Termglinchan, and J. C. Wu, "Human induced pluripotent stem cell-derived cardiomyocytes: insights into molecular, cellular, and functional phenotypes," *Circulation Research*, vol. 117, no. 1, pp. 80–88, 2015.

[79] T. Kamakura, T. Makiyama, K. Sasaki et al., "Ultrastructural maturation of human-induced pluripotent stem cell-derived cardiomyocytes in a long-term culture," *Circulation Journal*, vol. 77, no. 5, pp. 1307–1314, 2013.

[80] M. N. Hirt, J. Boeddinghaus, A. Mitchell et al., "Functional improvement and maturation of rat and human engineered heart tissue by chronic electrical stimulation," *Journal of Molecular and Cellular Cardiology*, vol. 74, pp. 151–161, 2014.

[81] D. K. Lieu, J.-D. Fu, N. Chiamvimonvat et al., "Mechanism-based facilitated maturation of human pluripotent stem cell-derived cardiomyocytes," *Circulation: Arrhythmia and Electrophysiology*, vol. 6, no. 1, pp. 191–201, 2013.

[82] P. Liang, F. Lan, A. S. Lee et al., "Drug screening using a library of human induced pluripotent stem cell-derived cardiomyocytes reveals disease-specific patterns of cardiotoxicity," *Circulation*, vol. 127, no. 16, pp. 1677–1691, 2013.

[83] C. Roma-Rodrigues and A. R. Fernandes, "Genetics of hypertrophic cardiomyopathy: advances and pitfalls in molecular diagnosis and therapy," *Application of Clinical Genetics*, vol. 7, pp. 195–208, 2014.

[84] M. Arad, J. G. Seidman, and C. E. Seidman, "Phenotypic diversity in hypertrophic cardiomyopathy," *Human Molecular Genetics*, vol. 11, no. 20, pp. 2499–2506, 2002.

[85] A. J. Marian and R. Roberts, "The molecular genetic basis for hypertrophic cardiomyopathy," *Journal of Molecular and Cellular Cardiology*, vol. 33, no. 4, pp. 655–670, 2001.

[86] M. Rao, "IPSC crowdsourcing: a model for obtaining large panels of stem cell lines for screening," *Cell Stem Cell*, vol. 13, no. 4, pp. 389–391, 2013.

[87] G. N. Stacey, J. M. Crook, D. Hei, and T. Ludwig, "Banking human induced pluripotent stem cells: lessons learned from embryonic stem cells?" *Cell Stem Cell*, vol. 13, no. 4, pp. 385–388, 2013.

[88] Y. Wang, P. Liang, F. Lan et al., "Genome editing of isogenic human induced pluripotent stem cells recapitulates long QT phenotype for drug testing," *Journal of the American College of Cardiology*, vol. 64, no. 5, pp. 451–459, 2014.

[89] S. Konermann, M. D. Brigham, A. E. Trevino et al., "Genome-scale transcriptional activation by an engineered CRISPR-Cas9 complex," *Nature*, vol. 517, no. 7536, pp. 583–588, 2015.

[90] O. Shalem, N. E. Sanjana, E. Hartenian et al., "Genome-scale CRISPR-Cas9 knockout screening in human cells," *Science*, vol. 343, no. 6166, pp. 84–87, 2014.

[91] A. K. Farraj, M. S. Hazari, and W. E. Cascio, "The utility of the small rodent electrocardiogram in toxicology," *Toxicological Sciences*, vol. 121, no. 1, pp. 11–30, 2011.

[92] S. Okata, S. Yuasa, T. Yamane, T. Furukawa, and K. Fukuda, "The generation of induced pluripotent stem cells from a patient with KCNH2 G603D, without LQT2 disease associated symptom," *Journal of Medical and Dental Sciences*, vol. 60, no. 1, pp. 17–22, 2013.

[93] G. Wang, M. L. McCain, L. Yang et al., "Modeling the mitochondrial cardiomyopathy of Barth syndrome with induced pluripotent stem cell and heart-on-chip technologies," *Nature Medicine*, vol. 20, no. 6, pp. 616–623, 2014.

[94] T. Yasuno, K. Osafune, H. Sakurai et al., "Functional analysis of iPSC-derived myocytes from a patient with carnitine palmitoyltransferase II deficiency," *Biochemical and Biophysical Research Communications*, vol. 448, no. 2, pp. 175–181, 2014.

[95] I. Itzhaki, L. Maizels, I. Huber et al., "Modeling of catecholaminergic polymorphic ventricular tachycardia with patient-specific human-induced pluripotent stem cells," *Journal of the American College of Cardiology*, vol. 60, no. 11, pp. 990–1000, 2012.

[96] N. Quarto, B. Leonard, S. Li et al., "Skeletogenic phenotype of human Marfan embryonic stem cells faithfully phenocopied by patient-specific induced-pluripotent stem cells," *Proceedings of the National Academy of Sciences of the United States of America*, vol. 109, no. 1, pp. 215–220, 2012.

[97] H.-P. Huang, P.-H. Chen, W.-L. Hwu et al., "Human Pompe disease-induced pluripotent stem cells for pathogenesis modeling, drug testing and disease marker identification," *Human Molecular Genetics*, vol. 20, no. 24, pp. 4851–4864, 2011.

17

The Relationship between Body Mass Index and the Severity of Coronary Artery Disease in Patients Referred for Coronary Angiography

Anne B. Gregory,[1] Kendra K. Lester,[1] Deborah M. Gregory,[1,2] Laurie K. Twells,[1,3] William K. Midodzi,[1,2] and Neil J. Pearce[2,4]

[1]*Department of Clinical Epidemiology, Faculty of Medicine, Memorial University of Newfoundland, St. John's, NL, Canada A1B 3V6*
[2]*Department of Medicine, Faculty of Medicine, Memorial University of Newfoundland, St. John's, NL, Canada A1B 3V6*
[3]*School of Pharmacy, Memorial University of Newfoundland, St. John's, NL, Canada A1B 3V6*
[4]*Eastern Health, St. John's, NL, Canada A1B 3V6*

Correspondence should be addressed to Deborah M. Gregory; dgregory@mun.ca

Academic Editor: Robert Chen

Background and Aim. Obesity is associated with an increased risk of cardiovascular disease and may be associated with more severe coronary artery disease (CAD); however, the relationship between body mass index [BMI (kg/m^2)] and CAD severity is uncertain and debatable. The aim of this study was to examine the relationship between BMI and angiographic severity of CAD. *Methods.* Duke Jeopardy Score (DJS), a prognostic tool predictive of 1-year mortality in CAD, was assigned to angiographic data of patients ≥18 years of age ($N = 8,079$). Patients were grouped into 3 BMI categories: normal (18.5–24.9 kg/m^2), overweight (25.0–29.9 kg/m^2), and obese (≥30 kg/m^2); and multivariable adjusted hazard ratios for 1-year all-cause and cardiac-specific mortality were calculated. *Results.* Cardiac risk factor prevalence (e.g., diabetes, hypertension, and hyperlipidemia) significantly increased with increasing BMI. Unadjusted all-cause and cardiac-specific 1-year mortality tended to rise with incremental increases in DJS, with the exception of DJS 6 ($p < 0.001$). After adjusting for potential confounders, no significant association of BMI and all-cause (HR 0.70, 95% CI .48–1.02) or cardiac-specific (HR 1.11, 95% CI .64–1.92) mortality was found. *Conclusions.* This study failed to detect an association of BMI with 1-year all-cause or cardiac-specific mortality after adjustment for potential confounding variables.

1. Introduction

Obesity is an independent risk factor for cardiovascular disease (CVD) [1–5] and is associated with advanced CVD requiring procedures such as percutaneous coronary intervention (PCI), reduction in life expectancy [6], and a higher mortality rate [3, 7, 8]. Weight loss has been associated with improvement in preexisting cardiovascular risk factors including hypertension (HTN), diabetes, and dyslipidemia and mortality [9–12]. Other studies have reported improved clinical outcomes in overweight and obese patients treated for CVDs compared to normal weight patients, suggesting a paradoxical survival benefit. This effect has been reported in patients with diabetes [13], end-stage renal disease [14], HTN [15], and other conditions traditionally associated with poorer outcomes [15–23]. Obesity was primarily measured using BMI in the studies. The mechanisms leading to this phenomenon, termed "obesity paradox," are unclear.

The quantification of coronary artery disease (CAD) severity can be captured using coronary angiography (CA) [24]. Historically CAD has been categorized as single, double, and triple vessel and left main disease, with luminal stenosis of either ≥50% (left main) or ≥70% (other major epicardial vessels) used to define significance [25]. Scoring systems to determine the severity of CAD and prognosis were developed to address the perceived limitations associated with stratification of patients with risk level variation [26–28].

Few studies have examined the association of body mass index (BMI) and CAD in patients undergoing CA. In a study by Rubinshtein et al. [29] obese patients referred for CA were younger and had a lower prevalence of left main disease. Niraj et al. [30] also found that obese patients referred for CA were younger and had a lower burden for CAD; however, the authors did not find obesity to be a significant predictor for severity of CAD after adjustment for confounders suggesting that younger age may influence the obesity paradox. Others have reported an inverse relationship between BMI and severity of CAD in a cross-sectional, prospective study of 414 patients with suspected CAD [31].

Obesity is an accepted risk factor for CAD; therefore, it may be assumed that obese patients have poorer outcomes than nonobese patients [32]. However, published findings contradict this supposition about the relationship between BMI and mortality in patients undergoing CA for suspected CAD. The influence of BMI on extent of coronary atherosclerosis and cardiac events in a cohort of patients at risk of CAD was examined by Rossi et al. [33]. BMI was not significantly associated with extent of coronary atherosclerosis and mortality confirming the findings of others [29, 34, 35].

Newfoundland and Labrador (NL), a Canadian province, has the highest rate of obesity in the country and it is estimated that 71% of the province's population will be either overweight or obese by 2019 [36]. The aim of the current study was to examine the relationship between BMI and severity of CAD and determine what impact, if any, BMI had on 1-year mortality in the NL patient population referred for CA at a single tertiary care centre.

2. Methods

2.1. Setting, Study Design, and Data Collection. Secondary analysis of deidentified data for all patients ≥18 years of age that had CA between January 1, 2008, and December 31, 2012, in NL, Canada was conducted using a large population-based clinical database. A clinical software application (i.e., Alberta Provincial Project for Outcome Assessment in Coronary Heart Disease [APPROACH]) is used to prospectively collect detailed demographic, clinical, and procedural data on all patients referred for and undergoing CA and coronary revascularization procedures. Details of the database and methods of collection have been previously described [37].

Patients undergoing CA were identified from the APPROACH-NL database. There were 13936 diagnostic CAs performed from January 1, 2008, to December 31, 2012. Eligible subjects included all residents of NL ≥ 18 years with a BMI ≥ 18.5 kg/m². The index CA and DJS were used; therefore, duplicate cases were excluded. The following patients were also excluded from the study: missing DJS data; missing BMI data or underweight; <18 years of age; missing indication code for CA or if the CA was performed for any reason other than the following: acute coronary syndrome, stable angina, unstable angina, atypical pain, serious arrhythmia, or presenting with cardiovascular symptoms not matching the above-mentioned common diagnostic categories. Since the focus of the study was on patients

with suspected but not yet confirmed CAD, patients with established CAD (i.e., history of CABG, PCI, or myocardial infarction) were excluded from the study. After exclusion criteria were applied, a final study sample of 8,079 patients having a first CA for suspected, but not yet confirmed, CAD was identified.

Weight and height were measured and documented by a nurse at the time of CA. If patients were unstable, self-reported weight and height were collected and BMI calculated. Patients were grouped according to three BMI categories using the World Health Organization classification system: normal (18.5–24.9 kg/m²), overweight (25.0–29.9 kg/m²), and obese class > 30 kg/m² [38] reflective of relative levels of risk to health [39]. Obese patients are much more likely to die from cardiac causes and lean patients are much more likely to die from noncardiac causes over a 10-year period following index myocardial infarction [40]. In the current study, the underweight BMI category (BMI < 18.5 kg/m²) was excluded because of the potential impact of comorbid conditions (e.g., advanced heart failure, cachexia) on outcome, conditions which are not captured in APPROACH-NL.

CA data were obtained from the Coronary Artery Reporting and Archiving Tool (CARAT), a graphic recording and communication application [41]. Detailed angiographic findings of all patients undergoing CA are automatically populated in APPROACH and a PDF file is created containing the anatomy of the coronary arteries according to the DJS [27] and becomes part of each patient's medical record. In the current study, severity and extent of obstructive CAD are based on the DJS. Dash et al. [27] developed the DJS, a prognostic tool predictive of 1-year mortality in patients with CAD, which was validated by Califf et al. [28] in 1985. The coronary tree is divided into 6 segments: the left anterior coronary artery (LAD), diagonal branches of the LAD, septal perforating branches, the circumflex coronary artery, obtuse marginal branches, and the posterior descending coronary artery. All segments with ≥75% stenosis, or ≥50% left main stenosis, are considered to be at risk. Each such segment is assigned 2 points. The maximum possible number of points is 12. A score from 0 to 12 is assigned to each CA based on the number of segments involved and automatically populated in APPROACH. The usefulness of the DJS as a simple score that is easy to use clinically as a prognostic tool has been confirmed in a large Canadian population cohort of >20,000 patients undergoing PCI or CABG [42]. Following PCI, there was no difference between DJSs 0 and 2; however, a stepwise increase in 1-year mortality with a DJS of >2 was found.

Mortality data stored in the NL Centre for Health Information (NLCHI) Mortality System was provided to the cardiac care program via a data linkage. The primary outcomes were 1-year all-cause and cardiac-specific mortality.

2.2. Ethical Considerations. All patients who had a CA during the time period under examination gave written, informed consent to the cardiac care program for data collection and follow-up observation after CA. The study was approved by the provincial Health Research Ethics Authority.

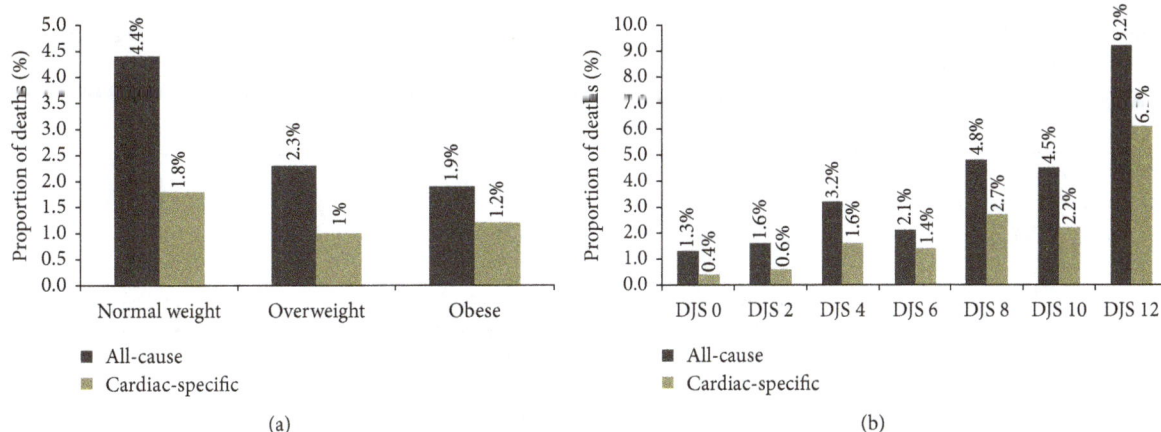

FIGURE 1: (a) Unadjusted 1-year all-cause and cardiac-specific mortality according to BMI. (b) Unadjusted 1-year all-cause and cardiac-specific mortality according to Duke Jeopardy Score.

2.3. Data Analysis. Analyses are based on 8,079 patients with a BMI $\geq 18.5 \, \text{kg/m}^2$ undergoing CA for the first time. Continuous variables are reported as mean ± standard deviation and were compared using ANOVA. Categorical variables are reported as number (%) and were compared using chi-square tests. After the assumptions of survival analysis were met, time-to-event outcomes were analyzed using Kaplan-Meier survival techniques. The final enrollment date was December 31, 2012, and patients without events were censored on December 31, 2013, the final date for which mortality data was available. Survival curves were compared using the log rank test. All factors that could potentially influence survival were included (see characteristics in Table 1) in addition to BMI and DJS. Univariate and multivariate-adjusted Cox regression models were performed to identify predictors of 1-year mortality and compute crude and multivariate-adjusted hazards ratios and 95% confidence intervals as a measure of the relative risk of death at one year for increasing BMI categories. Normal weight was the referent group ($18.5-24.9 \, \text{kg/m}^2$). Covariates included BMI, DJS, age, sex, HTN, diabetes, hyperlipidemia, smoking history, family history of premature CAD, left ventricular (LV) grade, peripheral vascular disease (PVD), chronic obstructive pulmonary disease (COPD), renal insufficiency, dialysis, chronic renal failure (CRF), congestive heart failure (CHF), and malignancy. A two-sided *p* value < 0.05 was considered statistically significant. In the model all independent variables were dichotomous with the exception of age and BMI. BMI was included both as a continuous variable [43] and as an ordinal variable. Obesity was defined as a BMI $\geq 30 \, \text{kg/m}^2$. All statistical analyses were performed using IBM SPSS Statistics for Windows, Version 22.0, Armonk, NY: IBM Corp.

3. Results

Baseline characteristics are presented in Table 1. Among 8,079 patients approximately 84% were overweight or obese: 1,297 (16.1%) had a normal BMI, 3,072 (38%) had a BMI indicating overweight, and 3,710 (45.9%) were classified as obese. The average weight in kilograms for the entire sample was 85.2 ± 17.8 and the average BMI was 30.3 ± 5.7. There were significant differences among BMI categories in terms of age, sex, HTN, diabetes, hyperlipidemia, and family history of premature CAD, COPD, PVD, and LV grade. Significantly higher proportions of males compared to females comprised all BMI categories. As expected, the prevalence of HTN, hyperlipidemia, and diabetes significantly increased with increasing BMI. Patients with obesity were significantly younger and had a higher rate of family history of CAD and COPD. Normal weight patients had a higher rate of PVD, renal insufficiency, dialysis, LV Grades III and IV, and lower rate of admission for acute coronary syndrome (ACS). BMI groups did not differ significantly with regard to smoking history, CRF, CVD, malignancy, or CHF. There were statistically significant differences in medications at time of referral for coronary angiography. Higher proportions of obese patients were taking ACE inhibitors, ARB antagonists, and CCB, and a lower proportion of obese patients were taking ticlopidine/clopidogrel compared to normal or overweight patients.

DJSs calculated during CA by BMI category are presented in Table 1. A score of 0, indicative of a normal angiogram or noncritical (<70%) stenosis in any of the coronary arteries, was assigned to 526 (40.6%) normal weight patients, 1,197 (39.0%) overweight patients, and 1,687 (45.5%) obese patients. Differences were observed among BMI categories and all DJS levels ($p < 0.001$), with the exception of DJS $\geq$ 10. Patients in the obese group tended to have lower scores indicating less CAD severity.

Within the first year of undergoing CA there were 199 deaths (2.5%) among 8,079 patients, of which 99 (1.2%) were cardiac-specific. A higher proportion of deaths due to any cause occurred in patients with normal BMI compared to overweight or obese patients ($p < 0.001$); however, there were no statistically significant differences observed for unadjusted cardiac-specific mortality among BMI categories (Figure 1(a)). Unadjusted mortality tended to rise with incremental increases in DJS scores ($p < 0.001$), with the exception of DJS 6 (Figure 1(b)).

TABLE 1: Baseline characteristics of study subjects undergoing coronary angiography in relation to BMI category and Duke Jeopardy Score (DJS) based on coronary angiographic findings in relation to BMI category ($N = 8079$).

Variable	Normal $n = 1297$	Overweight $n = 3072$	Obese $n = 3710$	p value[*]
Weight (kgs ± SD)	64.7 ± 8.8	78.8 ± 9.3	97.7 ± 16.0	0.000
BMI (mean ± SD)	22.9 ± 1.6	27.6 ± 1.4	35.0 ± 4.7	0.000
Age, years (mean ± SD)	63.4 ± 11.3	62.1 ± 10.6	59.7 ± 10.2	0.000
Male sex	744/1297 (57.4%)	2081/3072 (67.7%)	2249/3710 (60.6%)	0.000
HTN	735/1297 (56.7%)	1870/3069 (60.9%)	2629/3704 (71.0%)	0.000
Hyperlipidemia	991/1297 (76.4%)	2433/3068 (79.3%)	3022/3706 (81.5%)	0.000
Family history of premature CAD[†]	730/1295 (56.4%)	1925/3063 (62.8%)	2421/3695 (65.5%)	0.000
Current/former smoker	889/1295 (68.6%)	2105/3060 (68.8%)	2557/3693 (69.2%)	0.890
Diabetes	203/1297 (15.7%)	638/3069 (20.8%)	1279/3708 (34.5%)	0.000
Renal insufficiency	67/1296 (5.2%)	124/3069 (4.0%)	130/3705 (3.5%)	0.030
Dialysis	16/1296 (1.2%)	15/3069 (0.5%)	19/3705 (0.5%)	0.009
CRF	38/1296 (2.9%)	69/3069 (2.2%)	75/3705 (2.0%)	0.166
Malignancy	67/1296 (5.2%)	132/3069 (4.3%)	153/3705 (4.1%)	0.282
COPD	210/1297 (16.2%)	398/3069 (13.0%)	697/3705 (18.8%)	0.000
PVD	91/1297 (7.0%)	131/3069 (4.3%)	139/3705 (3.8%)	0.000
CHF	25/1296 (1.9%)	54/3069 (1.8%)	81/3705 (2.2%)	0.450
CVD	90/1296 (6.9%)	163/3069 (5.3%)	204/3705 (5.5%)	0.088
ACS ($n = 4359$)	842 (19.3)	1709 (39.2)	1808 (41.5)	
STEMI	243 (28.9)	426 (39.2)	419 (38.5)	
Non-STEMI	382 (45.4)	791 (46.3)	850 (47.0)	0.000
Unstable angina	217 (25.8)	492 (28.8)	539 (29.8)	
LV grade				
I (>50%)	1067/1286 (83.0%)	2557/3033 (84.3%)	3154/3668 (86.0%)	
II (35–50%)	136/1286 (10.6%)	334/3033 (11.0%)	353/3668 (9.6%)	0.003
III (20–34%)	52/1286 (4.0%)	110/3033 (3.6%)	110/3668 (3.0%)	
IV (<20%)	31/1286 (2.4%)	32/3033 (1.1%)	51/3668 (1.4%)	
DJS				
≥2	771/1297 (59.4)	1875/3072 (61.0)	2023/3710 (54.5)	0.000
≥4	542/1297 (41.8)	1229/3072 (40.0)	1303/3710 (35.1)	0.000
≥6	424/1297 (32.7)	966/3072 (31.4)	992/3710 (26.7)	0.000
≥8	248/1297 (19.1)	56/3072 (18.5)	593/3710 (16.0)	0.006
≥10	162/1297 (12.5)	369/3072 (12.0)	395/3710 (10.6)	0.096
12	91/1297 (7.0)	198/3072 (6.4)	188/3710 (5.1)	0.010
Medications at time of referral				
Aspirin	1162/1297 (89.6)	2780/3071 (90.5)	3294/3709 (88.8)	0.071
Beta blockers	990/1295 (76.4)	2313/3071 (75.3)	2806/3709 (75.7)	0.729
ACE inhibitors	514/1295 (39.7)	1279/3071 (41.6)	1651/3708 (44.5)	0.004
ARB antagonists	116/1295 (9.0)	357/3071 (11.6)	663/3708 (17.9)	0.000
CCB	161/1295 (12.4)	446/3071 (14.5)	619/3708 (16.7)	0.000
Statin therapy	972/1296 (75.0)	2382/3071 (77.6)	2897/3709 (78.1)	0.068
LA nitrates	264/1295 (20.4)	629/3071 (20.5)	769/3709 (20.7)	0.951
Ticlopidine/clopidogrel	800/1297 (61.7)	1603/3071 (52.2)	1699/3708 (45.8)	0.000

Values are means ± SD or % (n/N).

ACE = angiotensin converting enzyme; ACS = acute coronary syndrome; ARB = angiotensin receptor blocker; CAD = coronary artery disease; CCB = calcium channel blockers; CHF = congestive heart failure; COPD = chronic obstructive pulmonary disease; CRF = chronic renal failure; CVD = cerebrovascular disease; DJS = Duke Jeopardy Score; HTN = hypertension; LA = long-acting; PVD = peripheral vascular disease.

[†]Family history of CAD is positive if the patient has/had any direct blood relative (parent, siblings, and children) who have been diagnosed with angina, MI, or sudden cardiac death before age of 55 years.

Note. DJS, Duke Jeopardy Score, is a score from 0 to 12 which estimates the amount of myocardium at risk on the basis of particular location of stenosis. A score of 0 is indicative of a normal angiogram or noncritical (<70%) stenosis in any of the coronary arteries. A score of 0 was assigned to 526 (40.6%) normal weight patients, 1197 (39.0%) overweight patients, and 1687 (45.5%) obese patients.

[*]p value for chi-square for categorical variables or ANOVA for continuous variables.

TABLE 2: Correlates of 1-year all-cause mortality calculated by Cox proportional hazards multiple regression analysis.

	Overall n − 8079	β	SE	Wald χ^2	p value	HR	95% CI
Age	61.2 ± 10.6	.044	.008	26.802	0.000	1.04	1.03–1.06
DJS							
0 (referent category)	3410 (42.2%)			28.637	0.000		
2	1595 (19.7%)	−.021	.253	.007	0.932	.98	.60–1.61
4	692 (8.6%)	.296	.277	1.14	0.286	1.35	.78–2.31
6	973 (12.0%)	−.017	.286	.003	0.953	.98	.56–1.72
8	483 (6.0%)	.761	.268	8.088	0.004	2.14	1.27–3.62
10	449 (5.6%)	.662	.282	5.501	0.019	1.94	1.12–3.37
12	198 (6.4%)	.998	.239	17.415	0.000	2.71	1.70–4.33
BMI category							
Normal weight (referent category)	1297 (16.1)			4.213	0.122		
Overweight	3072 (38)	−.341	.189	3.255	0.071	.71	.49–1.03
Obese	3710 (45.9)	−.356	.194	3.37	0.066	.70	.48–1.02
LV Grade							
Grade I (referent category)	6778 (84.9)			50.146	0.000		
Grade II	823 (10.3)	.309	.216	2.038	0.153	1.36	.89–2.08
Grade III	272 (3.4)	1.226	.222	30.423	0.000	3.41	2.20–5.27
Grade IV	114 (1.4)	1.568	.280	31.337	0.000	4.80	2.77–8.31
Hypertension	5234 (64.9%)	−.040	.179	.050	0.823	.96	.68–1.37
Diabetes	342 (36.9%)	.175	.161	1.18	0.277	1.19	.87–1.63
Family history of premature CAD	5076 (63.0%)	−.170	.155	1.19	0.274	.84	.62–1.14
CHF	160 (2.0%)	.384	.259	2.193	0.139	1.47	.88–2.44
PVD	361 (4.5%)	.517	.223	5.361	0.021	1.68	1.08–2.60
CVD	457 (5.7%)	−.041	.232	.032	0.859	.96	.61–1.51
COPD	1305 (16.2%)	.585	.166	12.379	0.000	1.79	1.29–2.49
Malignancy	352 (4.4)	.559	.238	5.522	0.019	1.75	1.10–2.79
Renal insufficiency	321 (4.0%)	.666	.305	4.75	0.029	1.95	1.07–3.54
CRF	182 (2.3)	.355	.375	.898	0.343	1.43	0.89–4.28
Dialysis	50 (0.6)	.665	.402	2.738	0.098	1.95	0.68–2.97
Current/former smoker	5551 (69.0%)	.196	.174	1.26	0.262	1.22	.86–1.71

BMI = body mass index; CHF = congestive heart failure; CI = confidence interval; COPD = chronic obstructive pulmonary disease; CRF = chronic renal failure; CVD = cerebrovascular disease; DJS = Duke Jeopardy Score; HR = hazard ratio; LV = left ventricular; PVD = peripheral vascular disease; SE = standard error.

The unadjusted 1-year all-cause survival rates among the BMI categories revealed that the normal weight group had a higher mortality than the obese and overweight groups ($p < 0.001$) (Figure 2(a)). There were no significant differences among BMI categories for cardiac-specific mortality ($p = 0.106$) (Figure 2(b)).

Factors significantly associated with 1-year all-cause mortality during univariate analyses included age, HTN, diabetes, family history of premature CAD, CHF, PVD, CVD, COPD, malignancy, renal insufficiency, CRF, dialysis, DJS, and BMI as both categorical and continuous variable. The variables gender and hyperlipidemia were not significant. All statistically and clinically significant variables with p values < 0.20 were included in multivariate Cox proportional regression analysis. Significant correlates of 1-year all-cause mortality included age, diabetes, PVD, COPD, malignancy,

renal insufficiency, DJSs 8, 10, and 12, and LV Grades III and IV. BMI was not a statistically significant correlate of all-cause mortality (Table 2). Cox regression analysis was also performed using BMI as a continuous variable; however, it was not a significant factor associated with 1-year all-cause mortality (data not shown).

Significant correlates of 1-year cardiac-specific mortality included age, CHF, DJSs 4 to 12, and LV Grades III and IV, but not BMI (Table 3).

4. Discussion

Our study examined the relationship between BMI and CAD and 1-year mortality in a large cohort of patients undergoing CA for suspected, but not yet confirmed, CAD. 84% of

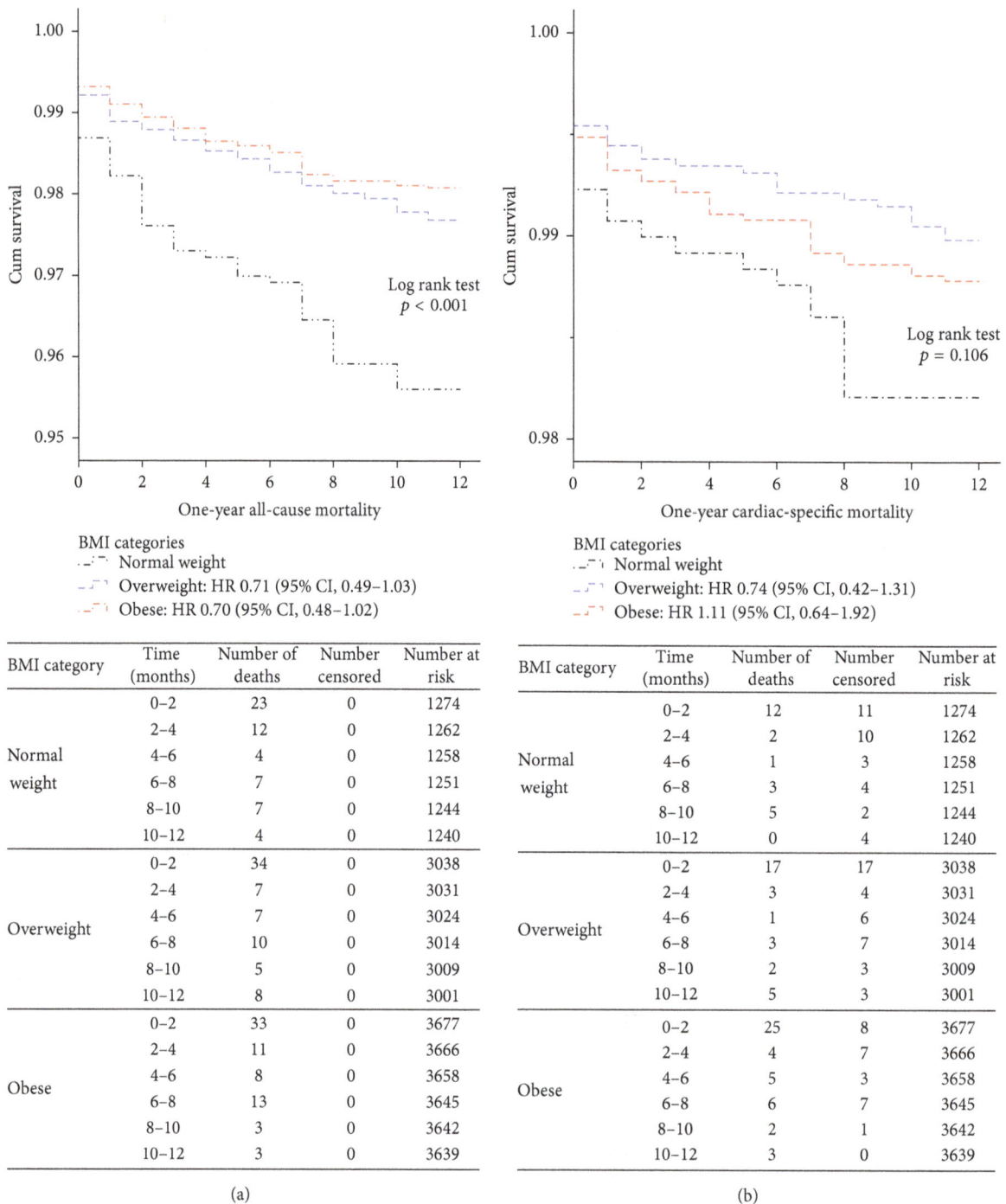

FIGURE 2: (a) Unadjusted Kaplan Meier and 1-year all-cause mortality in patients undergoing coronary angiography by BMI. (b) Unadjusted Kaplan Meier and 1-year cardiac-specific mortality in patients undergoing coronary angiography by BMI.

patients were overweight and obese. In the current study, obese patients were significantly younger (i.e., 3.7 years) than their nonobese counterparts and presented with less severe CAD based on DJSs despite having a higher prevalence of HTN, hyperlipidemia, and diabetes. Normal weight patients were older, had PVD, and had a history of renal insufficiency or were on dialysis.

Meta-analytic findings suggest a reverse J-shaped relationship between all-cause mortality and cardiovascular mortality and BMI in patients with established CAD [19, 20, 44]. However, very few studies have examined the association of BMI and CAD in patients undergoing CA for suspected, but unconfirmed, CAD. The current study findings support the findings of Rubinshtein et al. [29] and Niraj et al. [30].

TABLE 3: Correlates of 1-year cardiac-specific mortality calculated by Cox proportional hazards multiple regression analysis.

	Overall $n = 8079$	β	SE	Wald χ^2	p value	HR	95% CI
Age	61.2 ± 10.6	.046	.012	14.646	0.000	1.05	1.02–1.07
DJS							
0 (referent category)	3410 (42.2%)			30.545	0.000		
2	1595 (19.7%)	.242	.436	.307	0.579	1.27	.54–3.00
4	692 (8.6%)	1.012	.421	5.763	0.016	2.75	1.20–6.28
6	973 (12.0%)	.941	.401	5.513	0.019	2.56	1.17–5.62
8	483 (6.0%)	1.46	.407	12.854	0.000	4.31	1.94–9.57
10	449 (5.6%)	1.245	.432	8.317	0.004	3.47	1.49–8.09
12	198 (6.4%)	1.762	.367	23.023	0.000	5.83	2.84–11.99
BMI category							
Normal weight (referent category)	1297 (16.1)			2.72	0.257		
Overweight	3072 (38)	−.305	.293	1.083	0.298	.74	.42–1.31
Obese	3710 (45.9)	.100	.284	.126	0.722	1.11	.64–1.92
LV grade							
Grade I (referent category)	6778 (84.9)			37.607	0.000		
Grade II	823 (10.3)	.239	.320	.559	0.455	1.27	.68–2.38
Grade III	272 (3.4)	1.154	.320	12.987	0.000	3.17	1.69–5.94
Grade IV	114 (1.4)	1.98	.348	32.352	0.000	7.24	3.66–14.33
Hypertension	5234 (64.9%)	.112	.274	.167	0.682	1.12	.65–1.91
Diabetes	342 (36.9%)	.312	.225	1.93	0.165	1.37	.88–2.12
Family history of premature CAD	5076 (63.0%)	−.098	.222	.196	0.658	.91	.59–1.40
CHF	160 (2.0%)	.725	.340	4.56	0.033	2.07	1.06–4.02
PVD	361 (4.5%)	.510	.322	2.512	0.113	1.67	.89–3.13
CVD	457 (5.7%)	−.027	.329	.007	0.935	.97	.51–1.89
COPD	1305 (16.2%)	.275	.247	1.238	0.266	1.32	.81–2.14
Malignancy	352 (4.4)	−1.88	1.01	3.491	0.062	.150	.02–1.10
Renal insufficiency	321 (4.0%)	.466	.448	1.085	0.298	1.59	.66–3.83
CRF	182 (2.3)	.2925	.544	.288	0.591	1.34	.46–3.89
Dialysis	50 (0.6)	.422	.636	.440	0.507	1.53	.44–5.31
Current/former smoker	5551 (69.0%)	.272	.255	1.14	0.286	1.31	.86–1.71

BMI = body mass index; CHF = congestive heart failure; CI = confidence interval; COPD = chronic obstructive pulmonary disease; CRF = chronic renal failure; CVD = cerebrovascular disease; DJS = Duke Jeopardy Score; HR = hazard ratio; LV = left ventricular; PVD = peripheral vascular disease; SE = standard error.

Rubinshtein et al. [29] reported an inverse relationship between BMI and severity of CAD among 928 patients with CAD. Risk factors including diabetes, hyperlipidemia, and male gender were also correlated with severity of CAD. Niraj et al. [30] investigated the relationship between severity of CAD and BMI according to the DJS in a sample of 770 patients from the US. The authors also reported a paradoxical relationship. In both studies, obese patients were significantly younger than normal weight and overweight patients, leading to the conclusion that this association could be partly or completely explained by the increased likelihood of early physician referral of obese patients for cardiac catheterization and therefore at an earlier stage of CAD. The inverse relationship between BMI and severity of CAD was also reported most recently by Parsa and Jahanshahi [31] in a cross-sectional prospective study performed between September 2009 and March 2011 among 414 patients with suspected CAD undergoing CA.

After controlling for potential confounders such as other cardiovascular risk factors and comorbidities in our analyses, BMI did not emerge as an independent factor significantly associated with either all-cause or cardiac-specific mortality. Our study lacked the statistical power to support a potential doubling of cardiac-specific mortality or a 36% decrease among the obese group (HR 1.11, 95% CI .64–1.92).

It is important to note that, in the current study, significant proportions of overweight (39%) and obese (45.5%) patients who underwent CA did not have CAD based on angiographic generated DJSs. We were unable to examine the relationship between BMI and mortality in patients who had a CA but were not diagnosed with CAD due to low event rates (45 all-cause and 13 cardiac-specific deaths). An obesity paradox has been reported in patients who had CA with no CAD [19]. Two explanations were given for the unexpected finding: (1) other cardiac risk factors could classify these patients as having "preclinical" disease and that a higher BMI was protective and (2) referral and treatment bias in CAD since obesity is a "visible" risk factor that may predispose physicians to refer obese patients for CA earlier than those with a normal BMI. Niraj et al. [30] also suggested that the trend of normal or minimal change angiography in obese patients may have been due to a tendency of bias of physicians to refer obese patients for earlier angiography. Rubinshtein et al. [29] suggested that a younger age could be associated with a lower prevalence of high-risk coronary anatomy compared with nonobese older patients. This could partially explain the findings of the current study as well. Patients of normal weight were significantly older than their obese counterparts and had more angiographic severe CAD according to their DJSs.

Although the mechanism for the potential protective effect of obesity among patients with CAD remains unclear, a number of potential mechanisms have been proposed: greater metabolic reserves, less cachexia, younger presenting age, more aggressive medical therapy, more aggressive diagnostic and revascularization procedures, increased muscle mass and strength, possible improved cardiorespiratory fitness despite obesity, diminished hormonal response including the renin-angiotensin-aldosterone system, and unmeasured confounders, including selection bias [45]. It has been proposed that the apparent paradox that has been observed by other researchers may be the result of collider stratification, a source of selection bias that is common in epidemiology research [44]. According to Banack and Kaufman [46] the typical demonstration of this bias results from conditioning on a variable affected by exposure with the outcome (referred to as a collider). Distortion of the association between exposure and outcome as a result of this conditioning on a collider can therefore produce a spurious protective association between obesity and mortality in disease groups [46].

Study Strengths and Limitations. Our study has a number of strengths. We report on a large population-based cohort of consecutive patients undergoing CA at a single tertiary cardiac centre using APPROACH-NL prospectively collected data. Data quality assurance indicated that the amount of missing data was minimal (1.2%). Actual measures of weight and height were taken at the time of CA, unless the patients were unstable. In addition, although it is well documented that respondents have a tendency to underestimate their weight and/or overestimate their height, [47] self-reported height and weight are considered valid for identifying relationships in epidemiologic studies [48], with self-reported values being strongly correlated with measured values [49, 50]. We were able to assess the effect of BMI on 1-year all-cause and cardiac-specific mortality in patients with and without CAD using data linkage to up-to-date mortality data.

This study also has limitations. First, our study is an observational nonrandomized cohort study and therefore provides evidence of association not causation. Data from a clinical database was used and as such cannot account for potential residual or unmeasured confounders not captured in the database. Second, the study population was heterogeneous (i.e., included patients with variable levels of coronary artery disease severity ranging from acute coronary syndrome with cardiogenic shock to stable angina). Third, despite its widespread use, the use of BMI in terms of its accuracy to define obesity is controversial given its inability to differentiate lean mass and body fat [51–54]. BMI has been criticized as an inaccurate method to investigate body fatness because it is not as well correlated to CVD and death as other measures of obesity including waist circumference and waist-to-hip ratio [45], data that were unavailable in the APPROACH-NL clinical database. Fourth, BMI was collected at the time of the index CA only and potential changes in BMI were not accessed. Finally, this research examined BMI at an initial point in time and related it to mortality at 1 year. Comparisons were limited to three BMI groups: normal weight, overweight, and obese due to the relatively small sample size for patients and low event rates in the extreme ends of BMI classification.

5. Conclusions

This observational study failed to detect an association of BMI with 1-year all-cause or cardiac-specific mortality after adjustment for potential confounding variables.

Disclosure

Dr. A. Gregory, Kendra Lester, Dr. D. Gregory, Dr. Twells, and Dr. Midodzi have no disclosures to report. Dr. Pearce is the director of the APPROACH-NL cardiac care database, Division Head Cardiology, Eastern Health, and the former director of the Cardiac Catheterization Lab. This was an investigator initiated study.

Authors' Contributions

Anne B. Gregory, Deborah M. Gregory, Laurie K. Twells, and Neil J. Pearce were responsible for study concept and design. Anne B. Gregory, Kendra K. Lester, Neil J. Pearce, Laurie K. Twells, and William K. Midodzi were responsible for analysis and interpretation of the data. Anne B. Gregory and Deborah M. Gregory were responsible for drafting of the manuscript. Anne B. Gregory, Deborah M. Gregory, Kendra K. Lester, Neil J. Pearce, Laurie K. Twells, and William K. Midodzi were responsible for critical revision of the manuscript for important intellectual content. Anne B. Gregory, Deborah M. Gregory, Kendra K. Lester, and William K. Midodzi were responsible for statistical analysis. Deborah M. Gregory and William K. Midodzi had full access to all data in the study and take responsibility for the integrity of the data and the accuracy of the data analysis.

Acknowledgments

The authors gratefully acknowledge the Cardiac Care Program staff for data collection and entry, especially Jennifer Matthews, Program Coordinator of APPROACH-NL.

References

[1] S. W. Rabkin, F. A. L. Mathewson, and P.-H. Hsu, "Relation of body weight to development of ischemic heart disease in a cohort of young north American men after a 26 year observation period: the Manitoba study," *The American Journal of Cardiology*, vol. 39, no. 3, pp. 452–458, 1977.

[2] J. E. Manson, G. A. Colditz, M. J. Stampfer et al., "A prospective study of obesity and risk of coronary heart disease in women," *The New England Journal of Medicine*, vol. 322, no. 13, pp. 882–889, 1990.

[3] H. B. Hubert, M. Feinleib, P. M. McNamara, and W. P. Castelli, "Obesity as an independent risk factor for cardiovascular disease: a 26-year follow-up of participants in the Framingham Heart Study," *Circulation*, vol. 67, no. 5, pp. 968–977, 1983.

[4] Y. Chen, W. K. Copeland, R. Vedanthan et al., "Association between body mass index and cardiovascular disease mortality in east Asians and south Asians: pooled analysis of prospective data from the Asia Cohort Consortium," *British Medical Journal*, vol. 347, no. 7927, Article ID f5446, 2013.

[5] Y. Lu, K. Hajifathalian, M. Ezzati, M. Woodward, E. B. Rimm, and G. Danaei, "Metabolic mediators of the effects of body-mass index, overweight, and obesity on coronary heart disease and stroke: a pooled analysis of 97 prospective cohorts with 1.8 million participants," *The Lancet*, vol. 383, no. 9934, pp. 970–983, 2014.

[6] K. R. Fontaine, D. T. Redden, C. Wang, A. O. Westfall, and D. B. Allison, "Years of life lost due to obesity," *The Journal of the American Medical Association*, vol. 289, no. 2, pp. 187–193, 2003.

[7] E. E. Calle, M. J. Thun, J. M. Petrelli, C. Rodriguez, and C. W. Heath Jr., "Body-mass index and mortality in a prospective cohort of U.S. adults," *The New England Journal of Medicine*, vol. 341, no. 15, pp. 1097–1105, 1999.

[8] K. M. Flegal, B. K. Kit, H. Orpana, and B. I. Graubard, "Association of all-cause mortality with overweight and obesity using standard body mass index categories: a systematic review and meta-analysis," *The Journal of the American Medical Association*, vol. 309, no. 1, pp. 71–82, 2013.

[9] C. J. Lavie, R. V. Milani, and H. O. Ventura, "Obesity and cardiovascular disease. risk factor, paradox, and impact of weight loss," *Journal of the American College of Cardiology*, vol. 53, no. 21, pp. 1925–1932, 2009.

[10] C. J. Lavie, R. V. Milani, S. M. Artham, D. A. Patel, and H. O. Ventura, "The obesity paradox, weight loss, and coronary disease," *American Journal of Medicine*, vol. 122, no. 12, pp. 1106–1114, 2009.

[11] S. M. Artham, C. J. Lavie, R. V. Milani, and H. O. Ventura, "Value of weight reduction in patients with cardiovascular disease," *Current Treatment Options in Cardiovascular Medicine*, vol. 12, no. 1, pp. 21–35, 2010.

[12] J. Sierra-Johnson, A. Romero-Corral, V. K. Somers et al., "Prognostic importance of weight loss in patients with coronary heart disease regardless of initial body mass index," *European Journal of Cardiovascular Prevention and Rehabilitation*, vol. 15, no. 3, pp. 336–340, 2008.

[13] W. Doehner, E. Erdmann, R. Cairns et al., "Inverse relation of body weight and weight change with mortality and morbidity in patients with type 2 diabetes and cardiovascular co-morbidity: an analysis of the PROactive study population," *International Journal of Cardiology*, vol. 162, no. 1, pp. 20–26, 2012.

[14] K. Kalantar-Zadeh, E. Streja, M. Z. Molnar et al., "Mortality prediction by surrogates of body composition: an examination of the obesity paradox in hemodialysis patients using composite ranking score analysis," *American Journal of Epidemiology*, vol. 175, no. 8, pp. 793–803, 2012.

[15] S. Uretsky, F. H. Messerli, S. Bangalore et al., "Obesity paradox in patients with hypertension and coronary artery disease," *American Journal of Medicine*, vol. 120, no. 10, pp. 863–870, 2007.

[16] G. C. Fonarow, P. Srikanthan, M. R. Costanzo, G. B. Cintron, and M. Lopatin, "An obesity paradox in acute heart failure: analysis of body mass index and inhospital mortality for 108927 patients in the Acute Decompensated Heart Failure National Registry," *American Heart Journal*, vol. 153, no. 1, pp. 74–81, 2007.

[17] A. Oreopoulos, R. Padwal, C. M. Norris, J. C. Mullen, V. Pretorius, and K. Kalantar-Zadeh, "Effect of obesity on short- and long-term mortality postcoronary revascularization: a meta-analysis," *Obesity*, vol. 16, no. 2, pp. 442–450, 2008.

[18] A. Romero-Corral, V. M. Montori, V. K. Somers et al., "Association of bodyweight with total mortality and with cardiovascular events in coronary artery disease: a systematic review of cohort studies," *Lancet*, vol. 368, no. 9536, pp. 666–678, 2006.

[19] A. Oreopoulos, F. A. McAlister, K. Kalantar-Zadeh et al., "The relationship between body mass index, treatment, and mortality in patients with established coronary artery disease: a report from APPROACH," *European Heart Journal*, vol. 30, no. 21, pp. 2584–2592, 2009.

[20] A. P. Johnson, J. L. Parlow, M. Whitehead, J. Xu, S. Rohland, and B. Milne, "Body mass index, outcomes, and mortality following cardiac surgery in Ontario, Canada," *Journal of the American Heart Association*, vol. 4, no. 7, Article ID e002140, 2015.

[21] R. S. Jackson, J. H. Black III, Y. W. Lum et al., "Class I obesity is paradoxically associated with decreased risk of postoperative stroke after carotid endarterectomy," *Journal of Vascular Surgery*, vol. 55, no. 5, pp. 1306–1312, 2012.

[22] R. Barba, J. Bisbe, J. N. A. Pedrajas et al., "Body mass index and outcome in patients with coronary, cerebrovascular, or peripheral artery disease: findings from the FRENA registry," *European Journal of Preventive Cardiology*, vol. 16, no. 4, pp. 457–463, 2009.

[23] A. Blum, C. Simsolo, R. Sirchan, and S. Haiek, ""Obesity Paradox" in chronic obstructive pulmonary disease," *Israel Medical Association Journal*, vol. 13, no. 11, pp. 672–675, 2011.

[24] V. L. Roger, A. S. Go, D. M. Lloyd-Jones et al., "Heart disease and stroke statistics—2011 update: a report from the American Heart Association," *Circulation*, vol. 125, no. 1, pp. e2–e220, 2011.

[25] I. Ringqvist, L. D. Fisher, M. Mock et al., "Prognostic value of angiographic indices of coronary artery disease from the Coronary Artery Surgery Study (CASS)," *Journal of Clinical Investigation*, vol. 71, no. 6, pp. 1854–1866, 1983.

[26] G. G. Gensini, "A more meaningful scoring system for determining the severity of coronary heart disease," *The American Journal of Cardiology*, vol. 51, no. 3, article 606, 1983.

[27] H. Dash, R. A. Johnson, R. E. Dinsmore, and J. Warren Harthorne, "Cardiomyopathic syndrome due to coronary artery disease: I: relation to angiographic extent of coronary disease and to remote myocardial infarction," *Heart*, vol. 39, no. 7, pp. 733–739, 1977.

[28] R. M. Califf, H. R. Phillips III, M. C. Hindman et al., "Prognostic value of a coronary artery jeopardy score," *Journal of the American College of Cardiology*, vol. 5, no. 5, pp. 1055–1063, 1985.

[29] R. Rubinshtein, D. A. Halon, R. Jaffe, J. Shahla, and B. S. Lewis, "Relation between obesity and severity of coronary artery disease in patients undergoing coronary angiography," *American Journal of Cardiology*, vol. 97, no. 9, pp. 1277–1280, 2006.

[30] A. Niraj, J. Pradahan, H. Fakhry, V. Veeranna, and L. Afonso, "Severity of coronary artery disease in obese patients undergoing coronary angiography: "Obesity Paradox" revisited," *Clinical Cardiology*, vol. 30, no. 8, pp. 391–396, 2007.

[31] A. F. Z. Parsa and B. Jahanshahi, "Is the relationship of body mass index to severity of coronary artery disease different from that of waist-to-hip ratio and severity of coronary artery disease? Paradoxical findings," *Cardiovascular Journal of Africa*, vol. 26, no. 1, pp. 13–16, 2015.

[32] M. Shirzad, A. Karimi, S. Dowlatshahi et al., "Relationship between body mass index and left main disease: the obesity paradox," *Archives of Medical Research*, vol. 40, no. 7, pp. 618–624, 2009.

[33] R. Rossi, D. Iaccarino, A. Nuzzo et al., "Influence of body mass index on extent of coronary atherosclerosis and cardiac events in a cohort of patients at risk of coronary artery disease," *Nutrition, Metabolism and Cardiovascular Diseases*, vol. 21, no. 2, pp. 86–93, 2011.

[34] J. Auer, T. Weber, R. Berent et al., "Obesity, body fat and coronary atherosclerosis," *International Journal of Cardiology*, vol. 98, no. 2, pp. 227–235, 2005.

[35] S. D. Phillips and W. C. Roberts, "Comparison of body mass index among patients with versus without angiographic coronary artery disease," *American Journal of Cardiology*, vol. 100, no. 1, pp. 18–22, 2007.

[36] L. K. Twells, D. M. Gregory, J. Reddigan, and W. K. Midodzi, "Current and predicted prevalence of obesity in Canada: a trend analysis," *CMAJ Open*, vol. 2, no. 1, pp. E18–E26, 2014.

[37] D. Gregory, W. Midodzi, and N. Pearce, "Complications with Angio-Seal™ vascular closure devices compared with manual compression after diagnostic cardiac catheterization and percutaneous coronary intervention," *Journal of Interventional Cardiology*, vol. 26, no. 6, pp. 630–638, 2013.

[38] World Health Organization, *Obesity: Preventing and Managing the Global Epidemic*, World Health Organization, Geneva, Switzerland, 2000.

[39] Health Canada, "Canadian guidelines for body weight classification in adults. Quick reference tool for professionals," 2003, http://www.hc-sc.gc.ca/fn-an/nutrition/weights-poids/guide-ld-adult/cg_quick_ref-ldc_rapide_ref-table1-eng.php.

[40] A. Nigam, R. S. Wright, T. G. Allison et al., "Excess weight at time of presentation of myocardial infarction is associated with lower initial mortality risks but higher long-term risks including recurrent re-infarction and cardiac death," *International Journal of Cardiology*, vol. 110, no. 2, pp. 153–159, 2006.

[41] Alberta Provincial Project for Outcome Assessment in Coronary Heart Disease (APPROACH), "CARAT tutorials: history of coronary scoring," http://www.approach.org/support_pages/carat_tutorials/carat_coronary_scoring_tutorial.html.

[42] M. M. Graham, P. D. Faris, W. A. Ghali et al., "Validation of three myocardial jeopardy scores in a population-based cardiac catheterization cohort," *American Heart Journal*, vol. 142, no. 2, pp. 254–261, 2001.

[43] K. R. Fontaine and D. B. Allison, "Obesity and mortality rates," in *Handbook of Obesity: Etiology and Pathophysiology*, G. A. Bray, Ed., pp. 767–785, Marcel Dekker, New York, NY, USA, 2004.

[44] M. A. Hernán, S. Hernández-Díaz, and J. M. Robins, "A structural approach to selection bias," *Epidemiology*, vol. 15, no. 5, pp. 615–625, 2004.

[45] E. Jahangir, A. De Schutter, and C. J. Lavie, "The relationship between obesity and coronary artery disease," *Translational Research*, vol. 164, no. 4, pp. 336–344, 2014.

[46] H. R. Banack and J. S. Kaufman, "The 'obesity paradox' explained," *Epidemiology*, vol. 24, no. 3, pp. 461–462, 2013.

[47] M. Tjepkema, "Adult obesity in Canada: measured height and weight," Tech. Rep. 82-620-MWE, Statistics Canada, Ottawa, Canada, 2005.

[48] E. W. Gregg, Y. J. Cheng, B. L. Cadwell et al., "Secular trends in cardiovascular desease risk factors according to body mass index in US adults," *Journal of the American Medical Association*, vol. 293, no. 15, pp. 1868–1874, 2005.

[49] E. A. Spencer, P. N. Appleby, G. K. Davey, and T. J. Key, "Validity of self-reported height and weight in 4808 EPIC-Oxford participants," *Public Health Nutrition*, vol. 5, no. 4, pp. 561–565, 2002.

[50] J. Stevens, J. E. Keil, L. R. Waid, and P. C. Gazes, "Accuracy of current, 4-year, and 28-year self-reported body weight in an elderly population," *American Journal of Epidemiology*, vol. 132, no. 6, pp. 1156–1163, 1990.

[51] A. De Schutter, C. J. Lavie, and R. V. Milani, "The impact of obesity on risk factors and prevalence and prognosis of coronary heart disease—the obesity paradox," *Progress in Cardiovascular Diseases*, vol. 56, no. 4, pp. 401–408, 2014.

[52] A. Romero-Corral, V. K. Somers, J. Sierra-Johnson et al., "Diagnostic performance of body mass index to detect obesity in patients with coronary artery disease," *European Heart Journal*, vol. 28, no. 17, pp. 2087–2093, 2007.

[53] A. De Schutter, C. J. Lavie, K. Arce, S. G. Menendez, and R. V. Milani, "Correlation and discrepancies between obesity by body mass index and body fat in patients with coronary heart disease," *Journal of Cardiopulmonary Rehabilitation and Prevention*, vol. 33, no. 2, pp. 77–83, 2013.

[54] A. de Schutter, C. J. Lavie, J. Gonzalez, and R. V. Milani, "Body composition in coronary heart disease: how does body mass indexcorrelate with body fatness?" *Ochsner Journal*, vol. 11, no. 3, pp. 220–225, 2011.

18

Correlation between Doppler, Manual Morphometry, and Histopathology Based Morphometry of Radial Artery as a Conduit in Coronary Artery Bypass Grafting

Om Prakash Yadava,[1] **Vinod Sharma,**[2] **Arvind Prakash,**[3] **Vikas Ahlawat,**[1] **Anirban Kundu,**[1] **Bikram K. Mohanty,**[1] **Rekha Mishra,**[2] **and Amit K. Dinda**[4]

[1]*Department of Cardiothoracic Surgery, National Heart Institute, 49-50 Community Centre, East of Kailash, New Delhi 110065, India*

[2]*Department of Cardiology, National Heart Institute, 49-50 Community Centre, East of Kailash, New Delhi 110065, India*

[3]*Department of Cardiac Anesthesiology, National Heart Institute, 49-50 Community Centre, East of Kailash, New Delhi 110065, India*

[4]*Department of Pathology, All India Institute of Medical Sciences, New Delhi 110029, India*

Correspondence should be addressed to Anirban Kundu; dockundu@yahoo.com

Academic Editor: Michael S. Wolin

Background. Long-term graft patency is the major factor impacting survival after coronary artery bypass grafting. Arteries are superior in this regard. Radial artery is considered the second best conduit after internal mammary artery. Several studies have shown excellent radial artery patency. We evaluated the morphologic characteristics of radial artery by three modalities, (i) preoperative Doppler ultrasound, (ii) intraoperative manual morphometry, and (iii) postoperative histology-based morphometry, and compared these with the aim of validating Doppler as a noninvasive test of choice for preoperative assessment of radial artery. *Methods.* This was a prospective study involving 100 patients undergoing coronary artery bypass grafting in which radial artery was used. The radial artery was assessed using preoperative Doppler ultrasound studies, intraoperative morphometry, and postoperative histopathology and morphometry. The morphometric measurements included (i) luminal diameter, (ii) intimal and medial thickness, and (iii) intima-media thickness ratio. *Results.* Using Bland-Altman plots, there was a 95% limit of agreement between the preoperative Doppler measurements and the postoperative histopathology and morphometry. *Conclusion.* Doppler ultrasound is an accurate screening test for evaluation of radial artery, in terms of intimal/medial thickness and luminal diameter as a conduit in coronary artery bypass grafting and has been validated by both morphometric and histopathology based studies.

1. Introduction

Long-term bypass graft patency is the major factor impacting survival in patients after coronary artery bypass grafting (CABG). It has been proved that arterial grafts are superior to venous grafts in terms of long-term patency. Among the arterial grafts, radial artery (RA) is considered to be the best conduit next to internal mammary artery. Use of RA has been supported by the result of several angiographic studies that have shown excellent short-, medium-, and long-term patency rates. A good conduit has to be of good caliber and should be free from pathological wall thickening. In this study, we have evaluated the morphologic characteristics of RA like luminal diameter and wall thickness by three different modalities, namely, (i) preoperative Doppler ultrasound (USG), (ii) intraoperative manual morphometry, and (iii) postoperative histology-based morphometry, and have compared the measurements of these three modalities with the aim of validating Doppler as a noninvasive test of choice for preoperative measurements of RA morphology.

2. Patients and Methods

This prospective study included 100 patients undergoing CABG between September 2012 and February 2013 at the National Heart Institute, New Delhi, in whom RA was used as a conduit. The study was approved by the institutional Ethics Committee and informed written consent was obtained from all patients prior to start of the study. The suitability of RA was assessed by modified Allen's test in the nondominant forearm at the bedside using pulse oximeter. All the patients who had a negative modified Allen's test, which signified a complete palmar arch, were subjected to Doppler USG of RA, which was performed by a single experienced observer using PHILIPS–IE-33 with 7.5 MHz Phased Array Rectangular Vascular Probe. Thorough and complete scanning of the RA was done starting just after ulnar artery branching (proximally) up to the wrist (distally). The scanning evaluation included (i) luminal diameter, (ii) measurement of intimal thickness and medial thickness, and (iii) measurement of intima-media thickness ratio.

In the operating room, after the patient was anaesthetized, the RA was harvested with its pedicle using an open, no-touch technique simultaneously with sternotomy and harvesting of other conduits. Monopolar diathermy and clips were used in dissection. After the RA was exposed, visual assessment for any gross abnormality was made, along with diameter of the vessel. RA was palpated for assessment of wall thickness and calcification. After the RA was harvested, sections of 1 cm length from both ends were cut with fine scissors before hydrostatic dilatation and storage with heparinized saline. No vasodilator fluid was used for storage. The luminal diameter and thickness of arterial wall were measured using a Vernier caliper. After intraoperative morphometry measurements, specimens constituting the proximal and distal ends were preserved in 5% formaldehyde solution and sent for histopathology study. 5–20 sections were analyzed per segment of artery submitted for evaluation. These were cross-sectioned at 5 micrometers and stained with hematoxylin-eosin, Verhoef van Gieson's elastic stain, and Masson's Trichrome Stain. Histopathological assessments were followed by evaluation of the slides by another pathologist having expertise in morphometric measurements, who was blinded to the previous findings. The specimens were analyzed with a color image analysis system. The morphometric measurements included (i) luminal diameter, (ii) intimal and medial thickness, and (iii) intima-media thickness ratio. Any fibromyointimal proliferation between the endothelium and internal elastic lamina was considered as indicating intimal hyperplasia. An atherosclerotic lesion was defined by intimal lipid lying free as cholesterol clefts or in aggregates of foamy macrophages. Medial calcification was recorded if present.

2.1. Statistical Analysis.
Data was assessed and represented in mean values and association in categorical variables was evaluated by Fisher's exact/chi-square test. In case of continuous variables, two groups were compared by using t-test. Agreement in the two methods for the continuous variables was seen by Bland Altman Plot. Intraclass correlation was calculated with 95% confidence interval.

TABLE 1: Patient demographics.

Number of patients	100
Males : females	79 : 21
Mean age (years)	61.45
Mean Body Surface Area (m^2)	1.74
Mean left ventricular ejection fraction (%)	51.57
Double vessel disease	17
Triple vessel disease	83
Diabetes mellitus	54
Hypertension	69
Dyslipidemia	10
Smoking	33
Peripheral vascular disease	6
Stroke	3

3. Observations and Results

3.1. Patient Demography.
One hundred patients, who fulfilled the inclusion criteria of use of RA (on the basis of modified Allen's test) as a conduit in CABG, were included in this prospective study. Two patients were excluded as preoperative Doppler showed extensive calcification in one and luminal diameter <2 mm in another. There was no age bar. The minimum age of the patients was 44 years and the maximum age was 80 years, the mean being 61.45 years. 79 patients were males and 21 patients were females. The patient demographics are shown in Table 1.

3.2. Preoperative Radial Doppler Measurements.
The mean luminal diameter was 2.342 mm proximally and decreased serially distally with a reciprocal increase in intimal thickness, as we moved down towards the wrist. The IMT ratios in the proximal, mid, and distal segments were 0.530, 0.584, and 0.501, respectively (Ref. Table 2). Abnormal Intimal thickening was found in 10 patients.

3.3. Intraoperative Morphometry.
Radial artery was thick on palpation in 6 patients and intraoperative morphometric assessments revealed a mean arterial wall thickness of 0.502 mm and 0.548 mm at the proximal and distal ends of the harvested radial arteries, respectively. The respective proximal and distal arterial diameters were 2.30 mm and 2.18 mm.

3.4. Postoperative Histopathology Based Morphometry.
The findings of postoperative morphometry studies showed similar trends as preoperative morphometry (Table 3).

We observed that, as far as dimensions and measurements of RA are concerned, there was good correlation among the various modalities.

3.5. Correlation between Findings of Preoperative USG and Postoperative Morphometry.
A correlation was established among the preoperative Doppler USG and postoperative histopathology assessment and morphometric findings (Ref.

TABLE 2: Preoperative radial Doppler measurements; (Dia: diameter, D: distal, IMTR: intima-media thickness ratio, ITL intimal thickening, Lum: luminal, M: mid, MT: medial thickening, and P: proximal).

S. number	Findings	Mean value in mm (S. numbers 1–9)
1	Lum Dia (P)	2.342
2	Lum Dia (M)	2.264
3	Lum Dia (D)	2.164
4	IT (P)	0.064
5	IT (M)	0.075
6	IT (D)	0.1
7	MT (P)	0.137
8	MT (M)	0.174
9	MT (D)	0.211
10	IMTR (P)	0.530
11	IMTR (M)	0.584
12	IMTR (D)	0.501

TABLE 3: Postoperative histopathology.

S. number	Findings in mm (S. numbers 1, 2, and 4)	Proximal	Distal
1	Intimal thickness	0.065	0.105
2	Medial thickness	0.142	0.213
3	Intima-media thickness ratio	0.534	0.501
4	Luminal diameter	2.351	2.165

Table 4) and Bland Altman analysis plotted for intimal thickness (Ref. Figures 1 and 2), medial thickness (Ref. Figures 3 and 4), and intima-media thickness ratio (Figures 5 and 6).

We observed that as far as dimensions and measurements of radial artery are concerned, there was good correlation among the various modalities.

4. Discussion

RA is now well established as the best arterial conduit after the internal mammary artery and there exists strong and consistent evidence of the superior long-term patency of RA over the saphenous vein. There is also rapidly growing body of evidence that this superior patency of RA translates into improved clinical outcomes including mortality benefits [1, 2]. Indeed, the current authors recently published a study from the same cohort of patients showing that clinical profile of the patients was not a precluding factor in the use of this conduit [3]. However, it has also been seen that the RA has a significantly greater prevalence of intimal hyperplasia and atherosclerosis, reported variably from 5.3% [4] to 31.5% [5]. Further, there appears to be a difference in functional characteristics between the proximal and distal ends of RA with the proximal segment demonstrating more vasoreactivity and force of contraction in response to vasopressors [6].

Doppler has been validated against histological measurements for providing reliable data on luminal diameter and

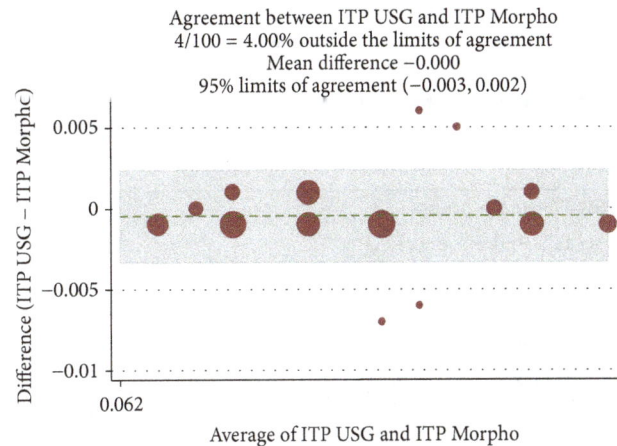

FIGURE 1: Intraclass Correlation Coefficient (ICC) was 0.91 with mean difference of −0.001; limit of agreement was 95% with upper and lower limits of −0.003 and 0.002. 4% values are above the limit of agreement, which means both of these methods are in agreement.

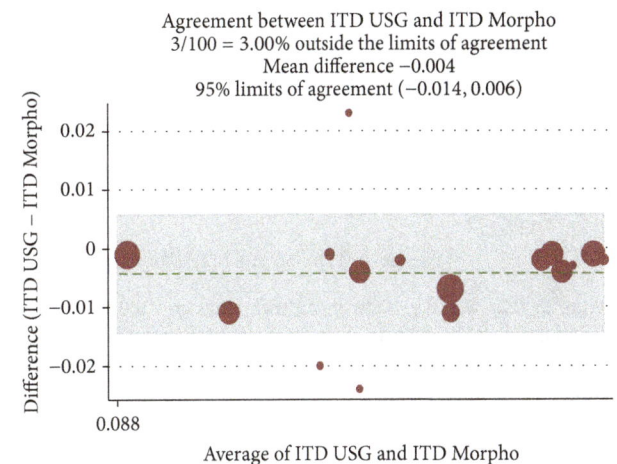

FIGURE 2: ICC was 0.90 with mean difference of −0.004; limit of agreement was 95% with upper and lower limits of −0.014 and 0.006. 3% values are above the limit of agreement, which means both methods are in agreement.

intima-media thickness of carotid arteries [7–9]. Doppler USG also has been used to assess the hand collateral circulation and to validate Allen's test [10]. However, though several authors have used preoperative USG and intraoperative morphometry for deciding the suitability of the use of the RA as a conduit in CABG, there is no data available validating the preoperative USG against postoperative histopathology examination and morphometry for radial arteries. In recent years, the possibility of measuring RA vessel wall abnormalities and measuring the intimal-medial thickness has gained interest. Kim et al. used high resolution USG for measuring the RA wall thickness (intima-media thickness) in haemodialysis patients and validated it with histology-based measurements on samples obtained during AV fistula creation at wrist ($r = 0.800$, $p < 0.001$) [11]. However, we could not locate a single paper in published English

TABLE 4: Comparison of USG and histology based morphometry; IMTRD: intima-media thickness ratio distal, IMTR: intima-media thickness ratio proximal, ITD: intimal thickness distal, ITP: intimal thickness proximal, MTD: medial thickness distal, and MTP: medial thickness proximal.

	Intraclass correlation coefficient (ICC)	Mean difference	Limit of agreement (upper and lower limit with 95% limits of agreement)
USG ITP and morpho-ITP	0.91	−0.001	−0.003 to 0.002
USG ITD and morpho-ITD	0.90	−0.004	−0.014 to 0.006
USG MTP and morpho-MTP	0.91	−0.004	−0.020 to 0.012
USG MTD and morpho-MTD	0.89	−0.002	−0.006 to 0.001
USG IMTRP and morpho-IMTRP	0.89	0.009	−0.039 to 0.057
USG IMTRD and morpho-IMTRD	0.92	−0.015	−0.063 to 0.033

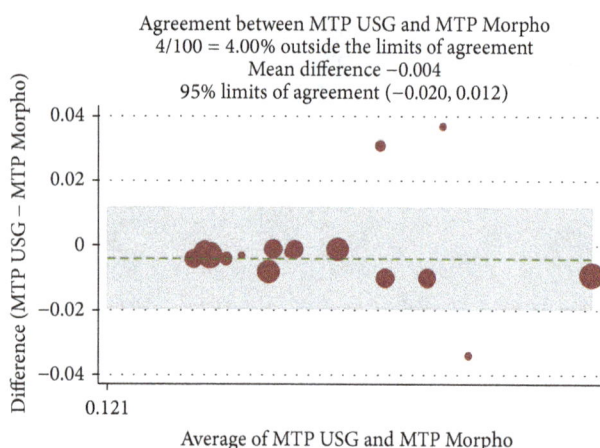

FIGURE 3: ICC was 0.91 with mean difference of −0.004; limit of agreement was 95% with upper and lower limit of −0.020 and 0.012. 4% values are above the limit of agreement, which means both of the methods are in agreement.

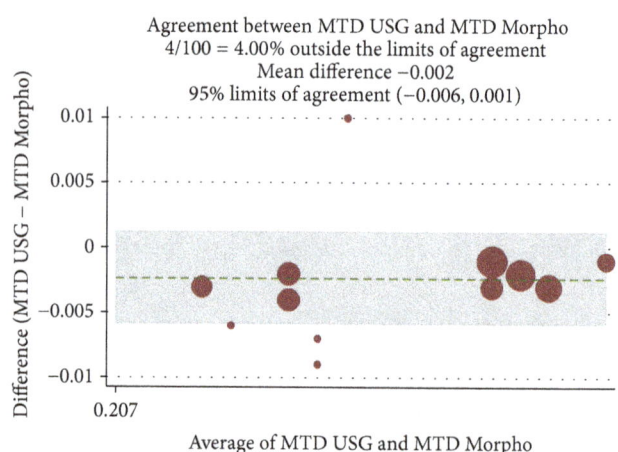

FIGURE 4: ICC was 0.89 with mean difference of −0.002; limit of agreement was 95% with upper and lower limits of −0.006 and 0.001. 4% values are above the limit of agreement, which means both of these methods are in agreement.

language literature comparing and validating preoperative RA ultrasonography against histopathology for use of RA as a conduit for CABG. To the best of our knowledge, this is the first paper on the subject. In our study, we found that the preoperative Doppler ultrasound, intraoperative and postoperative histopathology based morphometric measurements of intima-media thickness ratio, intimal hyperplasia, and luminal diameter showed good correlation and, when indicated, preoperative Doppler ultrasound could provide useful and reliable data on suitability of RA for its use as a conduit in CABG.

We found that the proximal ends of RA had a greater luminal diameter and less thicker wall than the distal ends. As we proceed distally, the wall thickness due to increased thickness of both intima and media, with the latter having a greater contribution, led to decreased IMT ratio compared to proximal end. This was also the finding of Bhan et al. [12] who found that the prevalence of atherosclerotic disease was higher at the distal end with comparative morphometric analysis revealing significantly smaller percentage of luminal narrowing, intimal thickness index, and intima to media ratios in the proximal segments compared with the distal

segments ($p > 0.001$). This has practical connotation, as the distal end of the RA is grafted to the coronary and at the time of doing the anastomosis to the aorta; the extra length of the RA conduit is excised and discarded which obviously comes from the proximal end of RA, which in fact is the better part. It is therefore suggested that near accurate length of the graft should be decided before the distal anastomosis and if any part of the conduit has to be discarded, it should be the distal and not the proximal end. On the contrary, Ueyama et al. [13], expressing the pathological index of arteriosclerosis as a ratio (internal luminal area/tunica media area), found no significant difference between the mean ratio of the proximal (0.177 ± 0.033) and the distal (0.258 ± 0.132) ends of the RAs. Although this did not achieve statistical significance, apparent trends are towards a higher degree of atherosclerosis in the distal end. Further, the proximal end was larger than the distal [13], thereby lending credence to our contention that the proximal segment of the RA should be preferred to the distal.

A confounding factor in this study is that the histological confirmation of Doppler findings was only possible in distal and proximal segments.

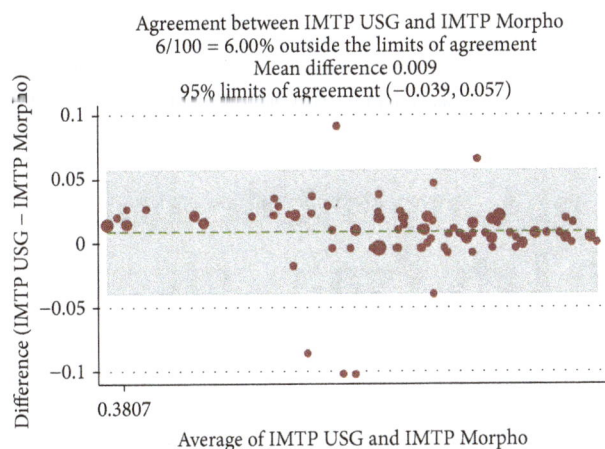

Agreement between IMTP USG and IMTP Morpho
6/100 = 6.00% outside the limits of agreement
Mean difference 0.009
95% limits of agreement (−0.039, 0.057)

FIGURE 5: ICC was 0.89 with mean difference of −0.009; limit of agreement was 95% with upper and lower limits of −0.039 and 0.057. 6% values are above the limit of agreement, which means both of these methods are in agreement.

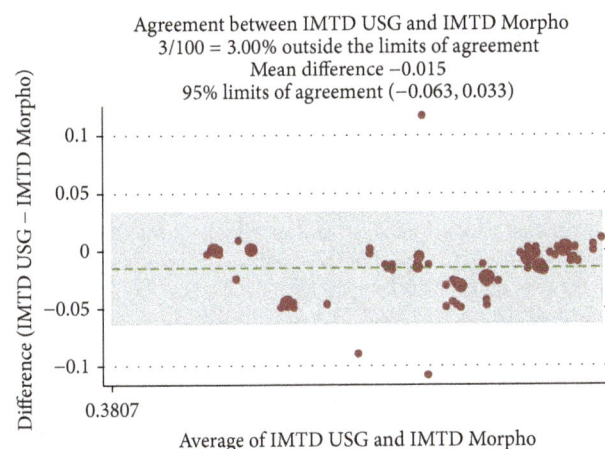

Agreement between IMTD USG and IMTD Morpho
3/100 = 3.00% outside the limits of agreement
Mean difference −0.015
95% limits of agreement (−0.063, 0.033)

FIGURE 6: ICC was 0.92 with mean difference of −0.015; limit of agreement was 95% with upper and lower limits of −0.063 and 0.033. 3% values are above the limit of agreement, which means both of these methods are in agreement.

5. Conclusions

Doppler USG is an accurate screening test for evaluation of the suitability of RA, in terms of intimal/medial thickness and luminal diameter as a conduit in CABG, and has been validated by both morphometric and histopathology based studies. However, that does not imply that a case can be made out for routine Doppler screening of all radial arteries prior to CABG [14]. Hence, preoperative Doppler scanning may be considered in cases with palpable radial disease, those with widespread peripheral vascular disease, or cases with a positive Allen's test where one is under pressure to use as many arterial grafts as possible [14].

References

[1] U. Benedetto and M. Codispoti, "Age cutoff for the loss of survival benefit from use of radial artery in coronary artery bypass grafting," *Journal of Thoracic and Cardiovascular Surgery*, vol. 146, no. 5, pp. 1078–1085, 2013.

[2] B. F. Buxton, W. Y. Shi, J. Tatoulis, J. A. Fuller, A. Rosalion, and P. A. Hayward, "Total arterial revascularization with internal thoracic and radial artery grafts in triple-vessel coronary artery disease is associated with improved survival," *The Journal of Thoracic and Cardiovascular Surgery*, vol. 148, no. 4, pp. 1238–1244, 2014.

[3] O. P. Yadava, V. Sharma, A. Prakash et al., "Does clinical profile preclude use of radial artery as a conduit in coronary artery bypass grafting?" *Journal of Clinical & Experimental Cardiology*, vol. 6, article 3, 2015.

[4] P. Ruengsakulrach, R. Sinclair, M. Komeda, J. Raman, I. Gordon, and B. Buxton, "Comparative histopathology of radial artery versus internal thoracic artery and risk factors for development of intimal hyperplasia and atherosclerosis," *Circulation*, vol. 100, article e139, 1999.

[5] P. Ruengsakulrach, M. Brooks, R. Sinclair, D. Hare, I. Gordon, and B. Buxton, "Prevalence and prediction of calcification and plaques in radial artery grafts by ultrasound," *Journal of Thoracic and Cardiovascular Surgery*, vol. 122, no. 2, pp. 398–399, 2001.

[6] A. H. Chester, A. J. Marchbank, J. A. A. Borland, M. H. Yacoub, and D. P. Taggart, "Comparison of the morphologic and vascular reactivity of the proximal and distal radial artery," *The Annals of Thoracic Surgery*, vol. 66, no. 6, pp. 1972–1976, 1998.

[7] I. Wendelhag, O. Wiklund, and J. Wikstrand, "Arterial wall thickness in familial hypercholesterolemia. Ultrasound measurement of intima-media thickness in the common carotid artery," *Arteriosclerosis and Thrombosis*, vol. 12, no. 1, pp. 70–77, 1992.

[8] D. H. O'Leary, J. F. Polak, R. A. Kronmal et al., "Distribution and correlates of sonographically detected carotid artery disease in the cardiovascular health study," *Stroke*, vol. 23, no. 12, pp. 1752–1760, 1992.

[9] M. L. Bots, P. G. H. Mulder, A. Hofman, G.-A. van Es, and D. E. Grobbee, "Reproducibility of carotid vessel wall thickness measurements. the rotterdam study," *Journal of Clinical Epidemiology*, vol. 47, no. 8, pp. 921–930, 1994.

[10] P. Pola, M. Serricchio, R. Flore, E. Manasse, A. Favuzzi, and G. F. Possati, "Safe removal of the radial artery for myocardial revascularization: a doppler study to prevent ischemic complications to the hand," *Journal of Thoracic and Cardiovascular Surgery*, vol. 112, no. 3, pp. 737–744, 1996.

[11] Y. O. Kim, J. I. Kim, Y. M. Ku et al., "Accuracy of Doppler ultrasonography in measuring radial artery wall thickness in hemodialysis patients: comparison with histologic examination," *Hemodialysis International*, vol. 8, no. 1, article 80, 2004.

[12] A. Bhan, V. Gupta, S. K. Choudhary et al., "Radial artery in CABG: could the early results be comparable to internal mammary artery graft?" *The Annals of Thoracic Surgery*, vol. 67, no. 6, pp. 1631–1636, 1999.

[13] K. Ueyama, G. Watanabe, K. Kotoh et al., "Pathological examination of radial artery—as a graft material for coronary artery bypass grafting," *Nihon Kyobu Geka Gakkai Zasshi*, vol. 45, no. 11, pp. 1816–1820, 1997.

[14] O. P. Yadava, A. K. Dinda, B. K. Mohanty, R. Mishra, V. Ahlawat, and A. Kundu, "Is radial artery Doppler scanning mandatory for use as coronary bypass conduit?" *Asian Cardiovascular and Thoracic Annals*, vol. 23, no. 7, pp. 822–827, 2015.

19

Comparison of the Effects of Carperitide and Tolvaptan on Patients with Left Ventricular Dysfunction

Chikahiko Koeda,[1] **Shohei Yamaya,**[2] **Maiko Hozawa,**[2] **Masayuki Sato,**[3] **Kazuhiro Nasu,**[3] **Tomohiro Takahashi,**[3] **and Katsutoshi Terui**[3]

[1]*Division of Cardioangiology, Department of Internal Medicine, Iwate Medical University, Iwate, Japan*
[2]*Department of Cardiology, Iwate Prefectural Kuji Hospital, Iwate, Japan*
[3]*Department of Emergency, Iwate Medical University, Iwate, Japan*

Correspondence should be addressed to Chikahiko Koeda; okihagoodman@yahoo.co.jp

Academic Editor: Stephan von Haehling

In patients with left ventricular (LV) dysfunction, diuretics can reduce blood pressure and lead to electrolyte abnormalities. The aim of this study was to compare the effects of tolvaptan (T group) and carperitide (C group) in these patients. Sixty-one consecutive patients admitted to the Iwate Prefectural Kuji Hospital or the Emergency Center of the Iwate Medical University between July 2011 and April 2015 were included in this study. These patients had acute heart failure (HF) and were initially treated with furosemide. Patients were excluded from the study if they received combined carperitide and tolvaptan, if they received tolvaptan or cardiotonic drugs prior to the study period, if their LV ejection fraction was ≥40%, and if they had renal dysfunction (serum creatinine > 2.0 mg/dL). There were no differences in the change in serum electrolytes in both groups, and none of the patients in the T group received supplementary dobutamine therapy. Oxygen administration was stopped successfully after a significantly shorter treatment period in the T group. These findings suggest that patients treated with tolvaptan did not require dobutamine as frequently as those treated with carperitide and indicated that tolvaptan may improve respiratory function more rapidly in patients with LV dysfunction.

1. Introduction

Diuretic drugs, including loop diuretics and natriuretic peptides, are used frequently as a conventional therapy in patients with acute heart failure (HF). Carperitide is a B-type natriuretic peptide that can produce therapeutic benefits because it has a diuretic effect and a vasodilator action and inhibits activation of the renin aldosterone system [1]. It is an important therapeutic agent for HF and is currently used in 69.4% of these cases in Japan [2]. However, older patients and those with a left ventricular (LV) ejection fraction of <35% may show reduced blood pressure (BP) after carperitide administration [3], and those with LV dysfunction were more likely to be nonresponders in the

COMPASS study of carperitide [4]. In a study of nesiritide, another B-type natriuretic peptide, approximately 80% of the participants had LV dysfunction and many showed dose-dependent decreases in BP, with no confirmed improvements in prognostic predictors [5]. Although B-type natriuretic peptides have significant therapeutic benefits, these agents do not currently provide sufficient effects in patients with LV dysfunction. Loop diuretic drugs activate neurohormonal factors, reduce BP, and reduce serum osmotic pressure. The associated hyponatremia limits their use in patients with HF because hyponatremia is recognized as an independent predictor of poor prognosis in patients with LV dysfunction [6]. Hyponatremia was reported in 33.7% of patients with an initial LV ejection fraction of <35% [7]. Thus many patients with LV dysfunction may show resistance to conventional carperitide therapy, which might negatively affect the results of the mega clinical trial.

Patients with LV dysfunction and hyponatremia showed increased levels of vasopressin, which has two functions, to constrict BP and to keep fluid in body, and decreases LV output. Many cases of congestion symptoms and electrolyte abnormalities due to fluid retention have been reported [8, 9]. Tolvaptan is a vasopressin receptor antagonist which affects hemodynamics favorably; recent studies have investigated its clinical efficacy in these patients [10, 11].

The aim of the present study was to evaluate the effects of tolvaptan on LV dysfunction retrospectively by comparing the clinical features of carperitide-treated patients (C group) with those of tolvaptan-treated patients (T group).

2. Materials and Methods

2.1. Patients. Sixty-one consecutive patients (37 male and 24 female patients) were enrolled in this retrospective study. These patients were admitted to the Iwate Prefectural Kuji Hospital or the Critical Care and Emergency Center of Iwate Medical University Hospital between July 2011 and April 2015 with acute HF and were initially treated with loop diuretics. Patients were excluded from the study if they had received combination therapy with carperitide and tolvaptan or if they had been treated with tolvaptan or cardiotonic drugs in an outpatient setting. They were also excluded if their LV ejection fraction was ≥40% or they showed signs of renal failure (serum creatinine > 2.0 mg/dL) on admission. In addition, there were no patients who underwent intubation and mechanical respiratory support.

2.2. Study Design and Data Collection. A retrospective cohort design was employed on the basis of a medical chart review. The following data were obtained at the time of admission and within 24 hours after drug administration: sex, age, anthropometric measures, New York Heart Association (NYHA) class, medical history, comorbidities, vital signs, laboratory data, echocardiographic findings, electrocardiogram, urine and intake volume, hospitalization, mortality, the number of days before beginning the combination of loop diuretic and target drug (carperitide or tolvaptan), use of cardiotonic drugs, and changes in serum electrolytes or vital signs. Furthermore, we investigated the number of days between beginning the test therapy and stopping oxygen administration because this can provide an objective measure of respiratory function.

2.3. Statistics. We compared clinical measures in the C and T groups on admission and after test drug administration. Statistical comparisons between the C and T groups were made using the unpaired t-test (parametric data) or Mann–Whitney U-test (nonparametric data). Categorical variables were analyzed using the chi-square test. All analyses were performed using the SPSS software package (Chicago, IL, USA), and a p value of <0.05 was considered to be statistically significant.

3. Results and Discussion

3.1. Results

3.1.1. Baseline Patient Characteristics. Table 1 shows the patient data prior to administration of carperitide or tolvaptan. The mean age of the C group ($n = 46$) was 6 years older than that of the T group ($n = 15$), although this difference was not statistically significant ($p = 0.15$). There were more males than females in both study groups. The mean body mass index of the T group was slightly higher than that of the C group ($p = 0.05$). The NYHA class was ≥III in all cases and there was no difference in the furosemide dose administered prior to carperitide or tolvaptan.

3.1.2. Medical History. There were no differences in the past histories of HF, hypertension, diabetes mellitus, brain infarction, or medication histories relating to angiotensin converting enzyme inhibitors, angiotensin II receptor blockers, antialdosterone compounds, or β-blockers. The patients with hyperlipidemia were higher in the T group ($p = 0.05$). The causes of HF in these patients are shown in Table 1; in patients where no definitive diagnosis was available ("Others"), hypertensive heart disease, takotsubo cardiomyopathy, and arrhythmia were suspected.

3.1.3. Vital Signs and Laboratory Data on Admission. As shown in Table 1, there were no differences in the systolic and diastolic BPs or heart rates of the study groups. The serum sodium level was slightly lower in the C group than in the T group ($p = 0.02$), while there were no significant group differences in the blood urea nitrogen or serum creatinine levels. Sinus rhythm on electrocardiogram was noted in 20 cases (43%) in group C and 8 cases (53%) in group T. There were no differences in LV ejection fraction between the two groups, but the LV end-diastolic dimension and the estimated LV volume were significantly higher in the T group than in the C group ($p < 0.05$ for both analyses). There were no significant group differences in the estimated stroke volumes or right ventricular pressures.

3.1.4. Vital Signs and Laboratory Data upon Initiation of Carperitide or Tolvaptan Administration. As shown in Table 2, there was a significantly shorter delay before therapy initiation in the C group than in the T group ($p < 0.001$). Immediately prior to therapy initiation, systolic and diastolic BPs were significantly lower in the T group than in the C group ($p < 0.05$ for both comparisons). The serum sodium level was significantly lower in the C group, as compared with the T group ($p = 0.03$).

After the initiation of carperitide or tolvaptan therapy, there were no significant differences in the durations of hospitalization or therapy administration in the C and T groups. The 5 fatalities all occurred in the C group (11%). There were no significant differences in the furosemide dose administered to the two study groups. In addition, the 28 cases in which dobutamine was used after a mean of 2.1 ± 5.4 days were all in the C group (61%). The time before

TABLE 1: Baseline characteristics. The values are expressed in mean (standard deviation) and median (interquartile range). NYHA = New York Heart Association; ACE = angiotensin converting enzyme; ARB = angiotensin II receptor blocker; LV = left ventricular.

	Carperitide	n	Tolvaptan	n	p value
Age (year)	82 (77–88)	46	74 (62–88)	15	0.15
Sex (male)	28 (61%)	46	9 (60%)	15	1
Body mass index (kg/m^2)	22.1 ± 3.9	40	24.8 ± 5.2	15	0.05
NYHA class					
III	7 (15%)	46	2 (13%)	15	1
IV	39 (85%)	46	13 (87%)	15	1
Furosemide dose (mg)	20 (0–40)	46	20 (0–40)	15	0.77
Previous therapies					
ACE inhibitors	9 (20%)	46	2 (13%)	15	0.72
ARBs	9 (20%)	46	5 (27%)	15	0.3
Aldosterone blockers	9 (20%)	46	2 (13%)	15	0.72
β-Blockers	15 (33%)	46	4 (27%)	15	0.76
Medical history					
Heart failure	31 (67%)	46	9 (60%)	15	0.76
Hypertension	26 (57%)	46	4 (27%)	15	0.07
Diabetes mellitus	8 (17%)	46	1 (7%)	15	0.43
Hyperlipidemia	2 (4%)	46	4 (27%)	15	0.05
Brain infarction	17 (37%)	46	2 (13%)	15	0.12
Type of heart failure					
Diastole cardiomyopathy	18 (39%)	46	3 (20%)	15	0.22
Ischemic heart disease	19 (41%)	46	3 (20%)	15	0.22
Hypertrophic cardiomyopathy	1 (2%)	46	0	15	1
Others	8 (17%)	46	9 (60%)	15	0.03
On admission					
Systolic blood pressure (mmHg)	144.3 ± 26.1	46	140.3 ± 22.4	15	0.59
Diastolic blood pressure (mmHg)	89.3 ± 14.5	46	93.1 ± 18.1	15	0.42
Heart rate (bpm)	100 (90–109)	46	101 (83–122)	15	0.67
Serum sodium (mEq/L)	139.9 ± 3.4	46	142.3 ± 2.9	15	0.02
Serum potassium (mEq/L)	4.3 ± 0.5	46	4.1 ± 0.3	15	0.56
Blood urea nitrogen (mg/dL)	28.2 ± 10.6	45	23.8 ± 8.7	15	0.16
Serum creatinine (mg/dL)	1.2 ± 0.4	46	1.0 ± 0.4	15	0.16
On initiation of therapy					
Systolic blood pressure (mmHg)	142.4 ± 24.6	46	121.9 ± 18.1	15	0.004
Diastolic blood pressure (mmHg)	88.7 ± 15.2	46	78.0 ± 13.2	15	0.02
Heart rate (bpm)	98 (90–105)	46	98 (84–119)	15	0.73
Serum sodium (mEq/L)	140.2 ± 3.7	46	142.5 ± 2.6	15	0.03
Serum potassium (mEq/L)	4.3 (4.2–4.3)	46	4.0 (3.9–4.2)	15	0.04
Blood urea nitrogen (mg/dL)	27.1 (19.2–38.0)	45	23.5 (19.1–31.0)	15	0.18
Serum creatinine (mg/dL)	1.2 ± 0.4	46	1.0 ± 0.3	15	0.12
Urine before combination therapy (mL)	1070 (650–1153)	5	1266 (858–1750)	7	0.29
Electrocardiogram					
Sinus rhythm	20 (43%)	46	8 (53%)	15	0.56
Echocardiography					
End-diastolic dimension (mm)	51.7 ± 9.8	42	56.7 ± 7.3	15	0.04
LV ejection fraction (%)	29.1 ± 7.3	46	26.9 ± 8.3	15	0.22
Diastolic LV volume (mL)	131.7 ± 42.5	17	183.3 ± 48.9	11	0.001
Systolic LV volume (mL)	93.4 ± 31.5	17	139.3 ± 40.7	11	0.001
Stroke volume (mL)	35.6 (20.7–48.8)	17	41.1 (28.7–51.0)	11	0.32
Right ventricle pressure (mmHg)	48.4 ± 11.5	40	49.6 ± 8.2	13	0.72

TABLE 2: After the initiation of carperitide or tolvaptan therapy. The values are expressed in mean (standard deviation) and median (interquartile range).

	Carperitide	n	Tolvaptan	n	p value
Hospitalization (day)	31 (20–43)	46	30 (21–34)	15	0.93
Duration of combination therapy (day)	9.0 ± 5.8	45	9.3 ± 5.6	14	0.87
Fatalities	5 (11%)	46	0	15	0.32
Combined furosemide dose	40 (20–60)	46	40 (20–60)	15	0.76
Time before combination therapy initiation	0.5 ± 1.3	46	2.9 ± 3.4	15	<0.001
Received dobutamine	28 (61%)	46	0	15	<0.001
After combination therapy initiation					
Time taken to stop oxygen administration (day)	11 (7–17)	38	9 (4–10)	14	0.04
Systolic blood pressure (mmHg)	118.7 ± 21.6	46	121.6 ± 17.7	15	0.64
Diastolic blood pressure (mmHg)	69 (62–77)	46	72 (62–81)	15	0.54
Heart rate (bpm)	88 (78–97)	46	86 (68–100)	15	0.9
Serum sodium (mEq/L)	142.6 ± 3.6	46	143.5 ± 2.8	15	0.4
Serum potassium (mEq/L)	3.9 ± 0.5	46	4.0 ± 0.4	15	0.63
Blood urea nitrogen (mg/dL)	23.1 (18.8–31.9)	46	22.1 (19.1–25.3)	15	0.44
Serum creatinine (mg/dL)	1.2 ± 0.4	46	1.0 ± 0.3	15	0.1
ΔSystolic blood pressure (mmHg)	-23.7 ± 17.2	46	-0.3 ± 12.8	15	<0.0001
ΔDiastolic blood pressure (mmHg)	16.0 (10.0–27.0)	46	3.0 (−2.0–11.0)	15	0.001
ΔHeart rate (bpm)	-10.7 ± 14.2	46	-7.1 ± 18.5	15	0.43
ΔSerum sodium (mEq/L)	2.5 ± 4.1	46	1.0 ± 4.0	15	0.21
ΔSerum potassium (mEq/L)	-0.3 ± 0.5	46	0 ± 0.5	15	0.09
ΔBlood urea nitrogen (mg/dL)	-3.9 ± 9.0	45	-1.5 ± 8.4	15	0.38
ΔSerum creatinine (mg/dL)	0 ± 0.3	46	0 ± 0.2	15	0.92
Urine volume (mean of 3 days) (mL)	1418 (1019–1813)	46	1833 (1183–4833)	11	0.03

successfully stopping oxygen administration was 20% shorter in the T group than in the C group ($p = 0.04$). There were no significant group differences in the change in renal function and the serum electrolytes. The C group showed a significantly greater decrease in systolic BP than the T group ($p < 0.001$), and the change in diastolic BP was also smaller in the T group than in the C group ($p = 0.001$). Although the mean urine volume in the 3 days after drug initiation was greater in the T group than in the C group, this difference was not statistically significant because the mean intake volume was unclear.

3.2. Discussion. This retrospective study of HF patients with an EF of <40% found that 61% of the C group received additional dobutamine within two days of carperitide therapy initiation, while those in the T group did not require dobutamine. There were no intergroup differences in the doses of furosemide and combination treatment in the two groups. Thus, the findings are comparable to those of studies comparing tolvaptan monotherapy and combination therapy with carperitide and dobutamine. The present study found no differences in serum electrolyte levels or renal function in the T and C groups. The time between therapy initiation and successful cessation of oxygen administration was significantly shorter in the T group than in the C group and none of the patients in the T group died during the study period, even though their heart expansion progressed. In contrast, 5 of the patients in the C group died during the study. These

results suggested that the therapeutic effects of monotherapy with tolvaptan may not be inferior to those of combined carperitide and dobutamine treatment in patients with LV dysfunction. The release of vasopressin positively correlated with HF stage [12], and the demand of tolvaptan may rise as HF stage progresses. Even though tolvaptan was not shown to produce prognostic improvements in a large-scale clinical trial [13], this compound may provide an effective treatment strategy for the subgroup of patients with LV dysfunction for the following reasons. First, it has been reported that aquaporin-defined responders may have a better prognosis with tolvaptan [14].

Second, although cardiac index remained unchanged, the pulmonary vascular resistance index decreased after tolvaptan treatment [15]. Finally, the result in this study indicated that tolvaptan use can reduce cardiotonic dose which is cause of the poor-prognosis factor.

Although 61% of the C group was treated with dobutamine, systolic BP showed a large decrease after carperitide infusion. In contrast, no significant change in BP was observed in the T group. The results of this study are consistent with those of a previous investigation of tolvaptan in patients with HF and reduced LV ejection fraction < 50% or systolic BP < 140 mmHg, who showed a greater effect of diuretics on BP than did patients with HF and a preserved ejection fraction [16]. However, these results may be influenced by the difference in the time delay prior to starting carperitide or tolvaptan therapy. The T group received only furosemide for approximately 3 days after hospitalization, allowing their stroke volumes and BP to decrease without dobutamine administration. On the other hand, the majority of the C group received carperitide on admission and yet 61% of these patients subsequently required dobutamine. There was a clear difference in group BPs at the time of treatment initiation, whereby the T group showed a significantly lower systolic BP than did the C group. Accordingly, this bias made it difficult to evaluate the effect of tolvaptan on BP.

There were limitations to this study related to the small number of cases and the retrospective analysis, although we aimed to minimize bias by using strict exclusion criteria. Bias affected normality in the baseline features of the study groups and this was difficult to correct for, even with an analysis of covariance. Furthermore, we wanted to reconsider our findings according to the various types of acute HF and compare tolvaptan responders and nonresponders; however, these were not possible due to the sample size. The larger number of patients in the C group indicated a tendency for clinicians to prescribe the more established therapy. These findings reflected the real-world use of tolvaptan, as a new drug.

4. Conclusions

The findings of this study indicated that tolvaptan use was associated with lower rates of dobutamine administration, as compared with carperitide, and that tolvaptan may improve respiratory function in patients with LV dysfunction. This indication that tolvaptan treatment may not be inferior to carperitide treatment in patients with LV dysfunction suggested that further examination of this was warranted in a future prospective study.

References

[1] N. Hata, Y. Seino, T. Tsutamoto et al., "Effects of carperitide on the long-term prognosis of patients with acute decompensated chronic heart failure: the PROTECT multicenter randomized controlled study," *Circulation Journal*, vol. 72, no. 11, pp. 1787–1793, 2008.

[2] N. Sato, K. Kajimoto, K. Asai et al., "Acute decompensated heart failure syndromes (ATTEND) registry. A prospective observational multicenter cohort study: rationale, design, and preliminary data," *American Heart Journal*, vol. 159, no. 6, pp. 949.e1–955.e1, 2010.

[3] M. Suwa, Y. Seino, Y. Nomachi, S. Matsuki, and K. Funahashi, "Multicenter prospective investigation on efficacy and safety of carperitide for acute heart failure in the 'real world' of therapy," *Circulation Journal*, vol. 69, no. 3, pp. 283–290, 2005.

[4] F. Nomura, N. Kurobe, Y. Mori et al., "Multicenter prospective investigation on efficacy and safety of carperitide as a first-line drug for acute heart failure syndrome with preserved blood pressure—COMPASS: carperitide effects observed through monitoring dyspnea in acute decompensated heart failure study," *Circulation Journal*, vol. 72, no. 11, pp. 1777–1786, 2008.

[5] C. M. O'Connor, R. C. Starling, and A. F. Hernandez, "Effect of nesiritide in patients with acute decompensated heart failure," *The New England Journal of Medicine*, vol. 365, no. 1, pp. 32–43, 2011.

[6] L. Klein, C. M. O'Connor, J. D. Leimberger et al., "Lower serum sodium is associated with increased short-term mortality in hospitalized patients with worsening heart failure: results from the outcomes of a prospective trial of intravenous milrinone for exacerbations of chronic heart failure (OPTIME-CHF) study," *Circulation*, vol. 111, no. 19, pp. 2454–2460, 2005.

[7] H. J. Milionis, G. E. Alexandrides, E. N. Liberopoulos, E. T. Bairaktari, J. Goudevenos, and M. S. Elisaf, "Hypomagnesemia and concurrent acid-base and electrolyte abnormalities in patients with congestive heart failure," *European Journal of Heart Failure*, vol. 4, no. 2, pp. 167–173, 2002.

[8] S. R. Goldsmith, G. S. Francis, A. W. Cowley Jr., T. B. Levine, and J. N. Cohn, "Increased plasma arginine vasopressin levels in patients with congestive heart failure," *Journal of the American College of Cardiology*, vol. 1, no. 6, pp. 1385–1390, 1983.

[9] K. Kinugawa, T. Imamura, and I. Komuro, "Experience of a vasopressin receptor antagonist, tolvaptan, under the unique indication in Japanese heart failure patients," *Clinical Pharmacology and Therapeutics*, vol. 94, no. 4, pp. 449–451, 2013.

[10] J. E. Udelson, W. B. Smith, G. H. Hendrix et al., "Acute hemodynamic effects of conivaptan, a dual V_{1A} and V_2 vasopressin receptor antagonist, in patients with advanced heart failure," *Circulation*, vol. 104, no. 20, pp. 2417–2423, 2001.

[11] T. Imamura, K. Kinugawa, D. Nitta, and I. Komuro, "Tolvaptan reduces long-term total medical expenses and length of stay in aquaporin-defined responders," *International Heart Journal*, vol. 57, no. 5, pp. 593–599, 2016.

[12] T. Imamura, K. Kinugawa, M. Hatano et al., "Low cardiac output stimulates vasopressin release in patients with stage d heart failure—its relevance to poor prognosis and reversal by surgical treatment," *The Journal of Heart and Lung Transplantation*, vol. 33, no. 4, p. S51, 2014.

[13] M. A. Konstam, M. Gheorghiade, J. C. Burnett Jr. et al., "Effects of oral tolvaptan in patients hospitalized for worsening heart failure: the EVEREST outcome trial," *Journal of the American Medical Association*, vol. 297, no. 12, pp. 1319–1331, 2007.

[14] T. Imamura, T. Fujino, T. Inaba et al., "Increased urine aquaporin-2 relative to plasma arginine vasopressin is a novel marker of response to tolvaptan in patients with decompensated heart failure," *Circulation Journal*, vol. 78, no. 9, pp. 2240–2249, 2014.

[15] K. Watanabe, K. Dohi, T. Sugimoto et al., "Short-term effects of low-dose tolvaptan on hemodynamic parameters in patients with chronic heart failure," *Journal of Cardiology*, vol. 60, no. 6, pp. 462–469, 2012.

[16] S. Suzuki, A. Yoshihisa, T. Yamaki et al., "Vasopressin V2 receptor antagonist tolvaptan is effective in heart failure patients with reduced left ventricular systolic function and low blood pressure," *International Heart Journal*, vol. 56, no. 2, pp. 213–218, 2015.

20

Impact of Body Mass Index on Short-Term Outcomes in Patients Undergoing Percutaneous Coronary Intervention in Newfoundland and Labrador, Canada

Anne B. Gregory,[1,2] Kendra K. Lester,[2] Deborah M. Gregory,[2,3] Laurie K. Twells,[2,4] William K. Midodzi,[2] and Neil J. Pearce[1,3]

[1]Eastern Health, St. John's, NL, Canada A1B 3V6
[2]Department of Clinical Epidemiology, Faculty of Medicine, Memorial University of Newfoundland, St. John's, NL, Canada A1B 3V6
[3]Department of Medicine, Faculty of Medicine, Memorial University of Newfoundland, St. John's, NL, Canada A1B 3V6
[4]School of Pharmacy, Memorial University of Newfoundland, St. John's, NL, Canada A1B 3V6

Correspondence should be addressed to Deborah M. Gregory; dgregory@mun.ca

Academic Editor: Mariantonietta Cicoira

Background and Aim. Obesity (BMI $\geq$ 30 kg/m^2) is associated with advanced cardiovascular disease requiring procedures such as percutaneous coronary intervention (PCI). Studies report better outcomes in obese patients having these procedures but results are conflicting or inconsistent. Newfoundland and Labrador (NL) has the highest rate of obesity in Canada. The aim of the study was to examine the relationship between BMI and vascular and nonvascular complications in patients undergoing PCI in NL. *Methods.* We studied 6473 patients identified in the APPROACH-NL database who underwent PCI from May 2006 to December 2013. BMI categories included normal, $18.5 \leq$ BMI < 25.0 ($n = 1073$); overweight, $25.0 \leq$ BMI < 30 ($n = 2608$); and obese, BMI ≥ 30.0 ($n = 2792$). *Results.* Patients with obesity were younger and had a higher incidence of diabetes, hypertension, and family history of cardiac disease. Obese patients experienced less vascular complications (normal, overweight, and obese: 8.2%, 7.2%, and 5.3%, $p = 0.001$). No significant differences were observed for in-lab (4.0%, 3.3%, and 3.1%, $p = 0.386$) or postprocedural (1.0%, 0.8%, and 0.9%, $p = 0.725$) nonvascular complications. After adjusting for covariates, BMI was not a significant factor associated with adverse outcomes. *Conclusion.* Overweight and obesity were not independent correlates of short-term vascular and nonvascular complications among patients undergoing PCI.

1. Introduction

Obesity is an independent risk factor for cardiovascular disease [1–5] and is associated with advanced cardiovascular disease requiring procedures such as percutaneous coronary intervention (PCI) and coronary artery bypass grafting (CABG), reduction in life expectancy [6], and a higher mortality rate [3, 7, 8]. A number of observational studies have reported improved clinical outcomes (i.e., increased survival benefit) in overweight and obese patients treated for cardiovascular diseases compared to normal weight patients, a phenomenon commonly referred to as "obesity paradox"

[9–14]. This phenomenon is considered to be counterintuitive, referred to as "reverse epidemiology," and reported in patients with hypertension [15], heart failure [16], coronary artery disease (CAD) [15, 17–19], CABG [17–20], and PCI [17–19]. The term "reverse epidemiology" was first used in a 2003 study by Kalantar-Zadeh et al. [21] which focused on cardiovascular risk factors including body mass index (BMI), serum cholesterol, and blood pressure in maintenance hemodialysis patients. Obesity, hypercholesterolemia, and hypertension were paradoxically associated with survival, the opposite of that observed in the general population. In 2004, Kalantar-Zadeh et al. also reported a protective role of conventional cardiovascular risk factors in chronic heart failure [22]. Use of the term "reverse epidemiology" and alternative terms including "risk factor reversal" and "altered risk factor patterns" [23] has continued in the research literature; however, some refer to the term as confusing, confounding, and inaccurate [24] and suggest it may be a "questionable concept." Inconsistent results have been reported regarding the association between BMI and short-term clinical outcomes (i.e., vascular complication, nonvascular in-lab and postprocedural complications) and/or mortality in patients undergoing PCI [9, 10, 13, 25–31]; therefore, it is not entirely clear whether an obesity paradox exists.

Obesity is a common and rapidly growing public health concern. Between 1985 and 2011, the prevalence of this disease in Canada increased by 200% from 6.1% to 18.3% equating to more than 4.8 million adults, with continued increases projected [32]. Newfoundland and Labrador (NL) has the highest rate of obesity in Canada. It is estimated that 71% of the province's population will be either overweight or obese by 2019 [32]. There is a paucity of data on the prevalence of obesity in patients undergoing PCI in the province. Furthermore, the relationship between short-term clinical outcomes and BMI has not been examined in patients undergoing PCI in NL. In the present study, we (1) examine the prevalence of obesity among patients undergoing PCI and the differences among BMI groups on demographic, clinical, and procedural findings and (2) examine the association between the most commonly used anthropometric parameter to assess adiposity (i.e., BMI) and short-term outcomes (vascular complication, nonvascular in-lab and postprocedural complications occurring within 48 hours).

2. Methods

2.1. Study Design. We performed a retrospective analysis of prospectively collected deidentified data for all patients 18 years of age and older who had a PCI between May 1, 2006, and December 31, 2013, in the province of NL, Canada, using a well-established clinical database (i.e., Alberta Provincial Project for Outcome Assessment in Coronary Heart Disease-Newfoundland and Labrador (APPROACH-NL)). Detailed prospective demographic, clinical, and procedural data on all patients undergoing diagnostic cardiac catheterization and/or percutaneous coronary intervention (PCI) and cardiac surgery since 2006 is collected by specifically trained clinical cardiac catheterization database nurses. Nurses collect and record, on an abstraction sheet, patient data provided by nurses responsible for the care of the patient which includes examination and assessment of the access site for potential vascular complications. The attending physician also examined the vascular access site. All data are verified by chart review until hospital discharge by these nurses. Prospectively collected data on each consecutive patient is entered into the APPROACH-NL clinical database. A research nurse is responsible for the management of the database including completeness of data entry and quality assurance activities. Details of the database and methods of collection have been previously described [33]. If patients are

not hospitalized, they remain in the local area for 24 hours and are advised to return to the emergency department (ER) if they encounter any problems. ER admissions are audited by a clerk in the cardiac catheterization laboratory in the event that a patient returns to the ER.

2.2. Study Population. For the current study, all consecutive PCIs (N = 6633) performed on patients 18 years of age and older between May 1, 2006, and December 31, 2013, at the Health Science Centre, Eastern Health, NL, were enrolled. PCI procedures performed on underweight (BMI < 18.5 kg/m^2) individuals (n = 47) or those with missing BMI data or unlikely valid BMI levels of >70 or <11 kg/m^2 (n = 113) were excluded. The remaining patients comprised the study cohort. Based on these selection criteria, 6,473 patients were included in the final analysis.

Weight and height were measured and documented by a nurse at the time of PCI. If patients were unstable, self-reported weight and height were collected and BMI was calculated. Patients were grouped according to three BMI categories using the World Health Organization classification system: normal (18.5–24.9 kg/m^2), overweight (25.0–29.9 kg/m^2), and obese ($\geq$30 kg/m^2) [34]. These categorizations reflect relative increasing levels of risk to health [35].

2.3. Clinical Outcomes and Definitions. The *primary outcome* was short-term complications occurring within 48 hours after the intervention. The clinical definitions for complications were as follows. *Vascular access complications* were defined as hematoma (>5 cm), pseudoaneurysm, arteriovenous fistula, vascular occlusion, access site bleeding, retroperitoneal bleed, loss of distal pulse, or occlusion. *Nonvascular complications* included in-lab events (abrupt coronary closure, emergency CABG, access site complications, death, ventricular tachycardia/ventricular fibrillation, pulmonary edema, shock, and dissection) and *postprocedural complications* included death, myocardial infarction, emergency CABG, abrupt coronary closure, hemorrhagic or ischemic CVA, and GI bleed. Each of the outcomes was a composite of the individual outcomes defined in each category.

2.4. Ethical Considerations. All patients who had a PCI during the time period under examination gave written informed consent to the cardiac care program for data collection and follow-up observation after PCI. The study protocol was approved by the Health Research Ethics Authority of Memorial University and Eastern Health.

2.5. Data Analysis. Demographic characteristics and clinical and procedural related variables were summarized. Continuous variables were expressed as mean ± standard deviation (SD). Categorical variables were expressed as frequencies and percentages. Continuous variables were compared using ANOVA, and the differences between categorical variables were examined using the χ^2 test and, where appropriate,

TABLE 1: Baseline characteristics of patients according to categories of BMI.

Variable	Total N	NW	OW	OB	p value*
Number of patients	6473	1073	2608	2792	
Age, years	6473	65.1 ± 11.1	63.1 ± 10.5	60.7 ± 10.1	$p < 0.001$
Male sex	6473	695 (64.8)	1975 (75.7)	1945 (69.7)	$p < 0.001$
Cardiovascular risk factors					
HTN	6462	658 (61.4)	1661 (63.8)	2066 (74.1)	$p < 0.001$
Hyperlipidemia	6462	905 (84.4)	2241 (86.1)	2434 (87.4)	$p = 0.050$
Diabetes	6464	226 (21.1)	637 (24.5)	1040 (37.3)	$p < 0.001$
Family history	6440	622 (58.3)	1627 (62.7)	1822 (65.5)	$p < 0.001$
Smoking status	6421				
Never	1719	298 (28.1)	698 (27.0)	723 (26.1)	$p = 0.441$
Smoking history	4702	763 (71.9)	1891 (73.0)	2048 (73.9)	
PVD	6460	91 (8.5)	172 (6.6)	156 (5.6)	$p = 0.005$
COPD	6459	156 (14.6)	335 (12.9)	479 (17.2)	$p < 0.001$

Values are presented as n (%) or mean ± SD, as indicated.
*p values for chi-squared or ANOVA tests.
BMI: body mass index; COPD: chronic obstructive pulmonary disease; NW: normal weight; OB: obese; OW: overweight; HTN: hypertension; PVD: peripheral vascular disease.

TABLE 2: Medications at time of referral for PCI by BMI category.

	Total N	NW	OW	OB	p value*
Number of patients	6473	1073	2608	2792	
Beta blockers	6431	863 (81.2)	2154 (83.1)	2318 (83.5)	$p = 0.220$
ACE inhibitors	6429	510 (48.0)	1296 (50.0)	1476 (53.2)	$p = 0.006$
ARB antagonist	6428	104 (9.8)	305 (11.8)	431 (15.5)	$p < 0.001$
CCB	6430	173 (16.3)	433 (16.7)	596 (21.5)	$p < 0.001$
LA nitrates	6430	307 (28.9)	729 (28.1)	869 (31.3)	$p = 0.032$
Statin therapy	6427	874 (82.3)	2199 (84.9)	2345 (84.5)	$p = 0.134$
Aspirin	6432	983 (92.5)	2402 (92.6)	2612 (94.1)	$p = 0.058$
Ticlopidine/clopidogrel	6432	806 (75.8)	1846 (71.2)	1925 (69.3)	$p < 0.001$
Coumadin	6429	15 (1.4)	47 (1.8)	59 (2.1)	$p = 0.329$
GP IIb/IIIa inhibitors	6437	5 (0.5)	14 (0.5)	13 (0.5)	$p = 0.924$
LMWH	6439	428 (40.2)	971 (37.4)	1003 (36.1)	$p = 0.068$
IV heparin	6439	220 (20.6)	497 (19.1)	579 (20.8)	$p = 0.268$
IV nitrates	6430	141 (13.3)	313 (12.1)	307 (11.1)	$p = 0.149$

Values are presented as n (%).
*p values for chi-squared tests.
ACE: angiotensin converting enzyme; ARB: angiotensin receptor blocker; BMI: body mass index; CCB: calcium channel blockers; LA nitrates: long-acting nitrates; LMWH: low molecular weight heparin; NW: normal weight; OB: obese; OW: overweight; PCI: percutaneous coronary intervention.

the Fisher exact test is reported. All p values were two-tailed, with statistical significance defined by a p value < 0.05. Comparisons were performed for a trend in increasing BMI categories using χ^2 test for trends. Univariate logistic regression analysis was performed to determine the odds ratio for vascular complications and nonvascular complications occurring in the cardiac care laboratory identified within 24–48 hours after PCI. Multivariate logistic regression analysis was used to examine independent predictors for each of the patient outcomes. Due to the low nonvascular postprocedural complication event rate, regression analyses were not performed. Variables identified in Tables 1–3 were selected for these models based on univariate p values < 0.20

and overall clinical significance. All statistical analyses were performed using IBM SPSS Statistics for Windows, Version 22.0 (IBM Corp., Armonk, NY) [36].

3. Results

A cohort of 6,473 patients was identified from the population of patients who had a PCI during the time period under examination. BMI values for normal weight, overweight, and obese patients from 2006 to 2013 are presented in Figure 1. Tables 1–3 show the baseline characteristics of patients according to categories of BMI, medications at

TABLE 3: Admitting clinical, angiographic, and procedural data for patients undergoing PCI according to BMI category.

	Total N	NW	OW	OB	p value*
Number of patients	6473	$n = 1073$	$n = 2608$	$n = 2792$	
Cardiovascular history					
Prior PCI	6462	226 (21.1)	543 (20.9)	627 (22.5)	$p = 0.318$
Prior CABG	6462	129 (12.0)	298 (11.5)	289 (10.4)	$p = 0.247$
Prior HF	6462	52 (4.9)	83 (3.2)	106 (3.8)	$p = 0.052$
Prior MI	6462	212 (19.8)	527 (20.3)	581 (20.8)	$p = 0.734$
CVD	6450	89 (8.3)	160 (6.2)	174 (6.3)	$p = 0.041$
Same sitting angioplasty	6473	864 (80.5)	2138 (82.0)	2321 (83.1)	$p = 0.149$
IABP/cardiogenic shock	6461	7 (0.7)	16 (0.6)	31 (1.1)	$p = 0.104$
Priority	6466				
Low risk	1861	220 (20.5)	783 (30.0)	858 (30.7)	
Emergency	397	72 (6.7)	170 (6.5)	155 (5.6)	$p < 0.001$
Urgent	4208	780 (72.7)	1654 (63.4)	1774 (63.5)	
PE	6216	8 (0.8)	13 (0.5)	15 (0.6)	$p = 0.641$
Thromboembolic history	6218	5 (0.5)	12 (0.5)	10 (0.4)	$p = 0.797$
DVT	6219	16 (1.6)	32 (1.3)	32 (1.2)	$p = 0.663$
Stable angina	1748	202 (18.9)	731 (28.1)	815 (29.3)	$p < 0.001$
ACS	4341	$n = 791$	$n = 1724$	$n = 1825$	
STEMI	1227	251 (31.7)	501 (29.1)	475 (26.0)	
Non-STEMI	1939	349 (44.1)	787 (45.6)	803 (44.0)	$p = 0.001$
Unstable angina	1174	191 (24.1)	436 (25.3)	547 (30.0)	
Thrombolytics contraindicated	4143	11 (1.5)	27 (1.6)	24 (1.4)	$p = 0.831$
Failed thrombolysis	4274	26 (3.4)	77 (4.5)	59 (3.3)	$p = 0.122$
Access site					
Radial/brachial	1172	193 (18.0)	468 (17.9)	511 (18.3)	$p = 0.938$
Femoral	5301	880 (82.0)	2140 (82.1)	2282 (81.7)	
Sheath size					
Sheath size 5 Fr	924	160 (14.9)	393 (15.1)	371 (13.3)	
Sheath size 6 Fr	5432	893 (83.2)	2171 (83.3)	2368 (84.9)	$p = 0.386$
Sheath size 7/8 Fr	114	20 (1.9)	43 (1.6)	51 (1.8)	
Closure device	6470	484 (45.1)	1359 (52.1)	1506 (54.0)	$p < 0.001$
GP IIb/IIIa inhibitors	6471	134 (12.5)	338 (13.0)	351 (12.6)	$p = 0.889$

Values are presented as n (%).
*p values for chi-squared tests.
ACS = acute coronary syndrome; BMI: body mass index; CABG: coronary artery bypass grafting; CVD: cerebrovascular disease; DVT= deep vein thrombosis; HF: heart failure; IABP: intra-aortic balloon pump; MI: myocardial infarction; NW: normal weight; OB: obese; OW: overweight; PCI: percutaneous coronary intervention; PE: pulmonary embolism; PVD: peripheral vascular disease; STEMI: ST elevation myocardial infarction.

time of referral, and admitting clinical angiographic and procedural data.

3.1. Baseline Characteristics.
Of the 6,473 patients, 16.6% were of normal weight ($n = 1073$), 40.3% were overweight ($n = 2608$), and 43.1% were obese ($n = 2792$). In each of the years examined, less than 19% of patients who had a PCI were of normal weight (Table 1 and Figure 1). The baseline characteristics of the study patients according to the three BMI categories are presented in Table 1. There were statistically significant differences between the groups on a number of characteristics. A higher proportion of overweight patients were male. Patients with obesity were younger, had

a higher incidence of coronary risk factors such as diabetes mellitus and hypertension, and had a family history of coronary artery disease. Patients with a higher BMI were also more likely to have COPD, whereas normal weight patients were more likely to have PVD. No significant differences were observed in smoking status.

Medications at the time of referral for PCI were examined. The details regarding the use of medications prior to PCI are presented in Table 2. No significant differences were found in the use of acetylsalicylic acid, coumadin, preprocedural GP IIb/IIIa inhibitors, beta blockers, LMWH, IV heparin, IV nitrates, or statin therapy between the groups. Patients with obesity were less likely to receive the antiplatelet medication ticlopidine/clopidogrel but were more likely to receive an

TABLE 4: Vascular and nonvascular complications occurring within 24 to 48 hours in patients undergoing PCI according to BMI category.

	NW ($n = 1073$)	OW ($n = 2608$)	OB ($n = 2792$)	p value[*]
Vascular complications	88 (8.2)	187 (7.2)	149 (5.3)	0.001
Nonvascular in-lab complications	43 (4.0)	87 (3.3)	87 (3.1)	0.386
Nonvascular postprocedural complications	11 (1.0)	20 (0.8)	25 (0.9)	0.725

Values are presented as n (%).
BMI: body mass index; NW: normal weight; OW: overweight; OB: obese; PCI: percutaneous coronary intervention.
[*] p values for chi-squared tests.
Vascular complications were defined as hematoma (>5 cm), pseudoaneurysm, arteriovenous fistula, vascular occlusion, access site bleeding, retroperitoneal bleed, loss of distal pulse, or occlusion.
Nonvascular complications occurring in-lab included abrupt coronary closure, emergency coronary artery bypass grafting (CABG), access site complications, death, ventricular tachycardia/ventricular fibrillation, pulmonary edema, shock, and dissection.
Nonvascular postprocedural complications included death, myocardial infarction, emergency CABG, abrupt coronary closure, hemorrhagic or ischemic CVA, and GI bleed.

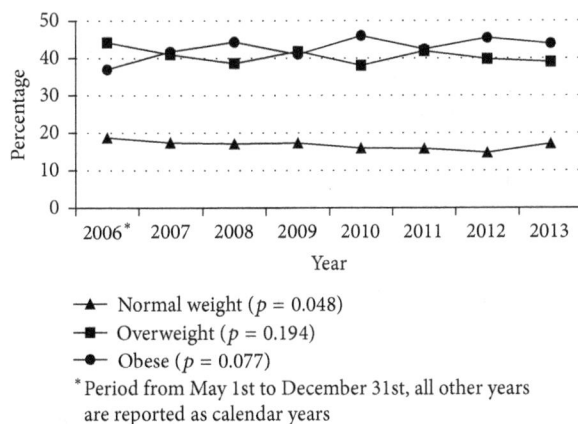

−▲− Normal weight ($p = 0.048$)
−■− Overweight ($p = 0.194$)
−●− Obese ($p = 0.077$)
[*]Period from May 1st to December 31st, all other years are reported as calendar years

FIGURE 1: Body mass index trends for normal weight, overweight, and obese patients from 2006 to 2013.

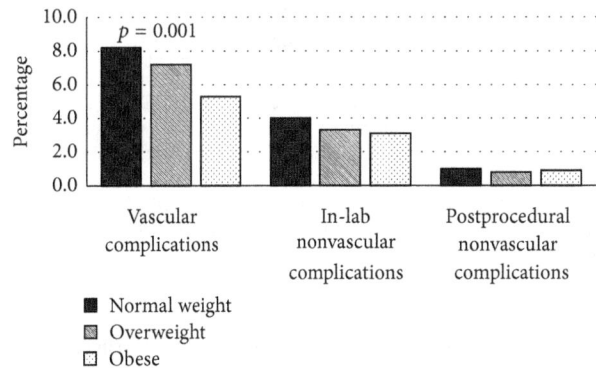

FIGURE 2: Prevalence of vascular and nonvascular complications (in-lab and postprocedural) by body mass index category.

angiotensin-converting enzyme inhibitor/angiotensin receptor blocker, calcium channel blockers, and long-acting nitrates.

3.2. Angiographic and Procedural Data. Admitting clinical, angiographic, and procedural data are shown in Table 3. Normal weight patients were significantly less likely to require a closure device ($p < 0.001$) compared to other BMI groups. However, there were no significant differences among the BMI categories in the prevalence of prior PCI, prior CABG, prior HF, prior MI, pulmonary embolism, thromboembolic history, deep vein thrombosis, same sitting angioplasty, IABP use at time of referral or during the procedure/cardiogenic shock at time of procedure, use of GP IIb/IIIa inhibitors, access site, and choice of sheath size. A greater proportion of normal weight patients presented as emergency/urgent cases, whereas more elective procedures were performed in overweight and obese patients. A greater proportion of obese patients presented with unstable angina, whereas a much lower proportion presented with a STEMI.

3.3. Complications Occurring within 24 to 48 Hours of PCI according to BMI. Complications occurring within 24 to 48 hours of PCI according to BMI category are presented in Table 4 and Figure 2. Obese subjects experienced a lower proportion of vascular complications (normal, overweight, and obese: 8.2%, 7.2%, and 5.3%, $p = 0.001$). No significant differences were observed for nonvascular complications either in-lab (4.0%, 3.3%, and 3.1%, $p = 0.386$) or postprocedural (1.0%, 0.8%, and 0.9%, $p = 0.725$).

We performed multivariate analyses to adjust for clinical and procedural characteristics. Independent factors associated with the primary outcomes of vascular complications and nonvascular in-lab complications are shown in Tables 5 and 6. Increasing age, GP IIb/IIIa inhibitor, and LMWH use during the procedure and the utilization of a femoral access site approach were significant factors associated with the occurrence of vascular complications. Males, patients with diabetes and patients who had a closure device, and PCIs performed in 2010 were less likely to have vascular complications. GI/liver disease, coumadin use, utilization of GP IIb/IIIa inhibitors or IV heparin during PCI, and older age were significant factors associated with the occurrence of nonvascular in-lab complications. Male sex and the use of a closure device were protective factors associated with

TABLE 5: Multivariate adjusted OR for vascular complications in patients undergoing PCI.

	OR	95% CI	p value
Age	1.02	1.01–1.03	0.001
Male	0.69	0.55–0.86	0.001
Diabetes	0.65	0.51–0.84	0.001
Sheath size 5 Fr	0.42	0.20–0.85	0.016
Procedural GP IIb/IIIa inhibitors	1.95	1.50–2.54	0.000
Preprocedural LMWH	1.29	1.03–1.61	0.029
Closure device	0.54	0.43–0.68	0.000
Femoral access	2.98	2.00–4.45	0.000
Year, 2010	0.49	0.30–0.80	0.005
BMI (referent category is normal weight)			
Overweight	1.01	0.76–1.33	0.967
Obese	0.83	0.62–1.11	0.219

Adjusted for access site, age, aspirin, BMI, closure device, diabetes, gender, GI/liver disease, LMWH in-lab, preprocedural LMWH, GP IIb/IIIa inhibitors in-lab, preprocedural GP IIb/IIIa inhibitors, preprocedural IV heparin, prior CVD, prior HF, prior PCI, sheath size, smoking status, ticlopidine/clopidogrel, and year.
BMI: body mass index; CVD: cardiovascular disease; GP: glycoprotein; HF: heart failure; LMWH: low molecular weight heparin; PCI: percutaneous coronary intervention.

TABLE 6: Multivariate adjusted OR for nonvascular in-lab complications in patients undergoing PCI.

	OR	95% CI	p value
Age	1.02	1.001–1.03	0.039
Male	0.64	0.47–0.87	0.005
GI/liver disease	1.53	1.02–2.27	0.038
GP IIb/IIIa inhibitors in-lab	4.99	3.65–6.81	0.000
IV heparin in-lab	1.70	1.14–2.52	0.009
Coumadin	2.38	1.14–4.98	0.021
Closure device	0.28	0.19–0.40	0.000
BMI (referent category is normal weight)			
Overweight	0.93	0.62–1.38	0.705
Obese	0.54	0.58–1.32	0.879

Adjusted for age, BMI, closure device, coumadin, diabetes, DVT, family history of premature CAD, GP IIb/IIIa inhibitors in-lab, gender, GI/liver disease, hypertension, IV heparin in-lab, LMWH in-lab, prior CABG, prior COPD, prior CVD, prior HF, prior PCI, prior PVD, pulmonary embolism, sheath size, and year.
BMI: body mass index; CAD: coronary artery disease; CABG: coronary artery bypass grafting; COPD: chronic obstructive pulmonary disease; CVD: cardiovascular disease; DVT: deep vein thrombosis; GP: glycoprotein; HF: heart failure; LMWH: low molecular weight heparin; PCI: percutaneous coronary intervention; PVD: peripheral vascular disease.

a less likelihood of nonvascular in-lab complications. BMI was not a significant factor associated with either vascular or nonvascular in-lab complications (Tables 5 and 6).

4. Discussion

The present study examined all adult patients who had a PCI procedure performed between 2006 and 2013 in one Canadian province to determine the prevalence of obesity in this patient population and trend in rates over time. A second objective was to examine the relationship between BMI and short-term vascular and nonvascular complications occurring within 48 hours and compare outcomes among three BMI categories (normal weight, overweight, and obese). The majority of patients (84.3%) were either overweight or obese. Our study findings are comparable to other studies that have used PCI registries [10, 11, 30]. In the current study, we found that over time there was a significant trend of decreasing prevalence for the normal weight category of patients undergoing PCI ($p = 0.048$). Similar to previous studies, the current study demonstrates that obese patients presented with more risk factors for CAD than overweight or normal weight patients. Obese patients were younger, diabetic, and hypertensive and had higher rates of hyperlipidemia and family history of CAD.

We hypothesized that BMI was an independent correlate of outcome in patients undergoing PCI; more specifically, obese patients would experience worse outcomes compared to normal and overweight patients. The obese patients in the present study were significantly younger and had higher incidence of coronary risk factors such as diabetes mellitus and hypertension and had a family history of coronary artery but based on the findings of the univariate analyses had a significantly lower rate of vascular complications (hematoma (>5 cm), pseudoaneurysm, arteriovenous fistula, vascular occlusion, access site bleeding, retroperitoneal bleed, loss of distal pulse, or occlusion) than their normal weight and overweight counterparts. There were no significant differences in the rates of nonvascular in-lab (acute coronary closure, emergency CABG, access site complications, death, ventricular tachycardia/ventricular fibrillation, pulmonary edema, shock, and dissection) and postprocedural complications (death, myocardial infarction, emergency CABG, abrupt coronary closure, hemorrhagic or ischemic CVA, and GI bleed) among the BMI categories.

After multiple logistic regression analysis, BMI was not a significant predictor of short-term outcomes (vascular complications or in-lab nonvascular complications). Our data regarding BMI in NL patients is consistent with one previous Canadian study but is contradictory to the findings of a 2009 study conducted by Byrne et al. [28]. Similar to our findings, Shubair et al. [10] evaluated the effect of BMI on in-hospital outcomes in a consecutive series of coronary artery disease patients undergoing PCI enrolled in a clinical database at the Hamilton Health Sciences in Ontario, Canada. The authors found that obesity was not associated with in-hospital postprocedural death, myocardial infarction, repeat PCI, CABG, or major adverse cardiac event defined as a composite of death, myocardial infarction, repeat PCI, and CABG. Using a large Canadian provincial registry, Byrne et al. [28] investigated the relationship between BMI, bleeding, and outcome (i.e., 1-year mortality) after PCI. The authors reported that lower BMI (≤18.5 kg/m^2) and higher BMI

($\geq 40 \, \text{kg/m}^2$) patients were at greater risk of bleeding and death after PCI. Other studies conducted in the western society have reported that underweight [9, 25, 28], normal weight [9, 25], and extremely obese [29–31] patients are at greater risk of adverse outcomes after PCI. Cox et al. [9] reported that the rate of vascular complications was the highest in extremely thin and morbidly obese patients and the lowest in moderately obese patients. In a study by Gruberg et al. [25], the authors reported that normal weight patients were at the highest risk of in-hospital complications (i.e., major bleeding, vascular complications, emergency CABG, and myocardial infarction) and cardiac death compared to overweight and obese patients. Two studies by Gurm et al. [26, 27] suggested that being moderately obese conferred a protective effect, referred to as an "obesity paradox," in relation to vascular complications and major adverse outcomes after PCI, a finding consistent with that reported by Cox et al. [9].

In other studies that have focused primarily on the comparison of normal weight and extremely obese ($\geq 40 \, \text{kg/m}^2$) patients undergoing PCI, researchers have reported that extremely obese patients have increased vascular complications [30] compared to normal weight individuals and higher rates of in-hospital mortality [29–31] compared to overweight individuals. In the current study, we were unable to examine the various classes of obesity due to the small numbers in each category.

Study Strengths and Limitations. Our study has a number of strengths. We report on a large population-based cohort of patients undergoing PCI at a single tertiary cardiac centre using APPROACH-NL prospectively collected data. Data quality assurance indicated that the amount of missing data was minimal (1.7%). Actual measures of height and weight were taken at the time of the procedure unless the patients were unstable.

This study also has a number of limitations. Our study is an observational nonrandomized cohort study with retrospective analysis. The current study design can only establish association and not causation. We used data from a clinical database and as such cannot account for confounders not captured in the database. The study population was heterogeneous (i.e., included patients with variable levels of coronary artery disease severity ranging from acute coronary syndrome with cardiogenic shock to stable angina). Patients with missing BMI data were excluded ($n = 113$) which may contribute to selection bias, but as missing data only accounted for 1.7% this is unlikely. Despite its widespread use, the use of BMI in terms of its accuracy to define obesity is controversial [37–39]. BMI is not as well correlated to cardiovascular disease and death as other measures including waist circumference and waist-to-hip ratio [40], data that were unavailable in the clinical database. A lack of underweight and severely obese patients meant that comparisons in our study were made between only three BMI groups: normal weight, overweight, and obese.

5. Conclusion

Overweight and obesity were not independent predictors of short term outcomes (vascular or nonvascular complications occurring within 24 to 48 hours) in patients undergoing PCI at our institution.

Competing Interests

Dr. Anne B. Gregory, Kendra K. Lester, Dr. Deborah M. Gregory, Dr. Laurie K. Twells, and Dr. William K. Midodzi have no competing interests to declare. Dr. Neil J. Pearce is the director of the APPROACH-NL cardiac care database, Division Head Cardiology, Eastern Health, and the former director of the Cardiac Catheterization Lab.

Authors' Contributions

Study concept and design were handled by Anne B. Gregory, Deborah M. Gregory, Laurie K. Twells, and Neil J. Pearce. Analysis and interpretation of the data were handled by Anne B. Gregory, Kendra K. Lester, Deborah M. Gregory, Neil J. Pearce, Laurie K. Twells, and William K. Midodzi. Drafting of the paper was handled by Anne B. Gregory and Deborah M. Gregory. Critical revision of the paper for important intellectual content was handled by Anne B. Gregory, Deborah M. Gregory, Kendra K. Lester, Neil J. Pearce, Laurie K. Twells, and William K. Midodzi. Statistical analysis was carried out by Anne B. Gregory, Deborah M. Gregory, Kendra K. Lester, and William K. Midodzi. Anne B. Gregory, Deborah M. Gregory, Kendra K. Lester, and William K. Midodzi had full access to all data in the study and take responsibility for the integrity of the data and the accuracy of the data analysis.

Acknowledgments

The authors gratefully acknowledge the cardiac care program staff for data collection and entry, especially Jennifer Matthews, Program Coordinator of APPROACH-NL, and staff from the Translational Personalized Medicine Initiative of Memorial University for their statistical consultation.

References

[1] S. W. Rabkin, F. A. L. Mathewson, and P.-H. Hsu, "Relation of body weight to development of ischemic heart disease in a cohort of young North American men after a 26 year observation period: the Manitoba study," *The American Journal of Cardiology*, vol. 39, no. 3, pp. 452–458, 1977.

[2] J. E. Manson, G. A. Colditz, M. J. Stampfer et al., "A prospective study of obesity and risk of coronary heart disease in women," *The New England Journal of Medicine*, vol. 322, no. 13, pp. 882–889, 1990.

[3] H. B. Hubert, M. Feinleib, P. M. McNamara, and W. P. Castelli, "Obesity as an independent risk factor for cardiovascular disease: a 26-year follow-up of participants in the Framingham Heart Study," *Circulation*, vol. 67, no. 5, pp. 968–977, 1983.

[4] Y. Chen, W. K. Copeland, R. Vedanthan et al., "Association between body mass index and cardiovascular disease mortality in east Asians and south Asians: pooled analysis of prospective data from the Asia Cohort Consortium," *British Medical Journal*, vol. 347, no. 7927, Article ID f5446, 2013.

[5] Y. Lu, K. Hajifathalian, M. Ezzati, M. Woodward, E. B. Rimm, and G. Danaei, "Metabolic mediators of the effects of body-mass index, overweight, and obesity on coronary heart disease and stroke: a pooled analysis of 97 prospective cohorts with 1·8 million participants," *The Lancet*, vol. 383, no. 9921, pp. 970–983, 2014.

[6] K. R. Fontaine, D. T. Redden, C. Wang, A. O. Westfall, and D. B. Allison, "Years of life lost due to obesity," *The Journal of the American Medical Association*, vol. 289, no. 2, pp. 187–193, 2003.

[7] E. E. Calle, M. J. Thun, J. M. Petrelli, C. Rodriguez, and C. W. Heath Jr., "Body-mass index and mortality in a prospective cohort of U.S. adults," *The New England Journal of Medicine*, vol. 341, no. 15, pp. 1097–1105, 1999.

[8] K. M. Flegal, B. K. Kit, H. Orpana, and B. I. Graubard, "Association of all-cause mortality with overweight and obesity using standard body mass index categories: a systematic review and meta-analysis," *The Journal of the American Medical Association*, vol. 309, no. 1, pp. 71–82, 2013.

[9] N. Cox, F. S. Resnic, J. J. Popma, D. I. Simon, A. C. Eisenhauer, and C. Rogers, "Comparison of the risk of vascular complications associated with femoral and radial access coronary catheterization procedures in obese versus nonobese patients," *The American Journal of Cardiology*, vol. 94, no. 9, pp. 1174–1177, 2004.

[10] M. M. Shubair, P. Prabhakaran, V. Pavlova, J. L. Velianou, A. M. Sharma, and M. K. Natarajan, "The relationship of body mass index to outcomes after percutaneous coronary intervention," *Journal of Interventional Cardiology*, vol. 19, no. 5, pp. 388–395, 2006.

[11] L. Mehta, W. Devlin, P. A. McCullough et al., "Impact of body mass index on outcomes after percutaneous coronary intervention in patients with acute myocardial infarction," *American Journal of Cardiology*, vol. 99, no. 7, pp. 906–910, 2007.

[12] C. E. Hastie, S. Padmanabhan, R. Slack et al., "Obesity paradox in a cohort of 4880 consecutive patients undergoing percutaneous coronary intervention," *European Heart Journal*, vol. 31, no. 2, pp. 222–226, 2010.

[13] T. Lancefield, D. J. Clark, N. Andrianopoulos et al., "Is there an obesity paradox after percutaneous coronary intervention in the contemporary era? An analysis from a multicenter australian registry," *Journal of the American College of Cardiovascular Interventions*, vol. 3, no. 6, pp. 660–668, 2010.

[14] M. Schmiegelow, C. Torp-Pedersen, G. H. Gislason et al., "Relation of body mass index to risk of stent thrombosis after percutaneous coronary intervention," *The American Journal of Cardiology*, vol. 110, no. 11, pp. 1592–1597, 2012.

[15] S. Uretsky, F. H. Messerli, S. Bangalore et al., "Obesity paradox in patients with hypertension and coronary artery disease," *American Journal of Medicine*, vol. 120, no. 10, pp. 863–870, 2007.

[16] G. C. Fonarow, P. Srikanthan, M. R. Costanzo, G. B. Cintron, and M. Lopatin, "An obesity paradox in acute heart failure: analysis of body mass index and inhospital mortality for 108,927 patients in the Acute Decompensated Heart Failure National Registry," *American Heart Journal*, vol. 153, no. 1, pp. 74–81, 2007.

[17] A. Oreopoulos, R. Padwal, C. M. Norris, J. C. Mullen, V. Pretorius, and K. Kalantar-Zadeh, "Effect of obesity on short- and long-term mortality postcoronary revascularization: a meta-analysis," *Obesity*, vol. 16, no. 2, pp. 442–450, 2008.

[18] A. Romero-Corral, V. M. Montori, V. K. Somers et al., "Association of bodyweight with total mortality and with cardiovascular events in coronary artery disease: a systematic review of cohort studies," *The Lancet*, vol. 368, no. 9536, pp. 666–678, 2006.

[19] A. Oreopoulos, F. A. McAlister, K. Kalantar-Zadeh et al., "The relationship between body mass index, treatment, and mortality in patients with established coronary artery disease: a report from APPROACH," *European Heart Journal*, vol. 30, no. 21, pp. 2584–2592, 2009.

[20] A. P. Johnson, J. L. Parlow, M. Whitehead, J. Xu, S. Rohland, and B. Milne, "Body mass index, outcomes, and mortality following cardiac surgery in Ontario, Canada," *Journal of the American Heart Association*, vol. 4, no. 7, Article ID e002140, 2015.

[21] K. Kalantar-Zadeh, G. Block, M. H. Humphreys, and J. D. Kopple, "Reverse epidemiology of cardiovascular risk factors in maintenance dialysis patients," *Kidney International*, vol. 63, no. 3, pp. 793–808, 2003.

[22] K. Kalantar-Zadeh, G. Block, T. Horwich, and G. C. Fonarow, "Reverse epidemiology of conventional cardiovascular risk factors in patients with chronic heart failure," *Journal of the American College of Cardiology*, vol. 43, no. 8, pp. 1439–1444, 2004.

[23] J. D. Kopple, "The phenomenon of altered risk factor patterns or reverse epidemiology in persons with advanced chronic kidney failure," *The American Journal of Clinical Nutrition*, vol. 81, no. 6, pp. 1257–1266, 2005.

[24] N. W. Levin, G. J. Handelman, J. Coresh, F. K. Port, and G. A. Kaysen, "Reverse epidemiology: a confusing, confounding, and inaccurate term," *Seminars in Dialysis*, vol. 20, no. 6, pp. 586–592, 2007.

[25] L. Gruberg, N. J. Weissman, R. Waksman et al., "The impact of obesity on the short-term and long-term outcomes after percutaneous coronary intervention: the obesity paradox?" *Journal of the American College of Cardiology*, vol. 39, no. 4, pp. 578–584, 2002.

[26] H. S. Gurm, D. M. Brennan, J. Booth, J. E. Tcheng, A. M. Lincoff, and E. J. Topol, "Impact of body mass index on outcome after percutaneous coronary intervention (The Obesity Paradox)," *The American Journal of Cardiology*, vol. 90, no. 1, pp. 42–45, 2002.

[27] H. S. Gurm, P. L. Whitlow, and K. E. Kip, "The impact of body mass index on short- and long-term outcomes in patients undergoing coronary revascularization. Insights from the Bypass Angioplasty Revascularization Investigation (BARI)," *Journal of the American College of Cardiology*, vol. 39, no. 5, pp. 834–840, 2002.

[28] J. Byrne, M. S. Spence, E. Fretz et al., "Body mass index, periprocedural bleeding, and outcome following percutaneous coronary intervention (from the British Columbia Cardiac Registry)," *The American Journal of Cardiology*, vol. 103, no. 4, pp. 507–511, 2009.

[29] S. R. Das, K. P. Alexander, A. Y. Chen et al., "Impact of body weight and extreme obesity on the presentation, treatment, and in-hospital outcomes of 50,149 patients with ST-segment elevation myocardial infarction: results from the NCDR (National Cardiovascular Data Registry)," *Journal of the American College of Cardiology*, vol. 58, no. 25, pp. 2642–2650, 2011.

[30] M. E. Buschur, D. Smith, D. Share et al., "The burgeoning epidemic of morbid obesity in patients undergoing percutaneous coronary intervention: insight from the blue cross blue shield of

Michigan cardiovascular consortium," *Journal of the American College of Cardiology*, vol. 62, no. 8, pp. 685–691, 2013.

[31] S. Payvar, S. Kim, S. V. Rao et al., "In-hospital outcomes of percutaneous coronary interventions in extremely obese and normal-weight patients. Findings from the NCDR (National Cardiovascular Data Registry)," *Journal of the American College of Cardiology*, vol. 62, no. 8, pp. 692–696, 2013.

[32] L. K. Twells, D. M. Gregory, J. Reddigan, and W. K. Midodzi, "Current and predicted prevalence of obesity in Canada: a trend analysis," *CMAJ Open*, vol. 2, no. 1, pp. E18–E26, 2014.

[33] D. Gregory, W. K. Midodzi, and N. J. Pearce, "Complications with Angio-Seal™ vascular closure devices compared with manual compression after diagnostic cardiac catheterization and percutaneous coronary intervention," *Journal of Interventional Cardiology*, vol. 26, no. 6, pp. 630–638, 2013.

[34] WHO Consultation on Obesity, "Obesity: preventing and managing the global epidemic. Report of a WHO consultation," World Health Organization Technical Report Series 894, WHO, 2000.

[35] Health Canada, "Canadian guidelines for body weight classification in adults. Quick reference tool for professionals," 2003, http://www.hc-sc.gc.ca/fn-an/nutrition/weights-poids/guide-ld-adult/cg_quick_ref-ldc_rapide_ref-table1-eng.php.

[36] *IBM SPSS Statistics for Windows, Version 22.0*, IBM Corp, Armonk, NY, USA, 2013.

[37] A. Romero-Corral, V. K. Somers, J. Sierra-Johnson et al., "Diagnostic performance of body mass index to detect obesity in patients with coronary artery disease," *European Heart Journal*, vol. 28, no. 17, pp. 2087–2093, 2007.

[38] A. Romero-Corral, V. K. Somers, J. Sierra-Johnson et al., "Accuracy of body mass index in diagnosing obesity in the adult general population," *International Journal of Obesity*, vol. 32, no. 6, pp. 959–966, 2008.

[39] A. De Schutter, C. J. Lavie, K. Arce, S. G. Menendez, and R. V. Milani, "Correlation and discrepancies between obesity by body mass index and body fat in patients with coronary heart disease," *Journal of Cardiopulmonary Rehabilitation and Prevention*, vol. 33, no. 2, pp. 77–83, 2013.

[40] M. Chrostowska, A. Szyndler, M. Hoffmann, and K. Narkiewicz, "Impact of obesity on cardiovascular health," *Best Practice and Research: Clinical Endocrinology and Metabolism*, vol. 27, no. 2, pp. 147–156, 2013.

21

Comparison of the Postprocedural Quality of Life between Coronary Artery Bypass Graft Surgery and Percutaneous Coronary Intervention

Kaneez Fatima,[1] Mohammad Yousuf-ul-Islam,[1] Mehreen Ansari,[1]
Faizan Imran Bawany,[1] Muhammad Shahzeb Khan,[1] Akash Khetpal,[1] Neelam Khetpal,[2]
Muhammad Nawaz Lashari,[3] Mohammad Hussham Arshad,[4]
Raamish Bin Amir,[5] Hoshang Rustom Kakalia,[5] Qaiser Hasan Zaidi,[5]
Sharmeen Kamran Mian,[5] and Bahram Kazani[6]

[1]MBBS-Dow University of Health Sciences (DUHS), Karachi 74100, Pakistan
[2]Kharadar General Hospital, Karachi, Pakistan
[3]Cardiology, Civil Hospital, DUHS, Karachi 74100, Pakistan
[4]Aga Khan University of Health Sciences, Karachi 74800, Pakistan
[5]Department of Biological Sciences, The Lyceum, Karachi 75600, Pakistan
[6]The Karachi Grammar School, Karachi 75600, Pakistan

Correspondence should be addressed to Mohammad Yousuf-ul-Islam; yousuf3220@gmail.com

Academic Editor: Piera Angelica Merlini

The treatment of choice between coronary artery bypass graft surgery (CABG) and percutaneous coronary intervention (PCI) has remained unclear. Considering quality of life (QOL) increases life expectancy, we believe QOL should be important in determining the optimum treatment. Thus the objective of this review was to illustrate the comparative effects of CABG and PCI on postprocedural QOL. *Methods.* We searched PubMed (Medline) and Embase from inception of the databases to May 2014 using "PCI versus CABG quality of life", "Percutaneous Coronary intervention versus Coronary artery bypass graft surgery Quality of life", "PCI versus CABG health status", "Angioplasty versus CABG", "Percutaneous coronary intervention versus coronary artery bypass surgery health status", and different combinations of the above terms. 447 articles were found. After applying strict exclusion criteria, we included 13 studies in this review. *Results.* From the 9 studies that compared QOL scores at 6 months after procedure, 5 studies reported CABG to be superior. From the 10 studies that compared QOL among patients at 1 year after procedure, 9 reported CABG to be superior. *Conclusion.* It can be established that CABG is superior to PCI in improving patient's QOL with respect to all scales used to determine quality of life.

1. Introduction

Coronary artery disease (CAD) is one of the leading causes of mortality and morbidity worldwide. Due to the high prevalence of CAD, both percutaneous coronary intervention (PCI) and coronary artery bypass graft surgery (CABG) are extremely common procedures [1]. Both techniques have proven to be safe and effective in treating CAD. Several studies have shown that both CABG and PCI can improve mortality and quality of life (QOL) significantly [2]. However

the treatment of choice between the two in certain commonly witnessed clinical scenarios such as unprotected left main CAD has remained uncertain for a long time.

Many randomized clinical trials have been conducted to compare the rates of mortality and myocardial infarction among CABG and PCI patients. Apart from the few studies [3, 4] that have established that CABG causes significant reduction in long term mortality and myocardial infarctions, many trials have demonstrated little difference [5–9]. We believe that in addition to mortality, QOL can be an important factor in deciding patient management especially among the indications where gray zones occur. QOL is a vital outcome after any medical procedure and for many people QOL is of equal significance, if not more, to increasing life expectancy. QOL is clearly the primary goal and benefit of any treatment plan [10].

Despite the several studies comparing QOL after CABG versus angioplasty among patients with CAD, the results have remained unclear. Moreover, very few systemic reviews have focused on QOL in deciding the better choice of treatment. The primary objective of this systematic review is to provide a complete picture of the comparative effects of CABG and PCI on postprocedural QOL.

2. Methods

2.1. The Literature Search. An extensive literature search was conducted using PubMed and Embase to find all published original articles comparing QOL after PCI and CABG from inception of the databases till May 2014. "PCI versus CABG quality of life", "Percutaneous Coronary intervention versus Coronary artery bypass graft surgery Quality of life", "PCI versus CABG health status", "Angioplasty versus CABG", "Percutaneous coronary intervention versus coronary artery bypass surgery health status", and different combinations of above terms were used for the retrieval of original articles. Due to inadequate resources, we had to limit our search parameters to English language only. The reference list of all the retrieved articles was also hand searched to spot any study that was missed during the database search.

2.2. Study Selection. 447 articles were found and subsequently reviewed by two authors in light of the exclusion criteria. Studies were excluded on the following basis (1) retrospective studies, (2) studies performed on animal models, (3) studies that were conducted without using a validated questionnaire to measure quality of life, (4) duplicate publication, (5) difficulty in extracting outcomes of interest from the study, and (6) studies which used minimally invasive coronary artery bypass graft surgery technique. Any dispute regarding exclusion of a study was settled by discussion and consensus. After deciding on the studies to be included, the data was extracted and verified by two authors. Considering the enormous heterogeneity, no attempt was made to pool the data. The selected studies were then summarized in a tabular form for easy reviewing (Table 2). Figure 1 shows the results of the literature search and study selection.

3. Results

Out of the total of 447 articles retrieved, 13 studies were incorporated in our systemic review. Table 1 shows the baseline characteristics of the patients from the included studies. From these 13 studies, 9 compared QOL scores at six months between CABG and PCI [1, 8, 11, 13–17, 20]. Out of these 9, 5 studies [1, 11, 13, 16, 20] reported that patients in the CABG group experienced better QOL six months after the procedure. The remaining four studies [8, 14, 15, 17] found QOL to be the same in both groups. Similarly, 10 studies

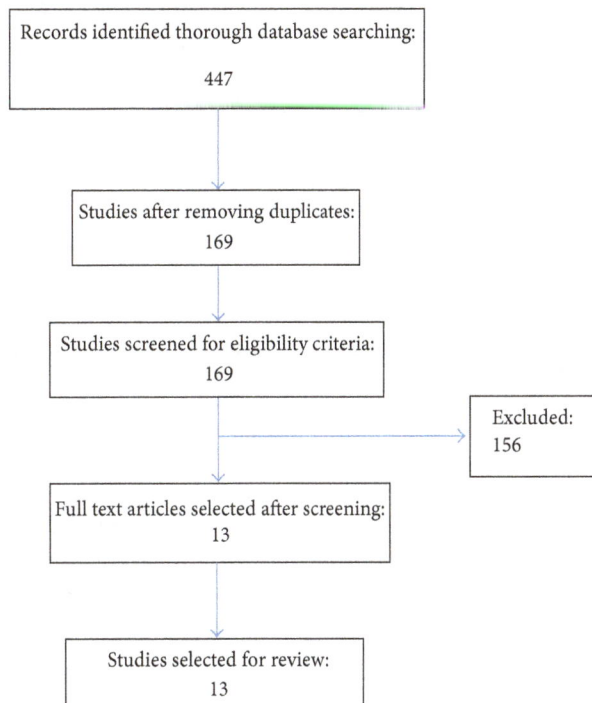

FIGURE 1: Showing the literature search results.

[2, 8, 11–16, 18, 19] were found that compared QOL among the two sets of patients at 1 year after the procedure. From these, 9 studies [8, 11–16, 18, 19] stated that QOL scores were significantly higher in the CABG group at 1 year after procedure while the remaining one study [2] found the QOL scores to be the same in both groups.

4. Discussion

4.1. Seattle Angina Questionnaire (SAQ). Five studies [11–15] were identified that had used SAQ for determining QOL. The SAQ is considered to be a superior assessor of clinical health status, with greater sensitivity and better interpretability than other health status scales, such as the SF-36. This scale is divided into 5 domains, namely, physical limitation score, angina frequency score, quality of life score, treatment satisfaction score, and angina stability score.

4.2. Physical Limitation. Borkon et al. reported that patients who had undergone CABG were able to achieve superior physical function one year after procedure as compared to the PCI patients, even though it had declined one month after revascularization. This decline was also reported by Cohen et al., with no significant differences at 6 months follow-up. Abdallah et al. found similar results as well, with physical function superiority by CABG following into the 2nd year of follow-up as well.

Another important finding by Borkon et al. was the effect of restenosis on physical function. Patients with restenosis reported a significant decrement in physical tasks, which at one month after procedure was comparable in degree to that observed in patients who had undergone CABG.

TABLE 1: Showing the studies included in the review.

Serial number	Author name/date	Scale	N (CABG/PCI)	Baseline mean age (CABG/PCI)	Males (% of patients) (CABG/PCI)
1	Zhang et al., 2003 [11]	SAQ	500/488	61.4/61.4	79.0/79.0
2	Spertus et al., 2005 [12]	SAQ	432/1027	66.0/66.1	74.0/70.0
3	Borkon et al., 2002 [13]	SAQ	223/252	67.0/64.0	66.0/68.0
4	Abdallah et al., 2013 [14]	SAQ	947/953	63.0/63.2	69.8/73.2
5	Cohen et al., 2011 [15]	SAQ and SF-36	897/903	65.0/65.2	78.9/76.4
6	van Domburg et al., 2008 [16]	SF-36	492/483	62.0/61.0	77.0/77.0
7	Rumsfeld et al., 2003 [17]	SF-36	196/193	67.3/67.6	98.5/98.9
8	Szygula-Jurkiewicz et al., 2005 [18]	Sf-36	104/392	62.4/61.8	71.2/66.3
9	Favarato et al., 2007 [19]	Sf-36	175/180	59.0/59.0	53.0/40.0
10	Währborg 1999 [2]	The Nottingham Health Profile	154	—	—
11	Pocock et al., 1996 [20]	Nottingham Health Profile	1011	—	—
12	Brorsson et al., 2001 [1]	Swedish Quality of Life Survey	252/349	62.8/59.8	77.8/75.1
13	Serruys et al., 2001 [8]	EuroQOL questionnaire	579/593	61.0/61.0	76.0/77.0

TABLE 2: A summary of the reviewed articles.

Serial number	Author name/date	Summary
1	Zhang et al., 2003 [11]	Quality of life scores were higher in patients opting for CABG at both 6 months and 1 year.
2	Spertus et al., 2005 [12]	1-year quality of life scores were significantly better for patients treated with CABG surgery as opposed to PCI.
3	Borkon et al., 2002 [13]	Patients undergoing CABG achieved greater quality of life at 6 and 12 months after their procedure.
4	Abdallah et al., 2013 [14]	For patients with diabetes and multivessel CAD, CABG surgery provided slightly better quality of life than PCI using drug-eluting stents. The magnitude of benefit was small, without consistent differences, beyond 2 years.
5	Cohen et al., 2011 [15]	Among patients with three-vessel or left main coronary artery disease, scores for quality of life were higher with PCI than with CABG, at 1 month. These differences were no longer apparent at 6 months. At 12 months, the score for quality of life was higher in the CABG group than in the PCI group.
6	van Domburg et al., 2008 [16]	Both stenting and CABG resulted in significant improvement in QOL of patients, up to one year, with CABG patients showing greater improvements.
7	Rumsfeld et al., 2003 [17]	High-risk patients with medically refractory ischemia randomized to PCI versus CABG surgery have equivalent six-month quality of life.
8	Szygula-Jurkiewicz et al., 2005 [18]	There is a significant difference in health-related quality of life, 12 months after percutaneous coronary intervention and coronary artery bypass graft surgery with the difference favoring the patients undergoing bypass.
9	Favarato et al., 2007 [19]	After 1 year of follow-up, the patients submitted to CABG were the ones that presented the greater improvement in QOL.
10	Währborg 1999 [2]	This study has shown that there is no general difference in health-related quality of life 1 year after bypass surgery or angioplasty.
11	Pocock et al., 1996 [20]	Both intervention strategies produce similar benefits for quality of life over several years.
12	Brorsson et al., 2001 [1]	Both bypass surgery and angioplasty lead to improved quality of life for patients with chronic stable angina and one- or two-vessel coronary artery disease. Bypass surgery is associated with better quality of life at 6 months, but by 48 months quality of life is similar for both sets of patients.
13	Serruys et al., 2001 [8]	A significantly better quality of life was reported with stenting, as compared to bypass surgery, after 1 month. No differences were reported between the two groups at 6 months and a slight difference in favor of surgery was found after 12 months.

Moreover, in spite of revascularization for restenosis, physical function score did not increase to the same degree as that observed in patients who had undergone fruitful PCI or CABG. Therefore, functional limitation in the PCI group was primarily due to the effect of restenosis. Zhang et al. however reported that because of repeat revascularization for restenosis in the PCI cohort, the degree of difference between the two groups decreased over time. Another finding worth mentioning was that the authors also studied the effect of repeat intervention on the relative benefit of CABG versus PCI. Average 6-month follow-up SAQ scores were low for those patients who required repeat intervention. The scores improved gradually between 6 and 12 months but did not increase to the same degree as that observed in patients who had undergone fruitful PCI or CABG.

4.3. Quality of Life. Borkon et al. showed that QOL score is significantly greater in the CABG group than in the PCI group at 6 and 12 months postoperatively ($p < 0.0001$), primarily due to restenosis in the PCI group. Repeat revascularization eventually increased the QOL score to the same level as that of patients who did not require repeat intervention, but less than that of CABG patients. In short, restenosis after PCI reduced the QOL scores over the 12-month period of study ($p < 0.0001$). Abdallah et al. had similar results as well in the QOL domain, with superior scores for CABG extending into 2-year follow-up.

Spertus et al. showed that CABG surgery resulted in greater 1-year QOL scores in patients with intermediate ($p = 0.0004$) and high ($p = 0.006$) risk of restenosis as compared to PCI. Similarly, Cohen et al. also demonstrated that QOL score was significantly higher in the CABG group than in the PCI group at 12 months (difference between groups = 2.4 points; $p = 0.03$).

4.4. Angina Frequency. Borkon et al. reported that CABG is associated with greater relief from angina than PCI ($p < 0.001$), primarily due to the effect of restenosis in the PCI group. Multivariable analysis confirmed the benefit of CABG over PCI ($p = 0.004$). The authors concluded that patients with restenosis had greater anginal distress over time than patients who underwent CABG or PCI without restenosis. Abdallah et al. reiterated the same results, with CABG associated with greater anginal relief as compared to PCI at 2-year follow-up (mean treatment benefit 1.3 [95% CI, 0.3–2.2], $p < 0.01$). Moreover, Spertus et al. concluded that CABG resulted in better anginal outcomes in patients with intermediate (difference in SAQ angina frequency scores favoring CABG = 6.1 ± 1.7 points, $p = 0.0003$) and high (SAQ angina frequency difference = 10.8 ± 4.2, $p = 0.01$) risk of restenosis as compared to PCI. Cohen et al. and Zhang et al. also found that CABG is associated with better anginal outcomes at both 6 and 12 months as compared to PCI.

Therefore, it can be safely concluded from these studies that CABG results in better physical function, QOL, and anginal outcomes during 1-year postoperative period in comparison to PCI. In addition, CABG yields in better anginal outcomes in patients with moderate or high risk for restenosis and restenosis is found to reduce QOL scores.

4.5. The Medical Outcomes Study Short Form 36 Health Survey. Five studies [15–19] in all were found to have used SF-36 in comparing the QOL between the two treatment procedures. The SF-36 is a generic written questionnaire comprising a total of 36 items that cover 8 health constructs: physical functioning, role limitations due to physical problems, bodily pain, energy and vitality, social functioning and role limitations due to emotional problems, and mental health. In the literature reviewed, two methods of reporting the results were found. In one form, the scores from these 8 original scales are aggregated into the Physical Component Summary (PCS) scores and the Mental Component Summary (MCS) scores reflecting the overall physical and mental health. In another form, the scores for individual items within each domain are summated and compared. We compare the effects of CABG and PCI in terms of physical and mental health.

4.6. Physical Health. Rumsfeld et al. investigated the health related quality of life (HRQL) outcomes in the Department of Veteran Affairs Angina with Extremely Serious Operative Mortality (AWESOME) study population at six months. No significant differences were reported at the end of the 6 months. However, diabetes was associated with a negative trend in PCS scores in the CABG surgery group. Furthermore diabetes, COPD, and elevated serum creatinine were identified as key predictors for worse physical health at six months.

Szygula et al. reported HRQL impairment in the PCS scores of the PCI group at 12 months in their investigation. This was attributed to worse outcomes in all four domains of physical health: physical functioning, role physical, bodily pain, and general health. A greater proportion of PCI patients were found to have unstable angina at twelve months, with substantially higher systolic and diastolic blood pressures. Similar to these results, the rate of repeat revascularization was also high in PCI over CABG surgery. It is worth mentioning here that a negative trend was found between systolic pressure and the PCS and MCS scores of only the PCI cohort.

Favarato et al. conducted a different study, in that they compared the effect of CABG surgery, PCI, and Medical Therapy (MT) on QOL in the study population of the Medicine, Angioplasty and Surgery Study (MASS-II) trial. At twelve months, a significant difference was found in the number of angina free patients with a higher proportion belonging to the CABG group (88%). In addition, only 0.5% of CABG patients were found to have undergone repeat revascularization as compared to a high number of PCI patients (13.3%). Overall, a positive trend in QOL assessment was found; though CABG showed worse scores at baseline in terms of physical functioning and vitality, it showed significant superiority over PCI and MT in vitality ($p = 0.0024$) and physical functioning ($p = 0.0029$) at six months. It is imperative to mention that no significant treatment difference was observed in any of the eight domains at twelve months. Though professional and occupational status (43.9% of the men were employed) was evaluated, no significant differences were reported based on choice of procedure at the end of the year. However, once the final scores were adjusted by their initial scores as covariable and other factors using a general linear model, it was observed that CABG was superior to PCI in terms of general health, a finding consistent with that of the Coronary Angioplasty versus Bypass Revascularization Investigation (CABRI) trial.

The Arterial Revascularization Therapy Study (ARTS) trial reported HRQL outcomes using the European QOL ED-5D at one and three years, but Domburg et al. also used the SF-36 survey and evaluated anginal status at baseline, 1, 6, 12, and 36 months. They made use of scale scores rather than the summary scores. At one month postop, similar to previous studies, a significant improvement was seen in the PCI group while the CABG patients showed a decrease in most SF-36 subscales. However from 1 month to 6 months, the CABG group showed a substantial increase. The only domain which showed a significant difference up till 6 months was bodily pain where PCI was superior to CABG, because of procedural effects. Between 6 and 12 months, the outcomes remained almost equal. Eventually three of the subdomain scores (physical functioning, social functioning, and general health) were substantially superior in CABG over PCI, where, with longer follow-up of 36 months, all scores decreased slightly to meet at the same level. A subgroup analysis showed that a greater proportion of PCI patients had angina at all times as compared to CABG. It is worth mentioning that this gap grew smaller with time. It is noteworthy that the prevalence of angina in those PCI patients who did not require another procedure is lesser than those who did but still greater than the CABG group. Furthermore, while diabetic PCI patients showed a decrease in general health scores at all-time points, physical functioning showed a steady decrease only with time.

The Synergy between PCI with Taxus and Cardiac Surgery (SYNTAX) trial differed from other studies because of its use of drug eluting stents in PCI. Like the ARTS study, it evaluated HRQL outcomes using EuroQOL ED-5D instrument and SF-36 survey, as well as SAQ. Similar to the findings of Favarato et al., Cohen et al. reported significant superiority of PCI over CABG in physical health status one month postop. However, except for role limitations because of physical problems, this difference did not persist at six months and, by twelve months, CABG gained significance over PCI in general health.

4.7. Mental Health. The AWESOME study yielded no significant difference in the MCS scores. As a result of the multivariable analyses, current smoking and hypertension were identified as worse outcome predictors at six months of mental health. The use of beta blockers was found to be associated with a better mental health outcome. Similarly, Szygula et al. reported no substantial difference in MCS scores between the two arms. With the MASS-II trial, Favarato et al. reported no significant difference in any of the three study arms in terms of mental and emotional functioning. However, a time effect was reported which showed an increase in these scores at six months postop in all three treatment arms which meant betterment of health. The authors commented that no significant pattern could be obtained because mental health poses a not so direct link to coronary artery disease. The ARTS and SYNTAX trials also

yielded no significant correlations or differences between the two procedures in terms of mental health status.

These studies yielded vague results, possibly owing to the generic nature of the SF-36 that simply evaluates the general health of the patients and is not disease-specific, and the varied composition of the study pools is included. Where Rumsfeld et al. reported no difference at 6 months after procedure, all others reported superiority of CABG over PCI at 12 months after revascularization. A high rate of repeat procedures was also reported for the PCI cohort and the difference in treatment procedures was found to decrease over time.

In terms of mental health, all authors ascertained that no correlation can be determined.

4.8. Other Scales Discussion. Our extensive literature search also yielded further four studies [1, 2, 8, 20] that used instruments apart from SAQ and SF-36 to assess health related quality of life of patients belonging to either of the treatment groups for comparison.

Pocock et al. utilized the Nottingham Health Profile (NHP) to assess the perception of health amongst the study population of the Randomized Intervention Treatment of Angina (RITA) trial. For this study, improvement in health status was quite substantial for both cohorts at 6 months and 2 years as compared to preop days without any significant difference. It can be mentioned though that the CABG patients were found to be slightly superior in all six dimensions (energy, pain, emotional reactions, social isolation, sleep, and physical mobility) at 6 months (mean difference of 1.21 points). Pocock et al. also found a slightly increased prevalence of health problems in the PTCA arm of the study at both end points by averaging the total number of life aspects adversely affected over the 6-month and 2-year visits (means, 0.87 and 1.07 aspects for CABG and PTCA groups, resp.; difference, 0.22; 95% CI, 0.00 to 0.39; $p = 0.05$). In terms of anginal status, no difference between the two cohorts could be found.

Similarly, Wåhrborg [2] investigated perception of health in the Coronary Angioplasty versus Bypass Revascularization Investigation (CABRI) trial study population but used 12 separate questions apart from the NHP. Overall betterment was reported for total life scores and separate dimension scores for both study groups, relative to baseline. These results were consistent with the findings of the RITA study. Wåhrborg [2] also commented on the energy difference they found to be in favor of CABG patients in NHP part 1 as well as in item 1 of the 12 separate questions. No other study commented on this trend. The authors attributed this trend to the CABRI trial protocol allowing incomplete revascularization of the PTCA patients and not excluding those patients who had totally occluded vessels. With respect to anginal status, no association could be made.

Brorsson et al. evaluated QOL and functional status using multiple standardized questionnaires. 33.5% of angioplasty patients had to undergo a repeat revascularization procedure within a 2-year follow-up. At 4-year follow-up, no significant difference in survival was found. Additionally, the frequency of angina symptoms was markedly less in both study arms by 6 months, with a great improvement in the CABG group (only 11.5% reporting symptoms). However it was found that the number of angina free patients and those who had not used sublingual nitrates was greater in the PTCA cohort at 6 months, though patients who had not used sublingual nitrates for a month were greater in the CABG group at 48 months. It is worth mentioning that the relative superiority of CABG over PTCA showed a decreasing trend over the follow-up period. With further analyses, it was found that a preop history of high anginal frequency at baseline was a strong predictor of high anginal frequency at follow-up. CABG surgery and history of positive stress test were found to be associated with lower anginal frequency at 6 months.

They also used the Swedish QOL survey (SWED-QUAL) to assess the well-being of the patients. A strong correlation between anginal frequency and both physical functioning and health perception was found, while that of anginal frequency and emotional well-being and sleep was not noteworthy. Preop QOL was the most constant predictor of postop QOL at 6 and 48 months for all 5 life scales. CABG patients saw greater improvement in physical functioning and general health status at 6 months than the PTCA group, but this was not present at 48 months. Male patients showed greater improvement in physical functioning and pain relief than women. Increasing age was also associated with low levels of physical functioning by 48 months but had no effect on any other scales. No differences in degree of improvement were found on the basis of history of smoking, COPD, hypertension, or positive stress test. No difference was also found on the basis of diabetes mellitus.

Serruys et al. evaluated angina status and QOL, using the EuroQOL questionnaire, as a secondary objective of their randomized control trial. A greater proportion of patients in the CABG group were found to be angina free throughout the study period. The QOL assessment initially yielded favorable results for PCI at 1 month, but this gap was reduced at 6 months and eventually became slightly significant in favor of CABG at 12 months. Elevated level of CK-MB was the main outcome predictor in the surgery group and diabetes mellitus in the stent group.

5. Limitations

There are several limitations in our systematic review that need to be considered. Firstly, using only one database and applying English language restriction may have resulted in some pertinent studies not being included. Secondly, there was significant heterogeneity among the sample populations considered in our review. However, we feel that regardless of this heterogeneity, the general pattern is very clear as shown by our review. In the future, a meta-analysis on this topic might help to elucidate and confirm the pattern as shown.

6. Conclusion

In this review we have summarized the major studies pertaining to the comparison of postprocedural QOL between CABG and angioplasty. Our review suggests that although angioplasty, through its less invasive nature, might provide better QOL within the first few months, CABG is superior in providing improved QOL at both 6 and 12 months after procedure and in the long run.

References

[1] B. Brorsson, S. J. Bernstein, R. H. Brook, and L. Werkö, "Quality of life of chronic stable angina patients 4 years after coronary angioplasty or coronary artery bypass surgery," *Journal of Internal Medicine*, vol. 249, no. 1, pp. 47–57, 2001.

[2] P. Währborg, "Quality of life after coronary angioplasty or bypass surgery. 1-year follow-up in the coronary angioplasty versus bypass revascularization investigation (CABRI) trial," *European Heart Journal*, vol. 20, no. 9, pp. 653–658, 1999.

[3] A. P. Kappetein, T. E. Feldman, M. J. MacK et al., "Comparison of coronary bypass surgery with drug-eluting stenting for the treatment of left main and/or three-vessel disease: 3-year follow-up of the SYNTAX trial," *European Heart Journal*, vol. 32, no. 17, pp. 2125–2134, 2011.

[4] I. Sipahi, M. H. Akay, S. Dagdelen, A. Blitz, and C. Alhan, "Coronary artery bypass grafting vs percutaneous coronary intervention and long-term mortality and morbidity in multivessel disease: meta-analysis of randomized clinical trials of the arterial grafting and stenting era," *JAMA Internal Medicine*, vol. 174, no. 2, pp. 223–230, 2014.

[5] S. N. Hoffman, J. A. TenBrook Jr., M. P. Wolf, S. G. Pauker, D. N. Salem, and J. B. Wong, "A meta-analysis of randomized controlled trials comparing coronary artery bypass graft with percutaneous transluminal coronary angioplasty: one- to eight-year outcomes," *Journal of the American College of Cardiology*, vol. 41, no. 8, pp. 1293–1304, 2003.

[6] The BARI Investigators, "Seven-year outcome in the Bypass Angioplasty Revascularization Investigation (BARI) by treatment and diabetic status," *Journal of the American College of Cardiology*, vol. 35, no. 5, pp. 1122–1129, 2000.

[7] S. B. King, A. S. Kosinski, R. A. Guyton, N. J. Lembo, and W. S. Weintraub, "Eight-year mortality in the Emory Angioplasty versus Surgery Trial (EAST)," *Journal of the American College of Cardiology*, vol. 35, no. 5, pp. 1116–1121, 2000.

[8] P. W. Serruys, F. Unger, J. E. Sousa et al., "Comparison of coronary-artery bypass surgery and stenting for the treatment of multivessel disease," *The New England Journal of Medicine*, vol. 344, no. 15, pp. 1117–1124, 2001.

[9] SoS Investigators, "Coronary artery bypass surgery versus percutaneous coronary intervention with stent implantation in patients with multivessel coronary artery disease (the Stent or Surgery trial): a randomised controlled trial," *The Lancet*, vol. 360, no. 9338, pp. 965–970, 2002.

[10] L. Noyez, M. J. de Jager, and A. L. P. Markou, "Quality of life after cardiac surgery: underresearched research," *Interactive Cardiovascular and Thoracic Surgery*, vol. 13, no. 5, pp. 511–514, 2011.

[11] Z. Zhang, E. M. Mahoney, R. H. Stables et al., "Disease-specific health status after stent-assisted percutaneous coronary intervention and coronary artery bypass surgery: one-year results from the Stent or Surgery trial," *Circulation*, vol. 108, no. 14, pp. 1694–1700, 2003.

[12] J. A. Spertus, R. Nerella, R. Kettlekamp et al., "Risk of restenosis and health status outcomes for patients undergoing percutaneous coronary intervention versus coronary artery bypass graft surgery," *Circulation*, vol. 111, no. 6, pp. 768–773, 2005.

[13] A. M. Borkon, G. F. Muehlebach, J. House, S. P. Marso, and J. A. Spertus, "A comparison of the recovery of health status after percutaneous coronary intervention and coronary artery bypass," *Annals of Thoracic Surgery*, vol. 74, no. 5, pp. 1526–1530, 2002.

[14] M. S. Abdallah, K. Wang, E. A. Magnuson et al., "Quality of life after PCI vs CABG among patients with diabetes and multivessel coronary artery disease: a randomized clinical trial," *The Journal of the American Medical Association*, vol. 310, no. 15, pp. 1581–1590, 2013.

[15] D. J. Cohen, B. Van Hout, P. W. Serruys et al., "Quality of life after PCI with drug-eluting stents or coronary-artery bypass surgery," *The New England Journal of Medicine*, vol. 364, no. 11, pp. 1016–1026, 2011.

[16] R. T. van Domburg, J. Daemen, S. S. Pedersen et al., "Short- and long- term health related quality-of-life and anginal status after randomisation to coronary stenting versus bypass surgery for the treatment of multivessel disease: results of the Arterial Revascularisation Therapy Study (ARTS)," *EuroIntervention*, vol. 3, no. 4, pp. 506–511, 2008.

[17] J. S. Rumsfeld, D. J. Magid, M. E. Plomondon et al., "Health-related quality of life after percutaneous coronary intervention versus coronary bypass surgery in high-risk patients with medically refractory ischemia," *Journal of the American College of Cardiology*, vol. 41, no. 10, pp. 1732–1738, 2003.

[18] B. Szygula-Jurkiewicz, M. Zembala, K. Wilczek, R. Wojnicz, and L. Polonski, "Health related quality of life after percutaneous coronary intervention versus coronary artery bypass graft surgery in patients with acute coronary syndromes without ST-segment elevation. 12-Month follow up," *European Journal of Cardio-Thoracic Surgery*, vol. 27, no. 5, pp. 882–886, 2005.

[19] M. E. Favarato, W. Hueb, W. E. Boden et al., "Quality of life in patients with symptomatic multivessel coronary artery disease: a comparative post hoc analyses of medical, angioplasty or surgical strategies-MASS II trial," *International Journal of Cardiology*, vol. 116, no. 3, pp. 364–370, 2007.

[20] S. J. Pocock, R. A. Henderson, P. Seed, T. Treasure, and J. R. Hampton, "Quality of life, employment status, and anginal symptoms after coronary angioplasty or bypass surgery. 3-year follow-up in the randomized intervention treatment of angina (RITA) trial," *Circulation*, vol. 94, no. 2, pp. 135–142, 1996.

22

Effect of Remote Ischemic Preconditioning on Perioperative Cardiac Events in Patients Undergoing Elective Percutaneous Coronary Intervention

Xiangming Wang,[1] **Na Kong,**[2] **Chuanwei Zhou,**[1] **Deeraj Mungun,**[1] **Zakaria Iyan,**[1] **Yan Guo,**[1] **and Zhijian Yang**[3]

[1]*Department of Geriatric Cardiology, The First Affiliated Hospital of Nanjing Medical University, Nanjing, China*
[2]*Reproductive Medicine Center, The Affiliated Drum Tower Hospital of Nanjing University, Nanjing, China*
[3]*Department of Cardiology, The First Affiliated Hospital of Nanjing Medical University, Nanjing, China*

Correspondence should be addressed to Zhijian Yang; zhijianyangnj@hotmail.com

Academic Editor: Robert Chen

Background. The main objective of this meta-analysis was to investigate whether remote ischemic preconditioning (RIPC) reduces cardiac and renal events in patients undergoing elective cardiovascular interventions. *Methods and Results.* We systematically searched articles published from 2006 to 2016 in PubMed, EMBASE, Web of Science, Cochrane Library, and Google Scholar. Odds ratios (ORs) with 95% confidence intervals (CIs) were used as the effect index for dichotomous variables. The standardized mean differences (SMDs) with 95% CIs were calculated as the pooled continuous effect. Sixteen RCTs of 2435 patients undergoing elective PCI were selected. Compared with control group, RIPC could significantly reduce the incidence of perioperative myocardial infarction (OR = 0.64; 95% CI: 0.48–0.86; $P = 0.003$) and acute kidney injury (OR = 0.56; 95% CI: 0.322–0.99; $P = 0.049$). Metaregression analysis showed that the reduction of PMI by RIPC was enhanced for CAD patients with multivessel disease (coef.: −0.05 [−0.09; −0.01], $P = 0.022$). There were no differences in the changes of cTnI ($P = 0.934$) and CRP ($P = 0.075$) in two groups. *Conclusion.* Our meta-analysis of RCTs demonstrated that RIPC can provide cardiac and renal protection for patients undergoing elective PCI, while no beneficial effect on reducing the levels of cTnI and CRP after PCI was reported.

1. Introduction

Percutaneous coronary intervention (PCI) is one of the most important treatments for coronary artery disease. In acute myocardial infarction, timely myocardial reperfusion therapy, such as PCI, CABG, and Thrombolysis, is an effective method to limit the myocardial infarct area, attenuate clinical symptoms, and improve the clinical prognosis. However, reperfusion may induce further damage to the myocardium itself [1, 2]. Myocardial ischemia-reperfusion injury (MIRI) is a common pathophysiological process that poses a serious threat to patients' health. Many studies have shown that elevated levels of cTnI after PCI are associated with a poor

prognosis in patients with coronary artery disease [3–7]. In recent years, many clinical studies have confirmed that RIPC provides effective myocardial protection in patients undergoing PCI, and RIPC is an important method to prevent MIRI.

While RIPC's cardioprotective effect has been seen in patients undergoing selective PCI, many clinical trials have examined whether RIPC has a protective effect on these patients [8–11]. Unfortunately, studies on the protective effects of RIPC in PCI patients are limited, and the results are controversial and contradictory because not all of the trials have observed the beneficial effects of RIPC. D'Ascenzo et al.'s meta-analysis showed that RIPC could reduce the incidence of PCI-related myocardial infarction, but PCI did not affect CRP after the procedure [12]. However, it is important to note that there were fewer studies included in the meta-analysis (5 studies with 731 subjects). A new meta-analysis reported by Pei et al. [13] in 2014, which included 11 studies and a total of 2,301 patients, demonstrated that RIPC could provide heart and kidney protection by reducing the incidence of MI and AKI in patients with selective PCI. In the past two years (2014–2016), new randomized controlled trials (RCTs) have been published; these findings suggest that the incidence of MI after PCI, the incidence of MACCE at 6 months after PCI, and the effect of PCI on renal function are different. These RCTs were not included in previous meta-analyses, and the role of RIPC in patients undergoing PCI needed to be reassessed. Thus, we conducted a comprehensive meta-analysis to study whether RIPC (compared with the controls) provided myocardial and renal protection for patients undergoing selective PCI.

2. Materials and Methods

2.1. Search Strategy. We performed this meta-analysis according to the PRISMA (Preferred Reporting Items for Systematic reviews and Meta-Analyses) statement [14] and the Cochrane Handbook for Systematic Reviews [15]. We systematically searched articles published from 2006 to 2016 in the following databases: PubMed, EMBASE, Web of Science, Cochrane Library, and Google Scholar. Our research was last updated on December 30, 2016. The following search phrases or keywords were used: "remote ischemic preconditioning," "ischemic preconditioning," "limb ischemic preconditioning," "elective percutaneous coronary intervention," "myocardial injury," and "cardioprotection."

2.2. Inclusion and Exclusion Criteria. The inclusion criteria were as follows: (1) RCTs published in English, (2) studies that involved patients undergoing elective PCI, (3) studies that reported the incidence of perioperative myocardial infarction or troponin levels after PCI or renal injury as endpoints, and (4) RIPC intervention regardless of the duration or number of cycles. The exclusion criteria were as follows: (1) repeated published literature, (2) trials that used RIPC in combination with another concomitant intervention, (3) incomplete original research data, (4) studies that included patients with ST-segment elevation myocardial infarction, (5) animal studies, and (6) nonrandomized clinical trials.

2.3. Data Extraction. Two researchers (WXM and ZI) independently screened the titles, abstracts, and the full articles as needed, and then they determined whether the studies met the inclusion criteria. When the researchers did not agree, the problems were resolved through a discussion or by a third-party reviewer (DM or KN) to make a determination. The researchers extracted the data from all of the qualifying articles and assessed the bias risk. If necessary, we directly contacted the original author for information. The main data extracted included basic research information (including the title, the first author, and the publication year), research characteristics (including sample size, age, gender, diabetes

mellitus, hypertension, heart failure, drugs, and vascular characteristics,), outcome indicators and the results of measurement data (i.e., the incidence of PMI, the incidence of AKI and MACCE, and serum or plasma cTns levels), and the key elements of bias risk assessment. We converted some of the original text in the "median and range" of the results of the indicators to "mean and standard deviation" through the O'Rourke method. The quality of the studies was assessed using Jadad et al.'s scoring system: randomization, blinding, and providing an explanation for withdrawals and dropouts [16]. Studies with a Jadad et al.'s score of greater than or equal to 3 points were considered to be high-quality trials.

2.4. Statistical Methods. The meta-analysis was performed using Stata software (version 12.1; StataCorp LP, College Station, TX, USA). Odds ratios (ORs) with 95% confidence intervals (CIs) were used as the effect index for dichotomous variables, such as the incidence of PMI and the incidence of AKI and MACCEs. The standardized mean differences (SMDs) with 95% CIs were calculated as the pooled continuous effect. Heterogeneity among studies was assessed by means of the chi-square-based Q test and the I^2 index [17]. $I^2 > 50\%$ or $P < 0.05$ indicated evidence of heterogeneity. When $I^2 < 50\%$, studies were considered to be heterogeneous, and fixed-effects models were used for analysis, whereas if heterogeneity was significant (I^2 value $\geq 50\%$ or $P < 0.05$), random-effects models were selected [18, 19]. To further investigate the possible sources of heterogeneity, subgroup analysis or metaregression analysis was performed. Forest plots were drawn to evaluate the effects of RIPC on every outcome. Sensitivity analyses were performed to assess the stability of the results. Publication bias was assessed using Begg's funnel plot and Egger's linear regression tests. A P value <0.05 indicated a statistically significant difference.

3. Results

3.1. Literature Search Results. A total of 306 citations were initially screened after searching the databases. We reviewed the article titles and extracts, and then we excluded the studies that did not meet the inclusion standards; the full texts of 31 trials were further evaluated. Of these, 15 trials were excluded: 8 due to study patients undergoing emergency PCI [20–27], 2 because endpoints were not evaluated, 3 because concomitant preconditioning treatments were used [28–30], and 2 because they were not RCTs. Lavi et al.'s trial [31] was divided into two independent studies because of the different preconditioning protocols (expressed as Lavi I and Lavi II). Finally, a total of 16 randomized controlled trials were included in the meta-analysis [8–11, 23, 31–40], with the literature screening process and results shown in Figure 1.

3.2. Study Characteristics. A total of 2,435 patients were enrolled (from 11 countries) in the included studies, with 1,215 patients randomized to the RIPC group and 1,220 patients to the control group. RIPC was performed by inflating a blood pressure cuff that was placed on the upper limb or leg to 200 mmHg or above the basic systolic pressure over 10 mmHg. The ischemic-reperfusion protocol [cycles $\times I/R$]

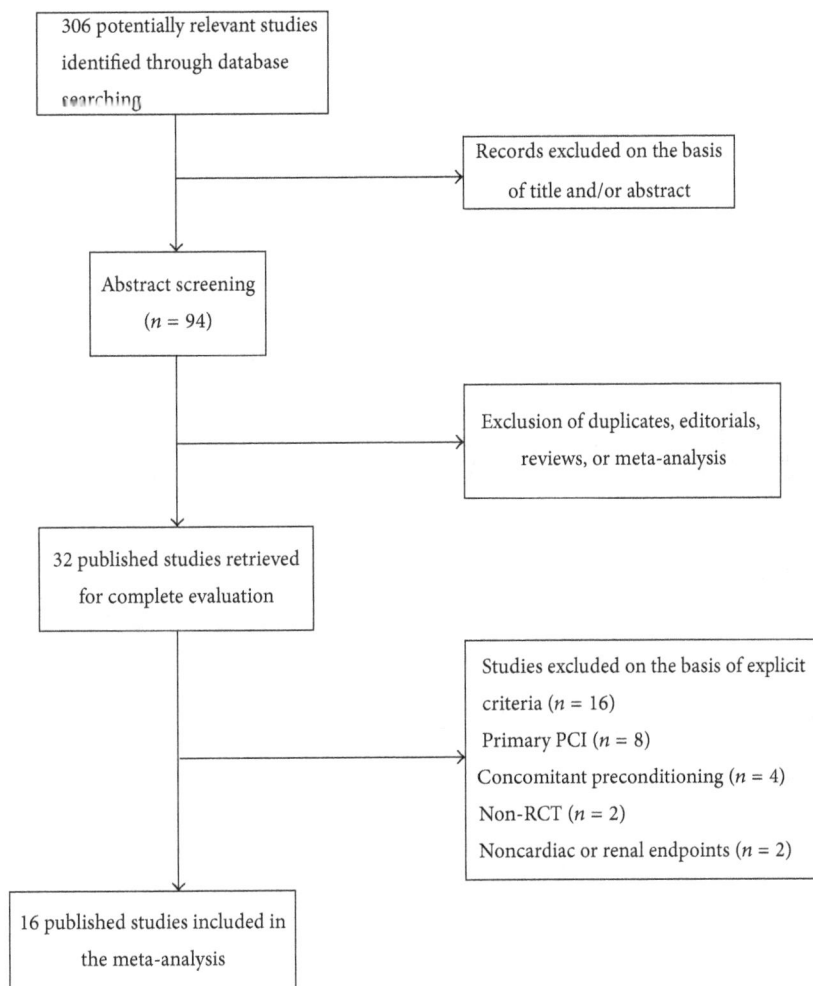

FIGURE 1: Flow chart of the studies identified with criteria for inclusion and exclusion.

was 3×5 min/5 min in 7 studies [8, 9, 11, 35, 36, 38, 39], 4×5 min/5 min in 1 study [32], 2×5 min/5 min in 1 study [34], 3×3 min/3 min in 3 studies [10, 34, 41], 1×5 min/5 min in 3 studies [31, 40], and 4×30 sec/30 sec in 1 study [23]. Among these trials, 11 studies reported the incidence of PMI [8–10, 31, 33, 35–38, 40], and 7 studies reported the incidence of AKI [10, 23, 31, 32, 35, 38]. There were 15 studies that reported the levels of myocardial injury biomarkers after PCI, with 10 trials using troponin I or T and 5 trials using CK-MB. The baseline characteristics were comparable between the RIPC group and the control group; their median age was 65.15 years and 69.2% of the patients were males. The percentages of patients with diabetes, hypertension, and dyslipidemia were 51.01%, 72.70%, and 63.05%, respectively. Of the patients, 61.81% were treated with angiotensin-converting enzyme inhibitors and 70.4% with beta-blockers; 31.1% of the patients presented with multivessel disease and 38.56% with a type C lesion. There were no statistically significant differences in patients' gender, their ages, and the preoperative eGFR levels between the two groups. The patients' baseline characteristics and the trial design of all of the included randomized trials are shown in

Tables 1 and 2. The quality of the included studies was assessed using Jadad et al.'s score as shown in Table 3. In terms of research quality, 12 studies had a Jadad et al.'s score ≥ 3 points, and 4 studies had Jadad et al.'s scores of <3 points.

3.3. Effects of RIPC on the Incidence of PMI. In 16 studies, 11 studies reported the incidence of PMI in patients. There was moderate heterogeneity in the 11 studies ($P = 0.101$, $I^2 = 44.4\%$), so we performed a meta-analysis using a random-effects model. The meta-analysis showed that the incidence of PMI in the RIPC group was significantly lower than that in the control group (OR = 0.64; 95% CI: 0.48–0.86; $P = 0.003$). The RIPC of the upper arm significantly prevented PMI (OR = 0.66; 95% CI: 0.49–0.88; $P = 0.005$; Figure 2); however, the incidence of PMI was not reduced by RIPC of the lower limb in patients (OR = 0.491; 95% CI: 0.11–2.11; $P = 0.339$). The leave-one-out sensitivity analysis, which removed individual studies one by one, showed that no single study significantly altered the overall effect of RIPC on reducing PMI (all $P < 0.05$, Figure 3(a)).

TABLE 1: Summarized patients' baseline characteristics of included randomized trials.

Study	Age	Male (%)	DM (%)	HT (%)	Dyslipidemia (%)	Previous MI (%)	Baseline LVEF (%)	Baseline renal function	ACEI (%)	β-Blockers (%)	Statins (%)	Multivessel disease (%)	Type C lesion (%)
Ahmed et al.	54	86.6	51.7	63.8	66.4	NA	NA	NA	55	81	72.5	25	15
Carrasco-Chinchilla et al.	65	68.1	42.1	75.6	62.2	NA	58.3	77.2	67.4	82.9	67.5	58.3	NA
Deftereos et al.	68	64	36	65	59	NA	56	75	68	17	36	55.1	NA
Er et al.	73	71	64	91	75	41	59.6	60	NA	82	NA	NA	NA
Ghaemian et al.	61	47.5	36.3	48.8	73.8	8.8	NA	NA	55	81.3	76.3	45	77
Hoole et al.	62	78.2	21.8	51.5	NA	55.4	50.2	NA	74	79.2	95	17	36
Iliodromitis et al.	62	55	34.1	NA	80.5	NA	55	NA	56.1	70.7	61	NA	NA
Lavi et al.	63.7	72.9	32.5	70	67	43	NA	Normal	NA	NA	NA	18.8	NA
Lavi II	64.3	74.2	29.5	70	65	42		Normal	NA	NA	NA	21.7	NA
Liu et al.	58	54.5	36	62.5	NA	NA	61.5	68.33	90.5	81	95.5	54	40.19
Luo et al.	60	76.1	27.8	65.9	NA	21.5	64	100	57	83	NA	28	NA
Melo et al.	NA	NA	NA	NA	NA	NA	NA	NA	NA	NA	NA	NA	NA
Prasad et al.	66	83.2	27.4	77.9	73.7	28.4	56	Normal	38	73	67.4	17	43
Singh et al.	68.9	48	100	85.3	48	7 (6.9)	59.3	47.66	55.9	32.4	80.4	29.4	NA
Xu	69	68	100	63.5	NA	23	63.7	Normal	NA	82.4	100	NA	100
Zografos et al.	61	88	19	82	71.5	20	56.4	88.4	NA	82	96	NA	NA

Table 2: Summarized trial design of the included randomized trials.

Study	Year	Country	Number of patients (RIPC/control)	Limb	Protocol of preconditioning	Definition of periproceduralmyocardial infarction	First cuff to balloon time
Ahmed et al.	2013	Egypt	77/72	Arm	200 mmHg × 3 cycles × 5 min	An increase of cTnT greater than 3 times the 99th percentile URL	Several minutes
Carrasco-Chinchilla et al.	2013	Spain	118/114	Arm	200 mmHg × 3 cycles × 5 min	An increase of cTnT greater than 3 times the 99th percentile URL	5 min after PCI
Defteros et al.	2013	Greece	113/112	Arm	200 mmHg × 4 cycles × 30 sec	NA	Several minutes before PCI
Er et al.	2012	Germany	26/26	Arm	50 mmHg > SBP × 4 cycles × 5 min	NA	40–85 min
Ghaemian et al.	2012	Iran	40/40	Leg	>SBP × 2 cycles × 5 min	An increase of cTnT greater than 3 times the 99th percentile URL	65 min
Hoole et al.	2009	UK	126/125	Arm	200 mmHg × 3 cycles × 3 min	An increase of cTnT greater than 3 times the 99th percentile URL	96 min
Iliodromitis et al.	2006	Greece	20/21	Arm	200 mmHg × 3 cycles × 3 min	NA	30 min
Lavi et al.	2014	Canada	120/120	Arm	200 mmHg or 50 mmHg > SBP × 1 cycle × 5 min	An increase of cTnT greater than 5 times the 99th percentile URL	Several minutes after PCI
Lavi II	2014	Canada	120/120	Leg	200 mmHg or 50 mmHg > SBP × 1 cycle × 5 min	An increase of cTnT greater than 5 times the 99th percentile URL	Several minutes after PCI
Liu et al.	2014	China	98/102	Arm	200 mmHg × 3 cycles × 5 min	An increase of cTnT greater than 5 times the 99th percentile URL	18–24 hours
Luo et al.	2013	China	101/104	Arm	200 mmHg × 3 cycles × 5 min	An increase of cTnT greater than 5 times the 99th percentile URL	<120 min
Melo et al.	2013	Brazil	9/20	Arm	200 mmHg × 3 cycles × 5 min	An increase of cTnT greater than 3 times the 99th percentile URL	NA
Prasad et al.	2013	USA	47/48	Arm	200 mmHg × 3 cycles × 3 min	An increase of cTnT greater than 3 times the 99th percentile URL	>18 min
Singh et al.	2016	Korea	51/51	Arm	200 mmHg × 3 cycles × 5 min	NA	30 min
Xu	2013	China	102/98	Arm	200 mmHg × 3 cycles × 5 min	An increase of cTnT greater than 3 times the 99th percentile URL	30–120 min
Zografos et al.	2014	Greece	47/47	Arm	200 mmHg × 1 cycle × 5 min	An increase of cTnT greater than 5 times the 99th percentile URL	4 min

TABLE 3: Jadad et al.'s scores of included studies.

Study	Randomization	Double-blinding	Withdrawals	Randomization methods	Double-blinding methods	Total score
Ahmed et al., 2013	1	0	1	0	0	2
Carrasco-Chinchilla et al., 2013	1	1	1	0	0	3
Deftereos et al.	1	0	1	1	0	5
Er et al., 2012	1	1	1	1	1	5
Ghaemian et al., 2012	1	1	1	1	1	4
Hoole et al., 2009	1	1	1	1	1	5
Iliodromitis et al., 2006	1	0	1	0	0	2
Lavi et al., 2014	1	1	1	1	1	5
Lavi II, 2014	1	1	1	1	1	5
Liu et al., 2014	1	0	1	0	0	3
Luo et al., 2013	1	0	1	0	0	3
Melo et al., 2013	N.A	N.A	N.A	N.A	N.A	N.A
Prasad et al., 2013	1	0	1	0	0	2
Singh et al., 2016	1	1	1	1	1	5
Xu, 2013	1	1	1	0	0	5
Zografos et al., 2014	1	1	1	0	1	3

3.4. Effect of Remote Ischemic Preconditioning on the Incidence of AKI. AKI after PCI was reported in 1,378 study subjects, and the overall incidence was 9.14% (45/698 in the RIPC group and 81/680 in the control group). This group of studies showed moderate heterogeneity ($P = 0.094$, $I^2 = 44.5\%$). The incidence of AKI in the remote preconditioned patients was significantly lower than that in the control groups (OR = 0.56; 95% CI: 0.32–0.99; $P = 0.049$; Figure 4). Sensitivity analysis revealed that our results were reliable and robust by excluding each included trial one at a time (all $P < 0.05$; Figure 3(b)).

3.5. cTnI Concentrations after PCI. Data about the cTnI concentrations after PCI were available in 13 of the trials. There were 10 studies that reported the cTnI levels at 24 h after PCI and 6 studies at 12 h after PCI. For the cTnI concentration at 12 h postoperatively, there was no significant difference between the RIPC group and the control group (SMD −0.11; 95% CI: −0.48–0.27; $P = 0.585$) with significant heterogeneity ($P < 0.001$, $I^2 = 92.6\%$; Figure 5(a)). Similarly, for the cTnI concentrations at 24 h postoperatively, there was also no significant difference between the RIPC group and the control group (SMD: −0.02; 95% CI: −0.43–0.39; $P = 0.934$; Figure 5(b)) with significant heterogeneity ($P < 0.001$, $I^2 = 93.2\%$).

3.6. Levels of CRP after PCI. There were 10 studies that reported CRP levels at 12–24 h after PCI. The studies about CRP had significant heterogeneity ($\chi^2 = 0.152$; $P < 0.001$; $I^2 = 86.1\%$), so we performed a meta-analysis with random-effects models. The results showed that there were no significant differences in the CRP concentrations after PCI

between the two groups (SMD: −0.24; 95% CI: −0.51–0.024; $P = 0.075$; Figure 6).

3.7. Publication Bias. Publication bias was evaluated by Begg's funnel plot and Egger's test (see Supplementary Figure 2 in Supplementary Material available online at https://doi.org/10.1155/2017/6907167). We found that there was no significant publication bias in the studies about the incidence of PMI ($P = 0.139$, Begg's test; $P = 0.065$, Egger's test; Figure 5) and the incidence of AKI ($P = 0.176$, Begg's test; $P = 0.116$, Egger's test). The shapes of the funnel plots seemed symmetrical for the levels of cTnT at 24 h after PCI ($P = 0.325$); this finding was also supported by Egger's test ($P = 0.853$). However, the results revealed that potential publication biases existed in the levels of cTnI 12 h after PCI ($P = 0.039$, Begg's test; $P = 0.006$, Egger's test) and in the CRP levels ($P = 0.009$, Begg's test; $P = 0.022$, Egger's test). All of Begg's funnel plots for the publication bias tests are presented in Figure 7 and Supplementary Figure 1.

3.8. Metaregression Analyses. Random-effects metaregression analysis showed that RIPC's protective effect was enhanced for patients with multivessel disease (coef.: −0.05 [−0.09; −0.01], $P = 0.022$). We did not find any significant relationship between the incidence of PMI and other confounding factors, such as age (coef.: 0.059 [−0.03; 0.15], $P = 0.118$), the percentage of patients being male (coef.: 0.002 [−0.039; 0.044], $P = 0.916$), the percentage of diabetes mellitus (coef.: −0.003 [−0.015; 0.015], $P = 0.960$), the percentage of hypertension (coef.: 0.017 [−0.019; 0.054], $P = 0.320$), the percentage of dyslipidemia (coef.: 0.093 [−0.195; 0.008], $P = 0.063$), the use of beta-blockers (coef.: −0.021 [−0.179; 0.138],

Study ID	OR (95% CI)	% weight
Arm		
Hoole et al. (2009)	0.70 (0.40, 1.22)	12.22
Ahmed et al. (2013)	0.42 (0.15, 1.19)	5.78
Carrasco-Chinchilla et al. (2013)	1.29 (0.75, 2.24)	12.36
Luo et al. (2013)	0.54 (0.31, 0.94)	12.18
Melo et al. (2013)	0.17 (0.03, 0.93)	2.54
Prasad et al. (2013)	0.80 (0.36, 1.81)	8.08
Xu (2013)	0.60 (0.34, 1.06)	12.01
Lavi et al. (2014)	0.83 (0.46, 1.51)	11.36
Zografos et al. (2014)	0.32 (0.13, 0.81)	6.78
Subtotal ($I^2 = 36.9\%$, $P = 0.124$)	0.66 (0.49, 0.88)	83.33
Leg		
Ghaemian et al. (2012)	0.21 (0.07, 0.66)	5.09
Lavi II (2014)	0.96 (0.53, 1.72)	11.58
Subtotal ($I^2 = 81.2\%$, $P = 0.021$)	0.49 (0.11, 2.11)	16.67
Overall ($I^2 = 44.4\%$, $P = 0.055$)	0.64 (0.48, 0.86)	100.00

Note. Weights are from random-effects analysis

.03   1   33.4

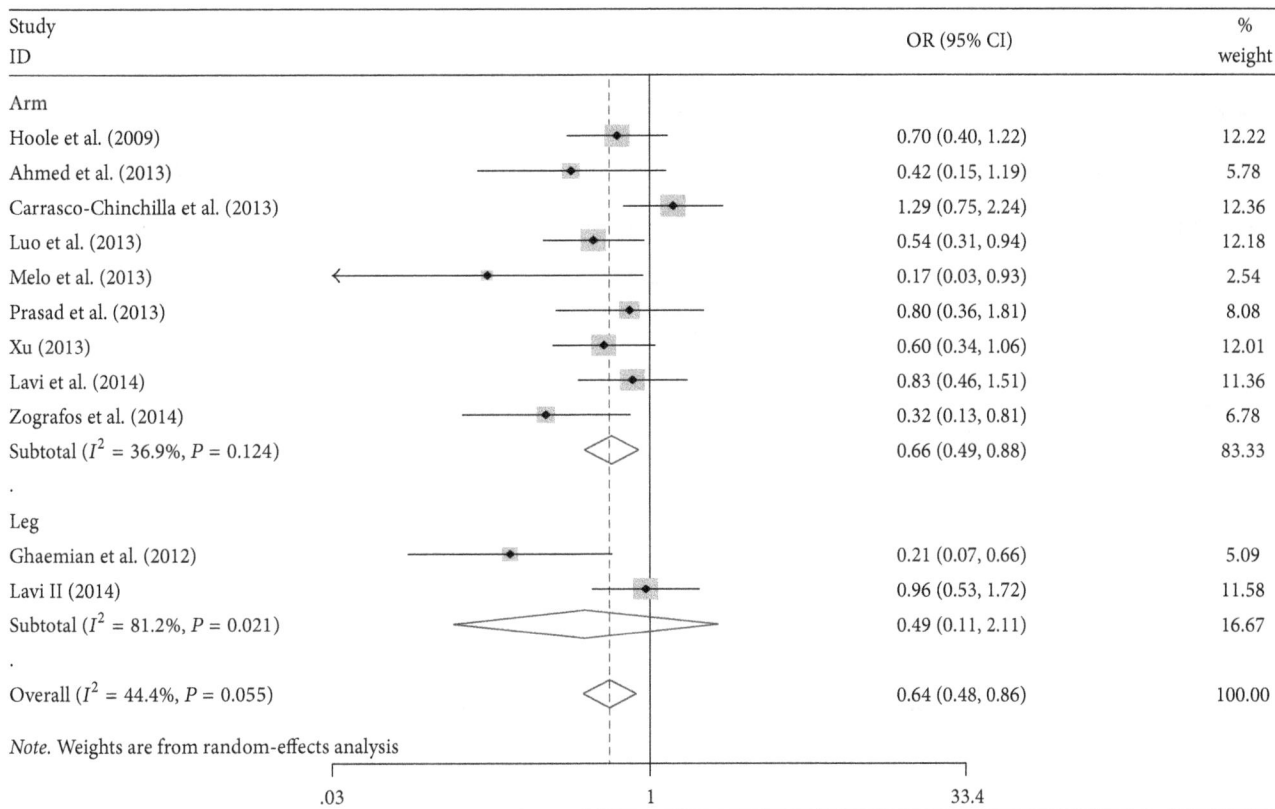

FIGURE 2: Forest plot for the incidence of perioperative myocardial infarction (PMI). RIPC: remote ischemic preconditioning; OR: odds ratio.

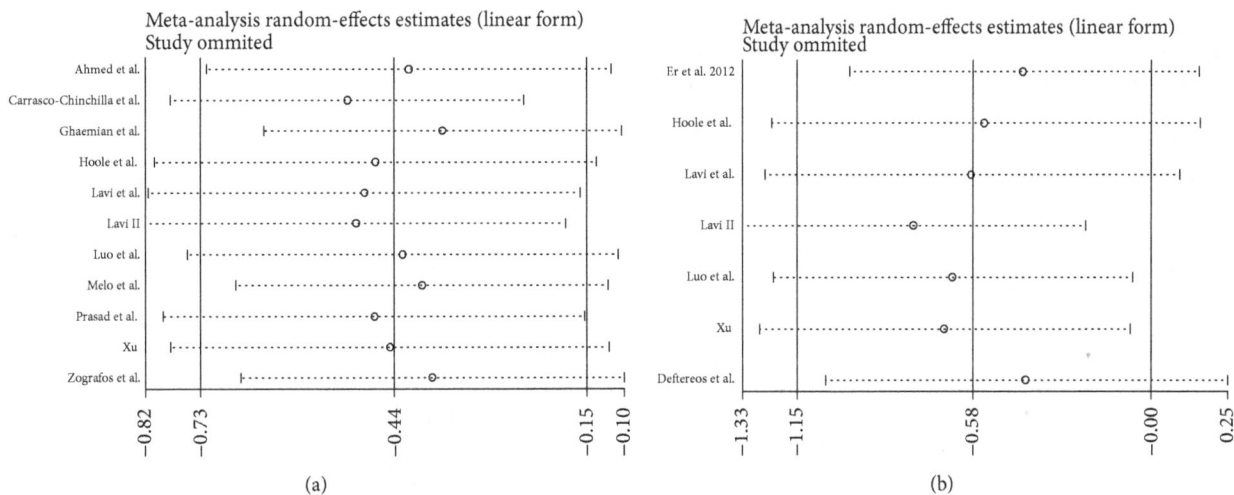

FIGURE 3: Sensitivity analysis of the effect of RIPC on PMI (a) and AKI (b).

$P = 0.759$), the use of statins (coef.: -0.05 [$-0.15; 0.05$], $P = 0.35$), and the use of angiotensin-converting enzyme inhibitors (coef.: 0.007 [$-0.049; 0.064$], $P = 0.697$). The results of the metaregression analysis are shown in Figure 8.

4. Discussion

In the present meta-analysis of 16 randomized trials that enrolled 2,435 adult patients who underwent elective PCI, we evaluated whether remote ischemic preconditioning can offer a protective effect by reducing cardiac and renal events.

Study ID		OR (95% CI)	% weight
Hoole et al. (2009)		0.54 (0.19, 1.54)	15.90
Er et al. 2012 (2012)		0.20 (0.07, 0.57)	16.37
Luo et al. (2013)		2.08 (0.19, 23.31)	4.86
Xu (2013)		1.29 (0.28, 5.93)	10.05
Deftereos et al. (2013)		0.31 (0.15, 0.63)	22.46
Lavi et al. (2014)		0.67 (0.21, 2.17)	14.00
Lavi II (2014)		1.25 (0.45, 3.48)	16.35
Overall ($I^2 = 44.5\%$, $P = 0.094$)		0.56 (0.32, 1.00)	100.00

Note. Weights are from random-effects analysis

.0429   1   23.3

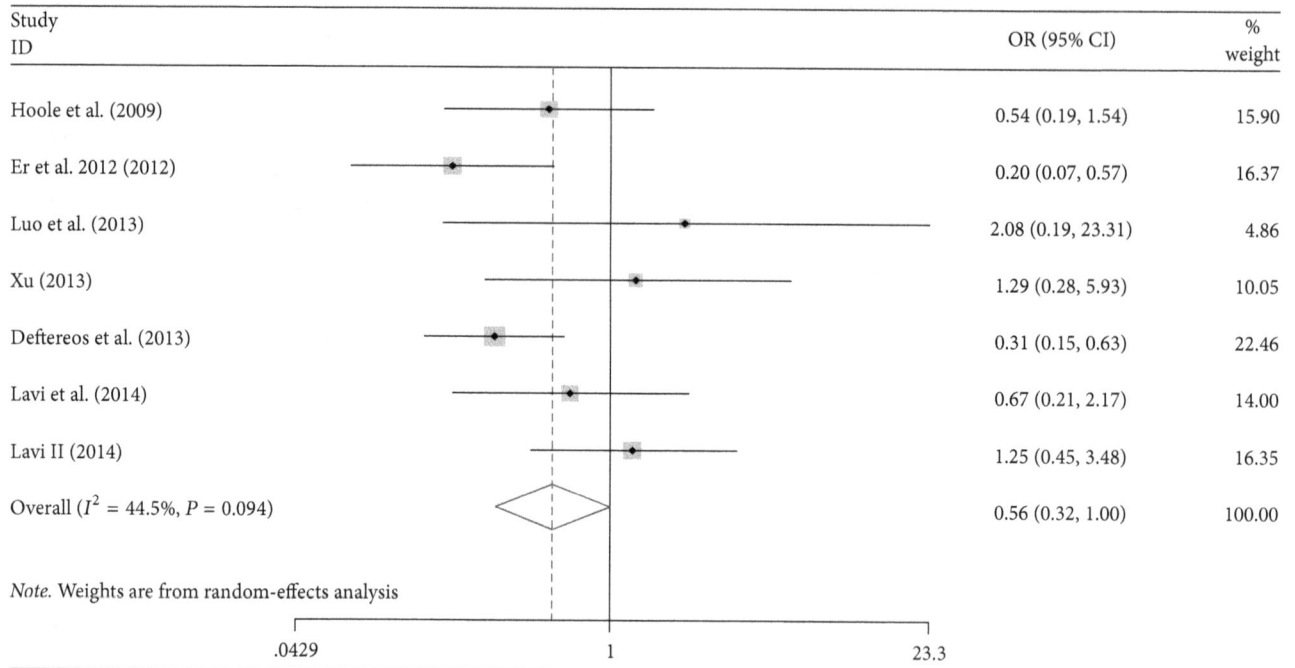

Figure 4: Forest plot for the incidence of acute kidney injury (AKI). RIPC: remote ischemic preconditioning; OR: odds ratio.

Coronary artery disease (CAD) is the most common cause of death in developed and some developing countries. Coronary revascularization with medical therapy and lifestyle alteration constitutes the modern management of patients with significant CAD. In acute myocardial infarction, timely myocardial reperfusion therapy, such as PCI, CABG, and Thrombolysis, is an effective method to limit the myocardial infarct area, attenuate clinical symptoms, and improve the clinical prognosis. However, a large number of studies have shown that reperfusion can lead to further damage to the heart itself [1, 2]. Myocardial ischemia-reperfusion injury (MIRI) is a common pathophysiological process, and it is a serious threat to patients' health.

Coronary revascularization by elective percutaneous coronary intervention (PCI) is the principal intervention in patients with stable CAD and acute coronary syndrome. Even though technical advances in PCI over the past two decades have resulted in a safe procedure with minimal complications, in several patients, the procedure is complicated by periprocedural injury, which can be detected by elevated values of myocardial necrosis biomarkers. Several studies have reported that periprocedural injury is associated with a worse prognosis [42, 43]. A high level of cTnI in patients undergoing PCI was an independent predictor of composite endpoint events (death, myocardial infarction, and revascularization) within 1 year [3–7]. With the progress of coronary heart disease intervention in the past two decades, surgical complications and long-term efficacy have been significantly improved; however, periprocedural myocardial infarction is still very common. Therefore, great efforts have been focused on the prevention of periprocedural complications in recent years.

Ischemic preconditioning (IPC) was first described in a study by Murray et al. in 1986 [44]. The cardioprotective effects of RIPC are also being explored in patients undergoing elective PCI. In 2009, Hoole et al. [10] extended the concept of RIPC to show that RIPC—induced by 3 5-minute blood pressure cuff inflations to 200 mmHg around the upper arm, interspersed with 5 minutes of reperfusion, before the patient's arrival in the catheterization laboratory for stenting—significantly reduced median troponin I concentrations at 24 h (0.06 ng/mL) compared with the control patients (0.16 ng/mL; $P < 0.04$). In the past, numerous clinical trials examined whether RIPC has a protective effect on PCI patients [8–11]; however, the studies regarding RIPC's protective effect in patients undergoing PCI were limited, and the results were controversial and contradictory.

The evidence from the present meta-analysis showed that RIPC can provide myocardial protection in patients undergoing PCI. In previous studies, RIPC has been shown to prevent myocardial ischemia-reperfusion injury in patients undergoing cardiovascular interventional procedures, and a number of meta-analyses showed that RIPC reduced myocardial injury markers and reduced perioperative myocardial infarction. The meta-analyses by D'Ascenzo et al. [12] and Pei et al. [13], which evaluated the effect of RIPC in the patients undergoing cardiac interventions, showed that the incidence of PMI was reduced by RIPC. Our latest study, which includes nearly two years of inclusion in a meta-analysis, also shows that RIPC is effective in preventing PMI, and it is consistent with previous meta-analyses. In the subgroup analysis, we compared preconditioning of upper and lower extremities and found that RIPC of the upper extremities had a statistically significant effect on protecting PMI; however,

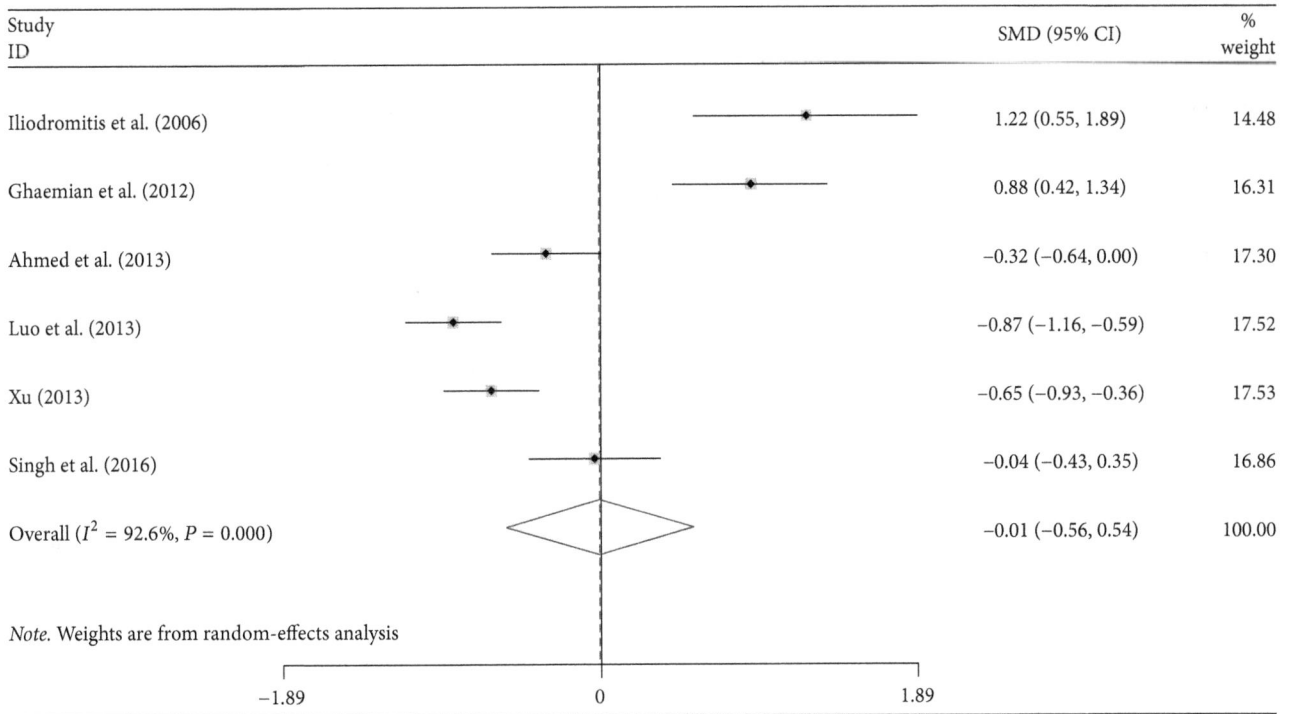

(a)

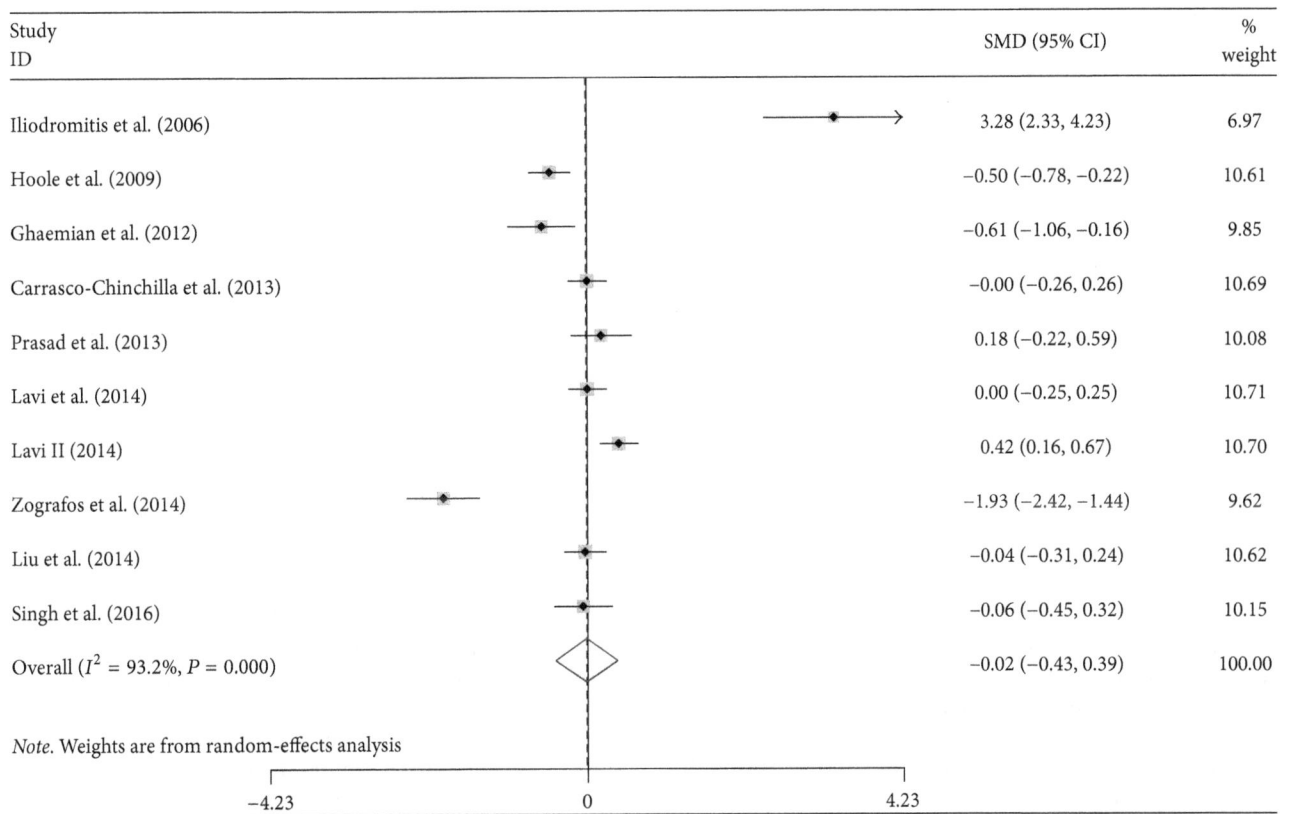

(b)

FIGURE 5: Forest plot for myocardial biomarkers expressed as SMD within 12 h (a) and 24 h (b) after PCI. SMD: standardized mean difference.

Study ID		SMD (95% CI)	% weight
Ahmed et al. (2013)		−0.12 (−0.44, 0.20)	10.24
Carrasco-Chinchilla et al. (2013)		−0.07 (−0.33, 0.18)	10.82
Hoole et al. (2009)		−0.03 (−0.30, 0.25)	10.66
Iliodromitis et al. (2006)		−0.57 (−1.20, 0.05)	7.21
Lavi et al. (2014)		0.16 (−0.10, 0.41)	10.86
Lavi II (2014)		0.02 (−0.23, 0.27)	10.86
Prasad et al. (2013)		−2.00 (−2.49, −1.51)	8.49
Xu (2013)		−0.16 (−0.44, 0.11)	10.64
Liu et al. (2014)		0.00 (−0.28, 0.28)	10.65
Singh et al. (2016)		−0.09 (−0.48, 0.30)	9.57
Overall ($I^2 = 86.1\%$, $P = 0.000$)		−0.24 (−0.51, 0.02)	100.00

Note. Weights are from random-effects analysis

−2.49   0   2.49

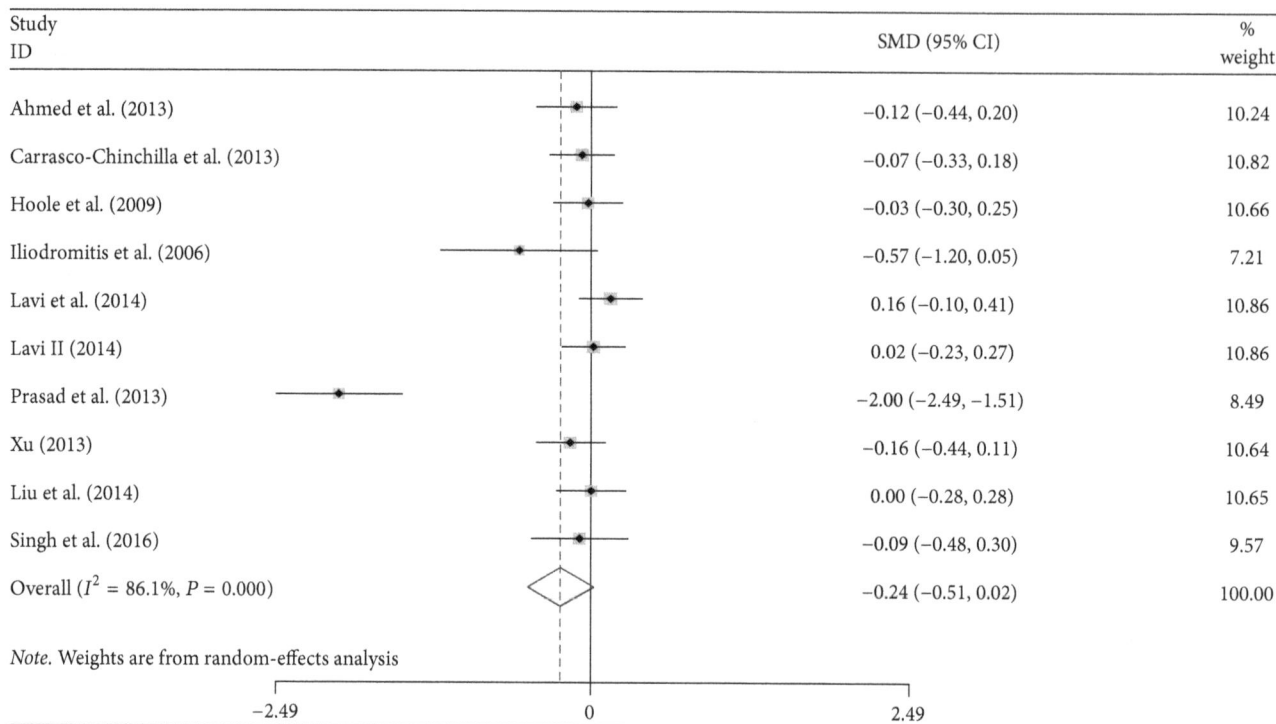

FIGURE 6: Forest plot for CRP as SMD after PCI. CRP: C-reactive protein; SMD: standardized mean difference.

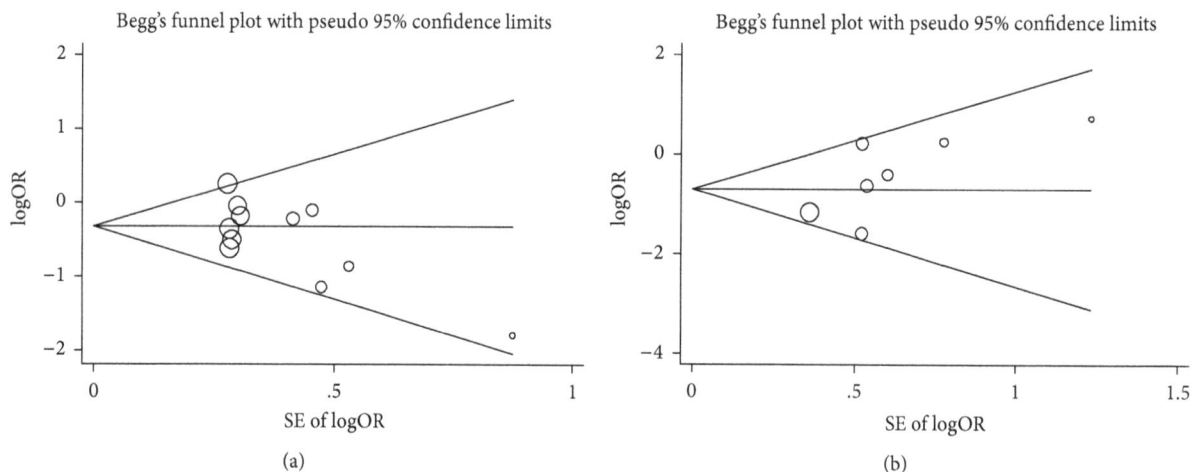

FIGURE 7: Begg's funnel plot for publication bias test. (a) The incidence of PMI and (b) the incidence of AKI.

RIPC with lower limb preconditioning cannot effectively reduce the incidence of PMI, which is inconsistent with the results of a meta-analysis by D'Ascenzo et al. In our analysis, there was greater heterogeneity in the clinical studies of limb preconditioning, particularly in Lavi et al.'s limb preconditioning procedure, which used only a 5-minute ischemia-reperfusion cycle, and the strength of the preconditioning could lead to a change in outcome. Previous studies have shown that the intensity of distal limb ischemia and protective effects are closely related [12]. The different mechanisms of RIPC between the upper arm and the lower limb remain

unclear. There are still a limited number of studies to evaluate whether RIPC with the upper arm is different from RIPC with the lower limb in relation to the protective effects for PMI. Therefore, future research is needed to compare these two types of RIPC to determine whether they exhibit different capacities for cardiac protection.

To further investigate the sources of heterogeneity, we performed metaregression analysis. We did not find any significant relationship between the incidence of PMI and other confounding factors, such as age, the percentage of male patients, the percentage of hypertension patients, the

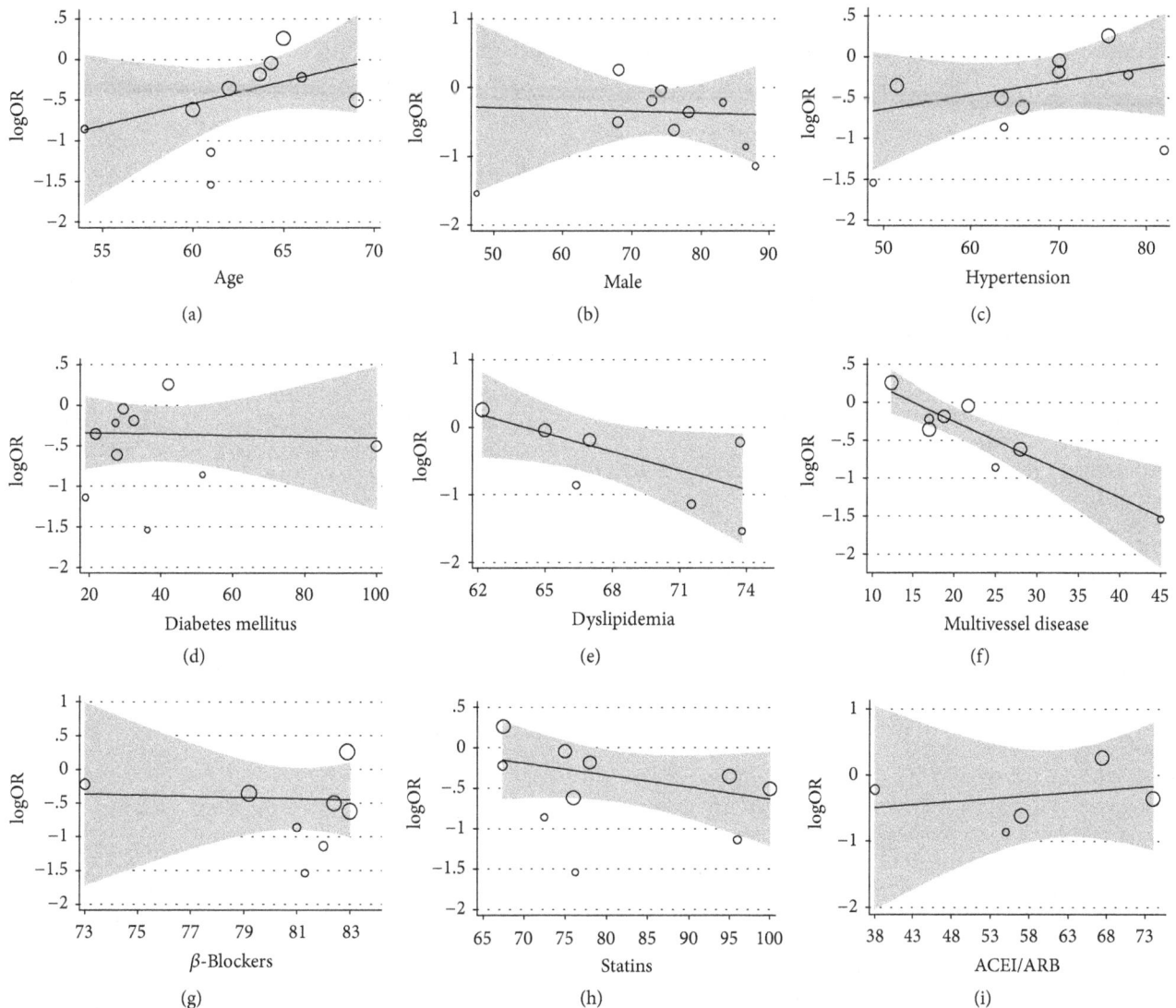

FIGURE 8: Metaregression results of reduction of PMI by RIPC. Metaregression of age (a), percentage of males (b), percentage of hypertension (c), percentage of diabetes mellitus (DM) (d), percentage of dyslipidemia (e), percentage of multivessel disease (f), percentage of β-blockers used (g), percentage of statins used (h), and percentage of ACEI/ARB used (i).

percentage of diabetes mellitus patients, the percentage of dyslipidemia patients, and their medication. Surprisingly, the reduction of PMI by RIPC was enhanced for patients with multivessel disease. These observations are consistent with previous published reports of RIPC in patients with diffuse coronary artery disease who underwent CABG surgery [45]. Our results may explain why some studies with a low sample size and a relatively low risk (a proportion of low diabetes mellitus and multivessel disease) failed to observe the effect of RIPC on PMI. In other words, the more the disease is diffused, the more significant RIPC's reduction of the effect of PMI is.

Many clinical observations have found that increased levels of myocardial injury markers, such as troponin T, troponin I, and CK-MB, are associated with adverse long-term prognosis after elective percutaneous coronary intervention

[41, 46, 47]. In the meta-analysis by Niu et al. [48], it was found that RIPC can reduce myocardial injury markers after PCI release; this protective effect was more obvious in STEMI patients, while in the elective PCI patients, RIPC cannot reduce myocardial injury markers, and the heterogeneity of the included studies was larger. To our knowledge, this is the first meta-analysis to explore whether RIPC could reduce the release of myocardial markers after PCI in patients with elective PCI. The results showed that RIPC was unable to reduce the concentration of cTnI at 12 h and 24 h after elective PCI (for 12 h, SMD: −0.11, 95% CI: −0.48–0.27, P = 0.585; for 24 h, SMD: −0.02, 95% CI: −0.43–0.39, P = 0.934), and there was a high degree of heterogeneity in the included studies (I^2 = 93.2%). We considered that the possible reason that there were no effective results in RIPC reduction of cTnI is because myocardial injury during elective

PCI is relatively minimal compared with that during acute myocardial infarction, which is mainly due to coronary artery side branch loss and distal embolization during balloon inflation or stent implantation [49, 50].

AKI is a serious postoperation complication in patients with cardiac and vascular interventions. Patients with postoperative acute kidney injury have significantly higher morbidity and mortality [44]. To date, whether RIPC can or cannot protect against kidney injury in patients undergoing percutaneous coronary intervention is still a controversial issue. Li et al. performed a meta-analysis in which they found that RIPC can reduce contrast-induced AKI in patients undergoing PCI/CAG [51]. Similarly, Alreja et al.'s meta-analysis [52] revealed that RIPC can also significantly reduce AKI incidence in patients undergoing cardiac or vascular interventions, but there was high heterogeneity among the 26 trials they analyzed. Conversely, D'Ascenzo et al. [12] and Brevoord et al. [53] also performed meta-analyses to evaluate the renal protective effect of RIPC in patients undergoing cardiac and vascular interventions, and the results of both showed that serum creatinine levels were not reduced by RIPC. These apparent inconsistencies may be due to limitations in the low number of studies, a small sample size, and different definitions of AKI. Our meta-analysis found that RIPC significantly decreased the incidence of AKI from 11.91% to 6.45% (OR: 0.494; 95% CI: 0.335–0.729; $P < 0.001$), confirming once again that RIPC has a protective effect on renal function in patients undergoing PCI. The causes of renal injury after PCI may include contrast-induced nephropathy and reperfusion injury. The mechanisms of contrast-induced AKI after PCI are still ill-defined and poorly understood, but potential mechanisms underlying CI-AKI include damage to the tubular epithelial cells and vascular endothelium, a change of renal hemodynamics with reduced effective arterial volume during the procedure, microemboli to the kidney, drug toxicity, regional hypoxia, and the production of oxygen free radicals that scavenge nitric oxide (NO) and blunt NO activity [54]. RIPC may promote endothelial oxide synthase to enhance the production of NO and reduce the production of reactive oxygen species, which is an important factor in the late phase of reperfusion, as it reduces damage to the tubular epithelial cells and vascular endothelium [55]. At present, the number of RIPC studies and the sample sizes are still small, so large randomized controlled trials that include a larger number of patients are required to confirm the efficacy of RIPC in AKI in patients undergoing PCI.

The mechanism of RIPC is very complex, but it is mainly concentrated in the mitochondrial ATP-sensitive potassium channel, protein kinase C, and the NF-kappa B molecular mechanism of signal transduction. The inflammatory response is an important mechanism for myocardial ischemia-reperfusion injury [56, 57]. Some studies have indicated that RIPC can protect the myocardium by inhibiting inflammation. In our meta-analysis, we found that RIPC cannot reduce the levels of CRP after PCI. This may be due to the fact that CRP is not a sensitive marker for assessing the inflammatory response of patients undergoing PCI. More sensitive inflammation markers, such as NF-kappa B, IL-6, HMGB1, are worth using to assess the inflammatory status in patients after PCI treatment. Further studies seeking to determine whether RIPC can reduce the inflammatory response after PCI are needed.

5. Limitations

Despite the overall robust statistical evidence produced by this analysis, some limitations should be pointed out. First, we were unable to access the individual patient data. The results of the meta-analysis were mainly based on the published merged patient data, such as the mean age, the proportion of males, the proportion of risk factors, and the proportion of various drugs used. Therefore, the effects of RIPC may be underestimated. Second, the RIPC protocol should impact its effects on clinical outcomes; however, we could not determine which protocol was superior to another (e.g., RIPC on arms or legs, different cycle times, etc.). Third, the definition of AKI varied among the individual studies, and this may influence the final incidence of AKI. However, there was no further study on the protective effect of RIPC on renal function in this analysis. Fourth, long-term morbidity and mortality were not evaluated in this meta-analysis because of insufficient data. Lastly, the studies included in this meta-analysis were only publications in English language, which may cause publication bias.

6. Conclusion

Our meta-analysis demonstrated that RIPC, using repeated brief episodes of limb ischemia-reperfusion, can provide cardiac and renal protection for patients undergoing elective PCI. RIPC has no beneficial effect on reducing the levels of cTnI and CRP after PCI. Future randomized clinical trials should be performed to apply optimal RIPC protocol and evaluate the long-term clinical outcomes.

Authors' Contributions

Xiangming Wang and Na Kong contributed equally to this work.

Acknowledgments

This study was supported by the National Natural Science Foundation of China (no. 81601246 to Dr. Na Kong). The authors acknowledge LetPub (http://www.letpub.com) for its linguistic assistance during the preparation of this manuscript.

References

[1] L. C. Becker and G. Ambrosio, "Myocardial consequences of reperfusion," *Progress in Cardiovascular Diseases*, vol. 30, no. 1, pp. 23–44, 1987.

[2] K. Matsumura, R. W. Jeremy, J. Schaper, and L. C. Becker, "Progression of myocardial necrosis during reperfusion of ischemic myocardium," *Circulation*, vol. 97, no. 8, pp. 795–804, 1998.

[3] T. Nageh, R. A. Sherwood, B. M. Harris, and M. R. Thomas, "Prognostic role of cardiac troponin I after percutaneous coronary intervention in stable coronary disease," *Heart*, vol. 91, no. 9, pp. 1181–1185, 2005.

[4] A. Ramirez-Moreno, R. Cardenal, C. Pera et al., "Predictors and prognostic value of myocardial injury following stent implantation," *International Journal of Cardiology*, vol. 97, no. 2, pp. 193–198, 2004.

[5] J. R. Kizer, M. R. Muttrej, W. H. Matthai et al., "Role of cardiac troponin T in the long-term risk stratification of patients undergoing percutaneous coronary intervention," *European Heart Journal*, vol. 24, no. 14, pp. 1314–1322, 2003.

[6] M. J. Ricciardi, C. J. Davidson, G. Gubernikoff et al., "Troponin I elevation and cardiac events after percutaneous coronary intervention," *American Heart Journal*, vol. 145, no. 3, pp. 522–528, 2003.

[7] W. J. Cantor, L. K. Newby, R. H. Christenson et al., "Prognostic significance of elevated troponin I after percutaneous coronary intervention," *Journal of the American College of Cardiology*, vol. 39, no. 11, pp. 1738–1744, 2002.

[8] R. M. Ahmed, E.-H. A. Mohamed, M. Ashraf et al., "Effect of remote ischemic preconditioning on serum troponin T level following elective percutaneous coronary intervention," *Catheterization and Cardiovascular Interventions*, vol. 82, no. 5, pp. E647–E653, 2013.

[9] F. Carrasco-Chinchilla, A. J. Muñoz-García, A. Domínguez-Franco et al., "Remote ischaemic postconditioning: Does it protect against ischaemic damage in percutaneous coronary revascularisation? Randomised placebo-controlled clinical trial," *Heart*, vol. 99, no. 19, pp. 1431–1437, 2013.

[10] S. P. Hoole, P. M. Heck, L. Sharples et al., "Cardiac remote ischemic preconditioning in coronary stenting (CRISP stent) study: a prospective, randomized control trial," *Circulation*, vol. 119, no. 6, pp. 820–827, 2009.

[11] G. B. Singh, S. H. Ann, J. Park et al., "Remote ischemic preconditioning for the prevention of contrast-induced acute kidney injury in diabetics receiving elective percutaneous coronary intervention," *PLoS ONE*, vol. 11, no. 10, Article ID e0164256, 2016.

[12] F. D'Ascenzo, C. Moretti, P. Omedè et al., "Cardiac remote ischaemic preconditioning reduces periprocedural myocardial infarction for patients undergoing percutaneous coronary interventions: A meta-analysis of randomised clinical trials," *EuroIntervention*, vol. 9, no. 12, pp. 1463–1471, 2014.

[13] H. Pei, Y. Wu, Y. Wei, Y. Yang, S. Teng, and H. Zhang, "Remote ischemic preconditioning reduces perioperative cardiac and renal events in patients undergoing elective coronary intervention: A meta-analysis of 11 randomized trials," *PLoS ONE*, vol. 9, no. 12, Article ID e115500, 2014.

[14] D. Moher, A. Liberati, J. Tetzlaff, and D. G. Altman, "Preferred reporting items for systematic reviews and meta-analyses: the PRISMA statement," *International Journal of Surgery*, vol. 8, no. 5, pp. 336–341, 2010.

[15] J. Higgins and S. Green, "Cochrane handbook for systematic reviews of interventions version 5.1. 0," *Cochrane database of systematic reviews (Online)*, vol. 2, p. S38, 2011.

[16] A. R. Jadad, R. A. Moore, D. Carroll et al., "Assessing the quality of reports of randomized clinical trials: is blinding necessary?" *Controlled Clinical Trials*, vol. 17, no. 1, pp. 1–12, 1996.

[17] J. P. T. Higgins and S. G. Thompson, "Quantifying heterogeneity in a meta-analysis," *Statistics in Medicine*, vol. 21, no. 11, pp. 1539–1558, 2002.

[18] N. Mantel and W. Haenszel, "Statistical aspects of the analysis of data from retrospective studies of disease," *Journal of the National Cancer Institute*, vol. 22, no. 4, pp. 719–748, 1959.

[19] R. DerSimonian and N. Laird, "Meta-analysis in clinical trials," *Controlled Clinical Trials*, vol. 7, no. 3, pp. 177–188, 1986.

[20] V. Manchurov, N. Ryazankina, T. Khmara et al., "Remote ischemic preconditioning and endothelial function in patients with acute myocardial infarction and primary PCI," *American Journal of Medicine*, vol. 127, no. 7, pp. 670–673, 2014.

[21] S. P. Hoole and D. P. Dutka, "Does remote ischemic conditioning salvage left ventricular function after successful primary PCI?" *Expert Review of Cardiovascular Therapy*, vol. 9, no. 5, pp. 563–566, 2011.

[22] T. Yamanaka, Y. Kawai, T. Miyoshi et al., "Remote ischemic preconditioning reduces contrast-induced acute kidney injury in patients with ST-elevation myocardial infarction: A randomized controlled trial," *International Journal of Cardiology*, vol. 178, pp. 136–141, 2015.

[23] S. Deftereos, G. Giannopoulos, V. Tzalamouras et al., "Renoprotective effect of remote ischemic post-conditioning by intermittent balloon inflations in patients undergoing percutaneous coronary intervention," *Journal of the American College of Cardiology*, vol. 61, no. 19, pp. 1949–1955, 2013.

[24] H. E. Bøtker, R. Kharbanda, M. R. Schmidt et al., "Remote ischaemic conditioning before hospital admission, as a complement to angioplasty, and effect on myocardial salvage in patients with acute myocardial infarction: a randomised trial," *The Lancet*, vol. 375, no. 9716, pp. 727–734, 2010.

[25] I. Rentoukas, G. Giannopoulos, A. Kaoukis et al., "Cardioprotective role of remote ischemic periconditioning in primary percutaneous coronary intervention," *JACC: Cardiovascular Interventions*, vol. 3, no. 1, pp. 49–55, 2010.

[26] G. Crimi, S. Pica, C. Raineri et al., "Remote ischemic post-conditioning of the lower limb during primary percutaneous coronary intervention safely reduces enzymatic infarct size in anterior myocardial infarction: a randomized controlled trial," *JACC: Cardiovascular Interventions*, vol. 6, no. 10, pp. 1055–1063, 2013.

[27] A. D. Sloth, M. R. Schmidt, K. Munk et al., "Improved long-term clinical outcomes in patients with ST-elevation myocardial infarction undergoing remote ischaemic conditioning as an adjunct to primary percutaneous coronary intervention," *European Heart Journal*, vol. 35, no. 3, pp. 168–175, 2014.

[28] F. Prunier, D. Angoulvant, C. Saint Etienne et al., "The RIPOST-MI study, assessing remote ischemic perconditioning alone or in combination with local ischemic postconditioning in ST-segment elevation myocardial infarction," *Basic Research in Cardiology*, vol. 109, no. 2, article no. 400, 2014.

[29] E. S. EL Desoky, A. K. M. Hassan, S. Y. Salem, S. A. Fadil, and A. F. Taha, "Cardioprotective effect of atorvastatin alone or in combination with remote ischemic preconditioning on the biochemical changes induced by ischemic/reperfusion injury in a mutual prospective study with a clinical and experimental animal arm," *International Journal of Cardiology*, vol. 222, pp. 866–873, 2016.

[30] I. Eitel, T. Stiermaier, K. P. Rommel et al., "Cardioprotection by combined intrahospital remote ischaemic perconditioning and postconditioning in ST-elevation myocardial infarction: The randomized LIPSIA CONDITIONING trial," *European Heart Journal*, vol. 36, no. 44, pp. 3049–3057, 2015.

[31] S. Lavi, S. D'Alfonso, P. Diamantouros et al., "Ischemic postconditioning during percutaneous coronary interventions: Remote ischemic postconditioning-percutaneous coronary intervention randomized trial," *Circulation: Cardiovascular Interventions*, vol. 7, no. 2, pp. 225–232, 2014.

[32] F. Er, A. M. Nia, H. Dopp et al., "Ischemic preconditioning for prevention of contrast medium-induced nephropathy: randomized pilot RenPro Trial (Renal Protection Trial)," *Journal of Vascular Surgery*, vol. 126, no. 3, pp. 296–303, 2012.

[33] A. Ghaemian, S. M. Nouraei, F. Abdollahian, F. Naghshvar, D. A. Giussani, and S. A. R. Nouraei, "Remote ischemic preconditioning in percutaneous coronary revascularization: A double-blind randomized controlled clinical trial," *Asian Cardiovascular and Thoracic Annals*, vol. 20, no. 5, pp. 548–554, 2012.

[34] E. K. Iliodromitis, S. Kyrzopoulos, I. A. Paraskevaidis et al., "Increased C reactive protein and cardiac enzyme levels after coronary stent implantation. Is there protection by remote ischaemic preconditioning?" *Heart*, vol. 92, no. 12, pp. 1821–1826, 2006.

[35] S. J. Luo, Y. J. Zhou, D. M. Shi, H. L. Ge, J. L. Wang, and R. F. Liu, "Remote ischemic preconditioning reduces myocardial injury in patients undergoing coronary stent implantation," *Canadian Journal of Cardiology*, vol. 29, no. 9, pp. 1084–1089, 2013.

[36] R. M. Melo, L. M. Costa, A. Uchida et al., "Prevention of myocardial injury after percutaneous coronary interventions with remote ischemic preconditioning. A comparative analysis with biomarkers and cardiac magnetic resonance," *European Heart Journal*, vol. 34, no. suppl 1, pp. P5487–P5487, 2013.

[37] A. Prasad, M. Gössl, J. Hoyt et al., "Remote ischemic preconditioning immediately before percutaneous coronary intervention does not impact myocardial necrosis, inflammatory response, and circulating endothelial progenitor cell counts: A single center randomized sham controlled trial," *Catheterization and Cardiovascular Interventions*, vol. 81, no. 6, pp. 930–936, 2013.

[38] X. Xu, Y. Zhou, S. Luo et al., "Effect of remote ischemic preconditioning in the elderly patients with coronary artery disease with diabetes mellitus undergoing elective drug-eluting stent implantation," *Angiology*, vol. 65, no. 8, pp. 660–666, 2014.

[39] Z. Liu, Y.-L. Wang, D. Xu, Q. Hua, Y.-Y. Chu, and X.-M. Ji, "Late remote ischemic preconditioning provides benefit to patients undergoing elective percutaneous coronary intervention," *Cell Biochemistry and Biophysics*, vol. 70, no. 1, pp. 437–442, 2014.

[40] T. A. Zografos, G. D. Katritsis, I. Tsiafoutis, N. Bourboulis, A. Katsivas, and D. G. Katritsis, "Effect of one-cycle remote ischemic preconditioning to reduce myocardial injury during percutaneous coronary intervention," *American Journal of Cardiology*, vol. 113, no. 12, pp. 2013–2017, 2014.

[41] E. Bignami, G. Landoni, G. Crescenzi et al., "Role of cardiac biomarkers (troponin I and CK-MB) as predictors of quality of life and long-term outcome after cardiac surgery," *Annals of Cardiac Anaesthesia*, vol. 12, no. 1, pp. 22–26, 2009.

[42] H. Idris, S. Lo, I. M. Shugman et al., "Varying definitions for periprocedural myocardial infarction alter event rates and prognostic implications," *Journal of the American Heart Association*, vol. 3, no. 6, Article ID 001086, 2014.

[43] H. Ishiia, T. Amano, T. Matsubara, and T. Murohara, "Pharmacological prevention of peri-, and post-procedural myocardial injury in percutaneous coronary intervention," *Current Cardiology Reviews*, vol. 4, no. 3, pp. 223–230, 2008.

[44] F. J. Abelha, M. Botelho, V. Fernandes, and H. Barros, "Determinants of postoperative acute kidney injury," *Critical Care*, vol. 13, no. 3, article no. R79, 2009.

[45] F. D'Ascenzo, E. Cavallero, C. Moretti et al., "Remote ischaemic preconditioning in coronary artery bypass surgery: a meta-analysis," *Heart*, vol. 98, no. 17, pp. 1267–1271, 2012.

[46] R. V. Milani, R. Fitzgerald, J. N. Milani, and C. J. Lavie, "The impact of micro troponin leak on long-term outcomes following elective percutaneous coronary intervention," *Catheterization and Cardiovascular Interventions*, vol. 74, no. 6, pp. 819–822, 2009.

[47] D. N. Feldman, R. M. Minutello, G. Bergman, I. Moussa, and S. C. Wong, "Relation of troponin I levels following nonemergent percutaneous coronary intervention to short- and long-term outcomes," *The American Journal of Cardiology*, vol. 104, no. 9, pp. 1210–1215, 2009.

[48] X. Niu, J. Zhang, D. Chen, G. Wan, Y. Zhang, and Y. Yao, "Remote ischaemic conditioning in percutaneous coronary intervention: A meta-analysis of randomised trials," *Postepy w Kardiologii Interwencyjnej*, vol. 10, no. 4, pp. 274–282, 2014.

[49] T. Yetgin, O. C. Manintveld, E. Boersma et al., "Remote Ischemic Conditioning in Percutaneous Coronary Intervention and Coronary Artery Bypass Grafting - Meta-Analysis of Randomized Trials -," *Circulation Journal*, vol. 76, no. 10, pp. 2392–2404, 2012.

[50] A. Prasad and J. Herrmann, "Myocardial infarction due to percutaneous coronary intervention," *New England Journal of Medicine*, vol. 364, no. 5, pp. 453–464, 2011.

[51] B. Li, X. Lang, L. Cao et al., "Effect of remote ischemic preconditioning on postoperative acute kidney injury among patients undergoing cardiac and vascular interventions: a meta-analysis," *Journal of Nephrology*, vol. 30, no. 1, pp. 19–33, 2017.

[52] G. Alreja, D. Bugano, and A. Lotfi, "Effect of remote ischemic preconditioning on myocardial and renal injury: meta-analysis of randomized controlled trials," *The Journal of invasive cardiology*, vol. 24, no. 2, pp. 42–48, 2012.

[53] D. Brevoord, P. Kranke, M. Kuijpers, N. Weber, M. Hollmann, and B. Preckel, "Remote ischemic conditioning to protect against ischemia-reperfusion injury: a systematic review and meta-analysis," *PLoS ONE*, vol. 7, no. 7, Article ID e42179, 2012.

[54] S. Tehrani, C. Laing, D. M. Yellon, and D. J. Hausenloy, "Contrast-induced acute kidney injury following PCI," *European Journal of Clinical Investigation*, vol. 43, no. 5, pp. 483–490, 2013.

[55] D. Russo, R. Minutolo, B. Cianciaruso, B. Memoli, G. Conte, and L. de Nicola, "Early effects of contrast media on renal hemodynamics and tubular function in chronic renal failure," *Journal of the American Society of Nephrology*, vol. 6, no. 5, pp. 1451–1458, 1995.

[56] P. K. Randhawa, A. Bali, and A. S. Jaggi, "RIPC for multiorgan salvage in clinical settings: evolution of concept, evidences and mechanisms," *European Journal of Pharmacology*, vol. 746, pp. 317–332, 2015.

[57] G. D. Katritsis, T. A. Zografos, and A. G. Katsivas, "Remote ischemic preconditioning for reduction of peri-procedural myocardial injury during percutaneous coronary intervention," *Hellenic Journal of Cardiology*, vol. 55, no. 3, pp. 245–255, 2014.

23

Renal Insufficiency and Early Bystander CPR Predict In-Hospital Outcomes in Cardiac Arrest Patients Undergoing Mild Therapeutic Hypothermia and Cardiac Catheterization: Return of Spontaneous Circulation, Cooling, and Catheterization Registry (ROSCCC Registry)

Anjala Chelvanathan,[1] David Allen,[1] Hilary Bews,[2] John Ducas,[1] Kunal Minhas,[1] Minh Vo,[1] Malek Kass,[1] Amir Ravandi,[1,2] James W. Tam,[1] Davinder S. Jassal,[1,2,3,4] and Farrukh Hussain[1]

[1]Section of Cardiology, Department of Internal Medicine, University of Manitoba, Winnipeg, MB, Canada R2H 2A6
[2]Institute of Cardiovascular Sciences, St. Boniface Research Centre, University of Manitoba, Winnipeg, MB, Canada R2H 2A6
[3]Section of Oncology, Department of Internal Medicine, University of Manitoba, Winnipeg, MB, Canada R2H 2A6
[4]Department of Radiology, University of Manitoba, Winnipeg, MB, Canada R2H 2A6

Correspondence should be addressed to Davinder S. Jassal; djassal@sbgh.mb.ca

Academic Editor: Firat Duru

Objective. Out of hospital cardiac arrest (OHCA) patients are a critically ill patient population with high mortality. Combining mild therapeutic hypothermia (MTH) with early coronary intervention may improve outcomes in this population. The aim of this study was to evaluate predictors of mortality in OHCA patients undergoing MTH with and without cardiac catheterization. *Design.* A retrospective cohort of OHCA patients who underwent MTH with catheterization (MTH + C) and without catheterization (MTH + NC) between 2006 and 2011 was analyzed at a single tertiary care centre. Predictors of in-hospital mortality and neurologic outcome were determined. *Results.* The study population included 176 patients who underwent MTH for OHCA. A total of 66 patients underwent cardiac catheterization (MTH + C) and 110 patients did not undergo cardiac catheterization (MTH + NC). Immediate bystander CPR occurred in approximately half of the total population. In the MTH + C and MTH + NC groups, the in-hospital mortality was 48% and 78%, respectively. The only independent predictor of in-hospital mortality for patients with MTH + C, after multivariate analysis, was baseline renal insufficiency (OR = 8.2, 95% CI 1.8–47.1, and $p = 0.009$). *Conclusion.* Despite early cardiac catheterization, renal insufficiency and the absence of immediate CPR are potent predictors of death and poor neurologic outcome in patients with OHCA.

1. Introduction

Over 350,000 out of hospital cardiac arrests (OHCA) occur each year in the United States, with around 45,000 cardiac arrests occurring each year in Canada [1]. Despite nearly 40 years of promotion of prehospital Advanced Cardiac Life Support (ACLS), long-term survival rates following OHCA remain dismal [2, 3]. In a recent meta-analysis, the aggregate survival rate for OHCA across various populations was reported at less than 8% [3]. In addition, postcardiac arrest complications, including severe anoxic brain injury (ABI), contributes to high morbidity and mortality rates for patients initially undergoing successful resuscitation [1]. As such, it remains an important goal to develop therapeutic strategies to improve survival in this patient population.

Mild therapeutic hypothermia (MTH) and targeted temperature management (TTM) afford long-term survival and neurologic benefits to comatose survivors of arrhythmia-induced cardiac arrest [1, 3–6]. More recently, studies have investigated the combination of early interventional strategies with MTH as a means of further improving long-term survival in resuscitated cardiac arrest patients with evolving evidence of ST elevation myocardial infarction (STEMI). A review of four nonrandomized case series involving STEMI patients who were successfully resuscitated from cardiac arrest and treated with both MTH and early coronary intervention demonstrated overall favorable outcomes [7–10]. Numerous other case series have illustrated that early coronary angiography and percutaneous coronary intervention (PCI), combined with MTH, produce the highest long-term survival rates among patients who remain comatose after resuscitated cardiac arrest [11–14]. As a result, in the ACCF/AHA 2013 STEMI Guidelines, MTH was endorsed as a class 1, level of evidence B recommendation [15]. Furthermore, immediate angiography and PCI as indicated were recommended in resuscitated OHCA patients whose initial ECG shows ST-segment elevation [15].

The objective of this retrospective study was to investigate the outcomes and predictors of mortality in individuals resuscitated from cardiac arrest who underwent MTH both with and without cardiac catheterization.

2. Methods

2.1. Study Design. A single-centre retrospective cohort study examining all consecutive adult patients who were successfully resuscitated following cardiac arrest who underwent either MTH with catheterization (MTH + C) or MTH without cardiac catheterization (MTH + NC) between January 1, 2006, and September 30, 2011, was performed. MTH was used at the discretion of the attending physician and the decision regarding need for cardiac catheterization was made by the treating cardiologist or intensivist. MTH was induced and maintained through a combination of surface cooling blankets and ice packs. Local institutional protocol stipulates that MTH should be initiated as soon as possible after return of spontaneous circulation (ROSC) to achieve a core temperature of 32–34°C within 6–8 hrs. This core temperature should be maintained for 24 hrs and followed by subsequent passive rewarming. The study was approved by the University of Manitoba and St. Boniface General Hospital research ethics boards.

2.2. Data Collection. Subjects were identified by searching the ICU quality-assurance database for an International Classification of Diseases-9 discharge diagnosis of cardiac arrest in addition to cointerrogation of the MACLAB cardiac catheterization database. Detailed demographics and prehospital data pertaining to the cardiac arrest, including location of cardiac arrest, duration of down time, bystander CPR, time to ROSC, and initial arrest rhythm, were collected. As cardiac rhythm monitoring was not always available during the pulseless period, the initial arrest rhythm was the first rhythm recorded either during or after the cardiac arrest. Cooling protocol and time data were noted. Detailed data

on cardiac interventions were recorded, including coronary anatomy, stent placement, coronary artery bypass grafting (CABG), mechanical circulatory support (MCS), and intra-aortic balloon pump (IABP) placement. Detailed data on complications within 1 week of hospitalization, in addition to patient outcomes, including in-hospital mortality, were abstracted.

2.3. Definitions. Cardiac arrest was defined as the absence of signs of circulation with the concomitant appearance of unconsciousness, apnea, or gasping and receipt of chest compressions or defibrillation for a pulseless arrhythmia as determined by a health care worker. Multivessel coronary disease was defined as ≥2 main (left anterior descending, right coronary artery, or circumflex) vessels with ≥70% stenosis. Early coronary angiogram was defined as receiving a coronary angiogram within 12 hours of arrival. A successful PCI was defined as residual stenosis ≤ 20% with TIMI 3 flow. Slow flow was defined as TIMI ≤ 2 flow in the intervened vessel. Angiographic, TIMI flow, and procedural success analysis was performed by local angiographic operators according to the aforementioned set criteria; there was no core lab available for analysis. The decision for PCI or CABG was at the operator's discretion, given the nature of a retrospective analysis.

Left ventricular ejection fraction (LVEF) was quantified using standard two-dimensional transthoracic echocardiography (TTE) or left ventriculography, whichever was available closer to index catheterization. The timing for TTE was variable, as this was a retrospective analysis and could include pre- or postrevascularization studies.

Cardiogenic shock was defined as systolic blood pressure (SBP) ≤ 90 mmHg for >30 minutes or the requirement of vasopressor/inotropic support to maintain SBP > 90 mmHg in addition to evidence of end organ hypoperfusion. Baseline renal insufficiency was defined as creatinine clearance (CrCl) < 60 mL/min. CrCl was calculated using the standard Cockgroft-Gault equation (CrCl = (140 − age) × wt (kg) × F/(plasma creatinine × 0.8136), where F = 1 if male and 0.85 if female). Report of anoxic brain injury (ABI) required chart documentation by the intensivist or neurologist in the ICU and/or CT brain evidence of ABI with a clinical agreement note.

The Glasgow-Pittsburgh Cerebral Performance Category (CPC) score was utilized to assess neurologic recovery [16]. The best CPC score achieved at hospital discharge was recorded by the treating neurologist or allied health personnel. A CPC score of 1 or 2 represented favorable functional neurologic recovery and was therefore defined as good neurologic outcome. A CPC score of 3, 4, or 5 reflected poor neurologic recovery.

2.4. Statistics. Descriptive statistical methods were used to summarize data. A negative binomial logistic regression model was utilized to identify univariate and multivariate predictors of in-hospital mortality. All univariate predictors with a p value < 0.05 were considered significant and were included into a stringent multivariable model to prevent

TABLE 1: Baseline clinical characteristics, prehospital arrest data, and cooling protocol of total population (n = 176).

Clinical characteristics	MTH + C (n = 66)	MTH + NC (n = 110)	p value
Age (yrs)	61 ± 12	61 ± 16	1.00
Sex (M)	52 (79)	77 (70)	0.22
Medical history			
Diabetes (%)	12 (18)	34 (31)	0.06
Smoking (%)	36 (55)	49 (45)	0.22
Hypertension (%)	36 (55)	65 (59)	0.63
Dyslipidemia (%)	27 (41)	39 (35)	0.42
Prior MI (%)	22 (33)	32 (29)	0.32
Prior PCI (%)	5 (8)	7 (6)	0.63
Baseline CRI (%)	17 (26)	12 (11)	0.24
Cardiac arrest			
OHCA (%)	50 (76)	89 (81)	0.44
Witnessed OHCA (%)	61 (92)	83 (75)	0.07
Immediate bystander CPR (%)	36 (55)	40 (45)	0.20
Duration of bystander CPR (min)	6.4 ± 4.1	7.5 ± 4.0	0.08
Time to ROSC from collapse (min)	28.0 ± 14.6	24.0 ± 14.8	0.10
Time from collapse to EMS (min)	8.0 ± 5.0	12.0 ± 12.0	<0.05
Total cooled time (min)	1671 ± 410	1625 ± 551	0.62
Initial arrest rhythm			
VF/pulseless VT	61 (92)	39 (35)	<0.05
PEA	5 (8)	61 (65)	<0.05
STEMI	45 (68)	0 (0)	<0.05
Mild therapeutic hypothermia			
Time from ROSC to cooling (min)	277 ± 110	211 ± 146	<0.05
Time to achieve 32–34°C from cooling (min)	252 ± 174	312 ± 466	0.30
Total cooled time (min)	1671 ± 410	1625 ± 551	0.56

Values are mean ± SD or n (%). MTH + C, mild therapeutic hypothermia with cardiac catheterization; OHCA, out of hospital cardiac arrest; MTH + NC, mild therapeutic hypothermia with no cardiac catheterization; yrs, years; m, males; MI, myocardial infarction; PCI, percutaneous coronary intervention; CRI, chronic renal insufficiency; CPR, cardiopulmonary resuscitation; min, minutes; ROSC, return of spontaneous circulation; EMS, emergency medical services; VF, ventricular fibrillation; VT, ventricular tachycardia; PEA, pulseless electrical activity; STEMI, ST elevation myocardial infarction.

model instability given our small sample size. SAS version 9.1.2 software was utilized to perform all analyses. Prespecified subgroup analyses were performed to identify univariate and multivariate predictors of good neurologic outcome.

3. Results

3.1. Study Population. A total of 176 consecutive patients (mean age 61 ± 13 years, 129 males) with a documented cardiac arrest who were admitted to a single tertiary care ICU and underwent MTH were the initial study population. A total of 66 patients underwent MTH + C at the discretion of the treating cardiologist or intensivist; the remaining 110 patients did not undergo cardiac catheterization (MTH + NC). Baseline demographics of the two study groups are outlined in Table 1. Despite the majority of patients in the MTH + C group having experienced a witnessed cardiac arrest (92%), only half of patients (55%) received immediate bystander CPR. Similarly, in the MTH + NC group, approximately 75% experienced a cardiac arrest, of which 45% received immediate bystander CPR. The mean duration of bystander CPR was similar at 6.4 ± 4.1 minutes and 7.5 ±

4.0 minutes for the MTH + C and MTH + NC groups, respectively. The median interval from the occurrence of cardiac arrest to ROSC was also similar at 28 ± 15 minutes and 24 ± 15 minutes for the MTH + C and MTH + NC groups, respectively. In the majority of patients who underwent MTH + C, ventricular fibrillation (VF)/pulseless ventricular tachycardia (VT) (92%) was the initial resuscitated cardiac rhythm, with 68% demonstrating evidence of STEMI. In patients who underwent MTH + NC, the initial cardiac rhythm was PEA or asystole in 65% of cases. The majority of patients in the entire population (>80%) were in cardiogenic shock requiring vasopressor or inotropic support within the first week of resuscitation following cardiac arrest. Baseline renal insufficiency was present in 26% of patients in the MTH + C group as compared to 11% in patients in the MTH + NC group (p = 0.8).

3.2. Mild Therapeutic Hypothermia (MTH). The parameters for MTH are listed in Table 1. The mean time from ROSC to initiation of MTH was 277 ± 110 minutes (4.6 ± 1.8 hrs) for the catheterization group and 211 ± 146 minutes (3.5 ± 2.4 hrs) for the no catheterization group. An average time of 252 ± 174

TABLE 2: Cardiac catheterization findings in study population who underwent MTH + C ($n = 66$).

Cardiogenic shock	53 (80)
Vasopressors	53 (80)
Inotropes	26 (40)
Duration of support (min)	52 ± 73
IABP use	24 (36)
ECMO use	3 (5)
Early catheterization (<12 hrs)	56 (86)
Time to catheterization from ROSC (min)	290 ± 333
STEMI (min)	212 ± 94
No STEMI (min)	465 ± 140
(1) Vessel CAD	24 (36)
(2) Vessel CAD	16 (24)
(3) Vessel CAD	14 (21)
Branch vessel disease or no culprit	12 (18)
PCI	45 (68)
Multivessel PCI	10 (22)
Stent deployment	43 (96)
Number of stents utilized	1.7 ± 1.1
Stent thrombosis	2 (4)
Successful PCI	40 (89)
Mean TIMI flow pre (min)	1.4 ± 1.4
Mean TIMI flow post (min)	2.9 ± 0.6
CABG	2 (3)
GPIIbIIIa inhibition	23 (51)

Values are mean ± SD or n (%). IABP, intra-aortic balloon pump; ECMO, extracorporeal membrane oxygenation; ROSC, return of spontaneous circulation; STEMI, ST elevation myocardial infarction; CAD, coronary artery disease; PCI, percutaneous coronary intervention; TIMI, thrombolysis in myocardial infarction; CABG, coronary artery bypass grafting.

minutes (4.2 ± 2.9 hrs) and 312 ± 465 minutes (5.2 ± 7.8 hrs) for the MTH + C and MTH + NC groups, respectively, from cooling initiation was required to achieve the target cooling temperature between 32 and 34°C. Total time at target cooling temperature was 1671 ± 410 minutes (27.9 ± 6.8 hrs) for the MTH + C group and 1625 ± 551 minutes (27.1 ± 9.2 hrs) for the MTH + NC group. MTH was initiated prior to cardiac catheterization in only 27% of patients in the MTH + C group.

3.3. Cardiac Interventions. Table 2 lists the cardiac interventions for the MTH + C patient population. Early cardiac catheterization (<12 hrs) was performed in the majority (86%) of patients. Although the overall mean time to catheterization from ROSC was 290 ± 333 minutes, STEMI patients received emergency coronary angiography sooner than patients without ECG changes (212 ± 94 minutes versus 465 ± 140 minutes). PCI was performed in two-thirds of patients and successful PCI was achieved in the majority of these cases (89%).

3.4. Outcomes. In patients who underwent MTH with and without cardiac catheterization, the in-hospital mortality was 48% and 78%, respectively. Among survivors in the MTH + C

TABLE 3: In-hospital outcomes for total population ($n = 176$).

Clinical characteristics	MTH + C ($n = 66$)	MTH + NC ($n = 110$)	p value
In-hospital mortality (%)	32 (48)	86 (78)	<0.05
Discharged home (%)	21 (32)	3 (3)	<0.05
Discharged to long term facility (%)	12 (20)	5 (5)	<0.05
CPC 1-2 neurological recovery (%)	32 (48)	10 (9)	<0.05
CPC 3–5 neurological recovery (%)	34 (52)	100 (91)	<0.05
Length of hospital stay (days)	12 ± 14	8 ± 8	<0.05
Length of ICU stay (days)	7 ± 6	5 ± 5	0.35

Values are mean ± SD or n (%). MTH + C, mild therapeutic hypothermia with cardiac catheterization; MTH + NC, mild therapeutic hypothermia with no cardiac catheterization; CPC, cerebral performance category; ICU, intensive care unit.

TABLE 4: Univariate predictors of in-hospital mortality for study population ($n = 176$).

Clinical characteristics	MTH + C ($n = 66$)	MTH + NC ($n = 110$)
Age	0.04	0.4
Diabetes	0.02	0.4
Dyslipidemia	0.02	0.6
Baseline CRI	0.003	0.6
Cardiogenic shock	0.05	0.04
Absence of cooling prior to cardiac catheterization	0.04	N/A
Use of dobutamine	0.04	0.06

MTH + C, mild therapeutic hypothermia with cardiac catheterization; MTH + NC, mild therapeutic hypothermia with no cardiac catheterization; CRI, chronic renal insufficiency.

group, only 48% of patients (32/66 patients) had good (CPC 1-2) neurologic recovery. On the contrary, among survivors in the MTH + NC group, only 13% of patients (14/110 patients) had good (CPC 1-2) neurologic recovery. Of those who survived in the MTH + C group, 20% patients were transferred to rehabilitation or referring hospital and one-third of the patients were successfully discharged home (Table 3). In the MTH + NC group, only 5% were transferred to a long-term facility, and only 3% were successfully discharged home.

3.5. Predictors of In-Hospital Mortality. Univariate predictors of in-hospital mortality for patients with MTH + C included increasing age, diabetes, dyslipidemia, baseline renal insufficiency postcardiac arrest, cardiogenic shock, use of dobutamine, and failure to initiate MTH prior to catheterization (Table 4). Multivariate analysis of these predictors identified baseline renal insufficiency as the only independent predictor of in-hospital mortality in patients with MTH + C (OR = 8.2, 95% CI 1.8–47.1, $p = 0.009$). In patients with MTH +

TABLE 5: Univariate negative predictors of good neurologic outcome in study population who underwent MTH + C ($n = 66$).

Variables	p value
Diabetes	0.03
Absence of immediate CPR	0.03
Collapse to ROSC time	0.02
Baseline renal insufficiency	0.006
Baseline pH	0.03
No cooling implemented before catheterization	0.02
Seizure	0.007

MTH + C, mild therapeutic hypothermia with cardiac catheterization; CPR, cardiac pulmonary resuscitation; ROSC, return of spontaneous circulation.

NC, shock was the only independent predictor of in-hospital mortality (OR = 3.5, 95% CI 1.0–11.3, $p = 0.04$).

3.6. Predictors of Neurologic Outcome. Diabetes, absence of immediate bystander CPR, increased collapse to ROSC time, baseline renal insufficiency, lower baseline pH, postcardiac arrest seizure, and failure to initiate MTH prior to catheterization were univariate negative predictors of good (CPC 1-2) neurologic outcome in patients with MTH + C (Table 5). Multivariate analysis identified baseline renal insufficiency (OR = 0.15, 95% CI 0.02–0.71, $p = 0.03$) and the absence of immediate bystander CPR (OR = 0.22, 95% CI 0.05–0.9, $p = 0.04$) as independent negative predictors of good neurologic outcome in patients with MTH + C. Univariate analysis for predictors of neurological outcome in patients with MTH + NC was not performed due to the small sample size of $n = 10$ who had good neurological outcome (CPC 1-2) in this study group.

4. Discussion

The current study describes the outcomes and predictors of increased mortality for patients resuscitated from cardiac arrest and treated with the combination of MTH and catheterization versus MTH with no cardiac catheterization. In-hospital mortality for the study population of MTH + C was high at 48%, with 97% of patient mortality attributed to brain death, as is typical for patients with ROSC [1, 3, 4]. Baseline renal insufficiency following resuscitation from cardiac arrest was determined to be the only independent predictor of in-hospital mortality in patients with MTH + C. Furthermore, independent negative predictors of neurologic outcome were determined to be baseline renal insufficiency and absence of immediate bystander CPR for patients with MTH + C.

Neurological outcomes after cardiac arrest are traditionally dismal. The poor prognosis is attributed to postcardiac arrest syndrome, which encompasses systemic ischemic-reperfusion injury with subsequent biochemical, structural, and functional insult [17, 18]. Ultimately, this leads to progressive cell destruction, postcardiac arrest brain injury, circulatory dysfunction, multiorgan failure, and death [17, 18]. The beneficial effects of MTH are based on the prevention of this

cascade, specifically, by reducing cellular metabolic needs and inhibiting temperature-sensitive pathways of the ischemia-reperfusion cascade to slow ongoing hypoxic neurological insult [13, 17, 18]. As such, a number of studies have demonstrated improved neurological outcomes with the use of MTH in the postcardiac arrest period. In a multicentre blinded randomized control trial involving patients resuscitated after cardiac arrest due to VT, 55% patients randomized to receive MTH had a favorable neurologic outcome, compared to 39% in the control group [5]. A recent study by Neilsen et al. also demonstrated that targeted temperature management at 36°C after OHCA conferred a similar benefit to MTH from a neurological function standpoint [6]. Our study corroborates that individuals who survive aggressive postresuscitative care are neurologically intact, with 48% of survivors having favorable neurological function at hospital discharge. The preservation of neurological function is an important treatment goal, as survival is correlated with neurologic status [13].

In addition to MTH, the role of early invasive strategies for postcardiac arrest patients has gained recent attention. In previous studies, 40–57% of OHCA patients without ST-segment elevation had pathological findings with therapeutic options on coronary angiography [11, 19]. A recent retrospective study involving a cohort of 435 patients with OHCA of presumed cardiac origin reported the poor predictive value of ST-segment elevation for coronary occlusion in the setting of cardiac arrest [11]. Furthermore, successful immediate coronary angioplasty was associated with a survival benefit regardless of ECG findings, suggesting that immediate catheterization may be warranted in the setting of resuscitated cardiac arrests even in the absence of ST-segment elevation [11]. This has led to an increased adoption of emergency coronary angiography for all patients with OHCA of suspected cardiac origin [20, 21]. In the current study of patients who underwent MTH + C, 32% did not have ST-segment elevation, 32% did not undergo PCI, and 18% had angiographically normal coronary arteries or nonocclusive coronary artery disease. Only patients with ST-segment elevation underwent emergent PCI after invasive angiography, raising question to the use of universal emergent angiography postcardiac arrest. This is an important consideration as there are inherent risks associated with coronary angiography and the ultimate goal is to reduce the number of patients undergoing an unnecessary procedure.

A contemporary approach to coordinated postresuscitative care by combining MTH with coronary angiography is associated with more favorable patient outcomes [13, 22, 23]. Sunde et al. reported 56% survival with favorable neurologic outcomes for patients randomized to a standardized postresuscitation protocol involving MTH and PCI, as compared to 26% in the control treatment arm [22]. Similarly, Stub et al. demonstrated that the combination of therapeutic hypothermia with early coronary intervention was associated with an improved survival of 64%, as compared to 39% in the control group [13]. The results of the current study are comparable to those previously stated. However, in our study over 80% of patients experienced cardiogenic shock within the first week after cardiac arrest and 36% required intra-aortic balloon pump counterpulsation, which is significantly higher than that reported in the previous literature [13]. Unlike previous studies, we did not exclude cardiogenic shock patients from the MTH protocol [5, 6, 9]. Although circulatory shock is still considered a relative contraindication for MTH, several recent studies including ours suggest that these patients may still derive benefit from MTH [24, 25].

Previous literature has identified key clinical characteristics to predict survival from OHCA: initial location of OHCA, witnessed cardiac arrest, prompt bystander CPR, ECG with shockable cardiac rhythm, early defibrillation, time to resuscitation, complete revascularization, hyperlactatemia, and presence of ABI [4, 6, 26–30]. In addition, renal insufficiency is a known predictor of mortality in the cardiogenic shock population [30]. Kidney function as assessed by CrCl appears to be a sensitive marker of poor tissue perfusion during cardiac arrest and perhaps an indirect marker of poor cerebral perfusion. Our findings confirmed the importance of renal function as an independent predictor of both in-hospital mortality and neurological outcome in the OHCA patient population who underwent MTH + C.

In addition to renal perfusion, bystander CPR improved 1-year survival with favorable neurological outcomes for OHCA patients in a study by Iwami et al. [29]. A similar study by Herlitz et al. further supported the survival benefit of bystander CPR afforded to this patient population [28]. Prompt provision of CPR may delay the degradation of tachyarrhythmias to asystole, explaining the positive impact on survival. Despite the majority of patients having experienced witnessed cardiac arrest, only half of patients had immediate bystander CPR in our population. The absence of immediate CPR was a potent independent negative predictor of good neurologic recovery, in keeping with previous studies. This stresses the critical importance of public awareness and education in early bystander CPR to improve the neurologic outcome for OHCA patients. The study population also experienced a longer median arrest time (low flow) (28 ± 15 min) as compared with other studies [5, 6]. A longer interval from collapse to ROSC has been associated with unfavorable neurologic outcomes, which is corroborated by our findings [6].

Although the correct population was cooled in the current study, the time to reach target temperature (32–34°C) from initiation of MTH was relatively prolonged at 8 hrs. The prolonged time to reach target temperature may be attributable to delayed initiation of the MTH protocol as a consequence of early coronary angiography, as less than 25% of our study population was cooled prior to catheterization. Of note, there was a trend towards less favorable outcomes in patients who had no cooling prior to coronary angiography, and it was a univariate predictor of in-hospital mortality and neurological outcome. This suggests the need for a well-planned and coordinated cooling protocol which is implemented prior to and during catheterization, such that early catheterization does not delay the initiation of MTH. Second, a transport based MTH protocol is required, in order to enable the implementation of MTH en route to central catheterization facilities. Finally, increased education for earlier MTH implementation in peripheral facilities (ER, ICU) will hopefully improve patient outcomes.

There are several limitations to the current study. This is a single-centre retrospective review and thus subject to potential confounders and selection bias. Data collection was limited by available documentation and not all measurements were made at exactly the same time intervals or course in hospital. We used the CPC score to assess neurologic recovery because of its ease of use and widespread reporting in the literature. However, this scoring system is not well validated and was retrospectively assigned based on clinical documentation at the time of discharge. Finally, our study does not include long-term outcome data and was limited to hospital discharge.

5. Conclusion

Although the outcome for patients resuscitated from cardiac arrest is traditionally low, it may be improved by the use of coordinated resuscitation protocols involving MTH and cardiac catheterization. Baseline renal insufficiency appears to be a potent predictor of in-hospital mortality and poor neurologic outcome in this population. The absence of immediate CPR also predicts poor neurologic recovery and this should be an impetus for widespread public education. Further multicentre registry collaboration may be indicated to study and refine outcomes in this severely ill patient population.

References

[1] Statistics Canada, *Mortality, Summary List of Causes 2008*, Statistics Canada, 2008.

[2] American Heart Association, "American Heart Association guidelines for cardiopulmonary resuscitation and emergency cardiovascular care," *Circulation*, vol. 112, pp. IV-1–IV-5, 2005.

[3] C. Sasson, M. A. M. Rogers, J. Dahl, and A. L. Kellermann, "Predictors of survival from out-of-hospital cardiac arrest a systematic review and meta-analysis," *Circulation: Cardiovascular Quality and Outcomes*, vol. 3, no. 1, pp. 63–81, 2010.

[4] J. Herlitz, A. Bång, J. Gunnarsson et al., "Factors associated with survival to hospital discharge among patients hospitalised alive after out of hospital cardiac arrest: change in outcome over 20 years in the community of Göteborg, Sweden," *Heart*, vol. 89, no. 1, pp. 25–30, 2003.

[5] Hypothermia after Cardiac Arrest Study Group, "Mild therapeutic hypothermia to improve the neurologic outcome after cardiac arrest," *The New England Journal of Medicine*, vol. 346, no. 8, pp. 549–556, 2002.

[6] N. Neilsen, J. Wetterslev, T. Cronberg et al., "Targeted temperature management at 33°C versus 36°C after cardiac arrest," *The New England Journal of Medicine*, vol. 369, no. 23, pp. 2197–2206, 2013.

[7] J. Hovdenes, J. H. Laake, L. Aaberge, H. Haugaa, and J. F. Bugge, "Therapeutic hypothermia after out-of-hospital cardiac arrest: experiences with patients treated with percutaneous coronary

intervention and cardiogenic shock," *Acta Anaesthesiologica Scandinavica*, vol. 51, no. 2, pp. 137–142, 2007.

[8] R. Knafelj, P. Radsel, T. Ploj, and M. Noc, "Primary percutaneous coronary intervention and mild induced hypothermia in comatose survivors of ventricular fibrillation with ST-elevation acute myocardial infarction," *Resuscitation*, vol. 74, no. 2, pp. 227–234, 2007.

[9] S. Wolfrum, C. Pierau, P. W. Radke, H. Schunkert, and V. Kurowski, "Mild therapeutic hypothermia in patients after out-of-hospital cardiac arrest due to acute ST-segment elevation myocardial infarction undergoing immediate percutaneous coronary intervention," *Critical Care Medicine*, vol. 36, no. 6, pp. 1780–1786, 2008.

[10] H. O. Peels, G. A. J. Jessurun, I. C. C. van der Horst, A. E. R. Arnold, L. H. Piers, and F. Zijlstra, "Outcome in transferred and nontransferred patients after primary percutaneous coronary intervention for ischaemic out-of-hospital cardiac arrest," *Catheterization and Cardiovascular Interventions*, vol. 71, no. 2, pp. 147–151, 2008.

[11] F. Dumas, A. Cariou, S. Manzo-Silberman et al., "Immediate percutaneous coronary intervention is associated with better survival after out-of-hospital cardiac arrest: insights from the PROCAT (Parisian Region Out of Hospital Cardiac Arrest) registry," *Circulation: Cardiovascular Interventions*, vol. 3, no. 3, pp. 200–207, 2010.

[12] P. Cronier, P. Vignon, K. Bouferrache et al., "Impact of routine percutaneous coronary intervention after out-of-hospital cardiac arrest due to ventricular fibrillation," *Critical Care*, vol. 15, article R122, 2011.

[13] D. Stub, C. Hengel, W. Chan et al., "Usefulness of cooling and coronary catheterization to improve survival in out-of-hospital cardiac arrest," *American Journal of Cardiology*, vol. 107, no. 4, pp. 522–527, 2011.

[14] V. B. Nanjayya and V. Nayyar, "Immediate coronary angiogram in comatose survivors of out-of-hospital cardiac arrest—an Australian study," *Resuscitation*, vol. 83, no. 6, pp. 699–704, 2012.

[15] P. T. O'Gara, F. G. Kushner, D. D. Ascheim et al., "2013 ACCF/AHA guideline for the management of st-elevation myocardial infarction: a report of the American College of Cardiology Foundation/American Heart Association Task Force on Practice Guidelines," *Journal of the American College of Cardiology*, vol. 61, no. 4, pp. e78–e140, 2013.

[16] I. Jacobs, V. Nadkarni, J. Bahr et al., "Cardiac arrest and cardiopulmonary resuscitation outcome reports: update and simplification of the Utstein templates for resuscitation registries. A statement for healthcare professionals from a task force of the international liaison committee on resuscitation (American Heart Association, European Resuscitation Council, Australian Resuscitation Council, New Zealand Resuscitation Council, Heart and Stroke Foundation of Canada, InterAmerican Heart Foundation, Resuscitation Council of Southern Africa)," *Resuscitation* , vol. 63, no. 3, pp. 233–249, 2004.

[17] W. L. Wright and R. G. Geocadin, "Postresuscitative intensive care: neuroprotective strategies after cardiac arrest," *Seminars in Neurology*, vol. 26, no. 4, pp. 396–402, 2006.

[18] V. A. Negovsky, "Postresuscitation disease," *Critical Care Medicine*, vol. 16, no. 10, pp. 942–946, 1988.

[19] C. M. Spaulding, L.-M. Joly, A. Rosenberg et al., "Immediate coronary angiography in survivors of out-of-hospital cardiac arrest," *The New England Journal of Medicine*, vol. 336, no. 23, pp. 1629–1633, 1997.

[20] L. M. Batista, F. O. Lima, J. L. Januzzi Jr., V. Donahue, C. Snydeman, and D. M. Greer, "Feasibility and safety of combined percutaneous coronary intervention and therapeutic hypothermia following cardiac arrest," *Resuscitation*, vol. 81, no. 4, pp. 398–403, 2010.

[21] J. C. Reynolds, C. W. Callaway, S. R. El Khoudary, C. G. Moore, R. J. Alvarez, and J. C. Rittenberger, "Coronary angiography predicts improved outcome following cardiac arrest: propensity-adjusted analysis," *Journal of Intensive Care Medicine*, vol. 24, no. 3, pp. 179–186, 2009.

[22] K. Sunde, M. Pytte, D. Jacobsen et al., "Implementation of a standardised treatment protocol for post resuscitation care after out-of-hospital cardiac arrest," *Resuscitation*, vol. 73, no. 1, pp. 29–39, 2007.

[23] M. Werling, A.-B. Thorén, C. Axelsson, and J. Herlitz, "Treatment and outcome in post-resuscitation care after out-of-hospital cardiac arrest when a modern therapeutic approach was introduced," *Resuscitation*, vol. 73, no. 1, pp. 40–45, 2007.

[24] A. O. Spiel, A. Kliegel, A. Janata et al., "Hemostasis in cardiac arrest patients treated with mild hypothermia initiated by cold fluids," *Resuscitation*, vol. 80, no. 7, pp. 762–765, 2009.

[25] R. Gal, M. Slezak, I. Zimova, I. Cundrle, H. Ondraskova, and D. Seidlova, "Therapeutic hypothermia after out-of-hospital cardiac arrest with the target temperature 34-35 degrees C," *Bratislavské Lekárske Listy*, vol. 110, no. 4, pp. 222–225, 2009.

[26] I. Lund-Kordahl, T. M. Olasveengen, T. Lorem, M. Samdal, L. Wik, and K. Sunde, "Improving outcome after out-of-hospital cardiac arrest by strengthening weak links of the local Chain of Survival: quality of advanced life support and post-resuscitation care," *Resuscitation*, vol. 81, no. 4, pp. 422–426, 2010.

[27] H. Hayashi and Y. Ujike, "Out-of-hospital cardiac arrest in Okayama City (Japan): outcome report according to the 'Utstein style'," *Acta Medica Okayama*, vol. 59, no. 2, pp. 49–54, 2005.

[28] J. Herlitz, L. Svensson, S. Holmberg, K.-A. Ängquist, and M. Young, "Efficacy of bystander CPR: intervention by lay people and by health care professionals," *Resuscitation*, vol. 66, no. 3, pp. 291–295, 2005.

[29] T. Iwami, T. Kawamura, A. Hiraide et al., "Effectiveness of bystander-initiated cardiac-only resuscitation for patients with out-of-hospital cardiac arrest," *Circulation*, vol. 116, no. 25, pp. 2900–2907, 2007.

[30] F. Hussain, R. K. Philipp, R. A. Ducas et al., "The ability to achieve complete revascularization is associated with improved in-hospital survival in cardiogenic shock due to myocardial infarction: manitoba cardiogenic SHOCK Registry investigators," *Catheterization and Cardiovascular Interventions*, vol. 78, no. 4, pp. 540–548, 2011.

24

Avoiding the Learning Curve for Transcatheter Aortic Valve Replacement

Sergey Gurevich,[1] Ranjit John,[1] Rosemary F. Kelly,[1] Ganesh Raveendran,[1] Gregory Helmer,[1] Demetris Yannopoulos,[1] Timinder Biring,[1] Brett Oestreich,[1] and Santiago Garcia[1,2]

[1]University of Minnesota-Fairview Medical Center, Minneapolis, MN, USA
[2]Minneapolis VA Healthcare System, Minneapolis, MN, USA

Correspondence should be addressed to Santiago Garcia; santiagogarcia@me.com

Academic Editor: Robert Chen

Objectives. To evaluate whether collaboration between existing and new transcatheter aortic valve replacement (TAVR) programs could help reduce the number of cases needed to achieve optimal efficiency. *Background.* There is a well-documented learning curve for achieving procedural efficiency and safety in TAVR procedures. *Methods.* A multidisciplinary collaboration was established between the Minneapolis VA Medical Center (new program) and the University of Minnesota (established program since 2012, $n = 219$) 1 year prior to launching the new program. *Results.* 269 patients treated with TAVR (50 treated in the first year at the new program). Mean age was 76 ($\pm$18) years and STS score was 6.8 ($\pm$6). Access included transfemoral ($n = 35, 70\%$), transapical ($n = 8$, 16%), transaortic ($n = 2, 4\%$), and subclavian ($n = 5, 10\%$) types. Procedural efficiency (procedural time 158 ± 59 versus 148 ± 62, $p = 0.27$), device success (96% versus 87%, $p = 0.08$), length of stay (5 ± 3 versus 6 ± 7 days, $p = 0.10$), and safety (in hospital mortality 4% versus 6%, $p = 0.75$) were similar between programs. We found no difference in outcome measures between the first and last 25 patients treated during the first year of the new program. *Conclusions.* Establishing a partnership with an established program can help mitigate the learning curve associated with these complex procedures.

1. Introduction

The introduction of a novel technology is usually accompanied by a period of learning in which operators develop and refine new skills until they achieve a "steady state" characterized by high efficiency and procedural success with low complications [1, 2]. In the Placement of Aortic Transcatheter Valve (PARTNER) trial, 26 cases were required to achieve a sustained level of procedural performance and safety profile with transfemoral (TF) transcatheter aortic valve replacement (TAVR) [3].

The number of new TAVR procedures in the US has doubled in fiscal year (FY) 2013 from the previous year, with 10,599 total Medicare claims in FY 2013 as compared to 5,400 claims in FY 2012 [4]. The number of TAVR programs is also rapidly proliferating, from 228 in FY 2012 to 336 in FY 2013. The results of PARTNER 2A and SAPIEN 3 registry

in intermediate-risk patients suggest that these trends will accelerate in the near future as TAVR indications expand to lower risk patients [5, 6].

In this context, it is important to develop strategies and partnerships that allow initiation of new TAVR programs that can produce efficacy and safety results that are comparable to existing national benchmarks in a reasonable period of time. In this manuscript, we describe our experience during the launch of a new TAVR program at the Minneapolis VA Medical Center. This program was launched after 1 year of close collaboration, proctorship, and hands-on experience with the University of Minnesota Medical Center.

2. Methods

The Minneapolis VA Healthcare System (MVAHCS) is a tertiary, 250-bed hospital within the VA Midwest Heath Care

Network (Veterans Integrated Service Network VISN 23). The network serves more than 440,000 enrolled Veterans residing in the states of Iowa, Minnesota, Nebraska, North Dakota, and South Dakota and portions of Illinois, Kansas, Missouri, and Wyoming. The MVAHCS is the only approved TAVR program in an eight-state area and has an academic affiliation with the University of Minnesota. The University of Minnesota Medical Center (UMMC) has an existing TAVR program since 2012 and had performed 140 TAVR procedures prior to mentoring the MVAHCS program.

2.1. Mentorship Plan. Prior to launching the TAVR program, an institutional collaboration agreement was established between MVAHCS (new program) and UMMC (established program) with the goal of launching the new program with high success and low complications rates that were comparable to national benchmarks.

Specific interventions included the following: (1) common weekly TAVR video conference to discuss patients by a multidisciplinary team of interventional cardiologist, cardiac surgeons, anesthesiologists, and cardiac imaging, (2) privileging and hands-on training of lead interventional cardiologist and cardiac surgeon (total of 20 cases each, 7 as second operator and 13 as primary), (3) observation of UMMC cases by MVAHCS heart team members including anesthesiologists, perfusionists, and operating room and cardiac catheterization laboratory personnel, and (4) sharing of order sets and imaging protocols (i.e., CTA for annular sizing).

2.2. Patients and Outcomes. We included 219 patients treated with TAVR at UMMC since 2012 and 50 patients treated at MVAHCS during the first year of the program (April 2015–April 2016). We excluded patients that underwent transcatheter valve replacement in a nonaortic position (i.e., mitral valve in valve procedures or pulmonary). Patients that underwent TAVR procedures for off-label indications (bicuspid valve and aortic insufficiency) and/or valve in vale (VIV) procedures were included in the analysis.

Outcomes measures included procedural efficiency, as assessed by procedural time and contrast volume. Contrast volume included contrast used for peripheral angiography at the end of the procedure, which is routinely used in both programs. Procedural time was the time from arterial puncture or surgical incision until the end of the procedure. Measures of procedural success (device success) and safety (stroke, vascular complications, pacemaker requirement, and in-hospital mortality) were assessed in both groups using Valve Academic Research Consortium (VARC) definitions [7].

2.3. Statistical Methods. Comparisons between groups were made using Student's t-test (expressed as mean value standard deviation) for continuous variables. Indices were tested for normality of distribution, with nonnormally distributed data compared using 2-sample t-tests after initial logarithmic transformation. Categorical variables were compared using chi-square or, when there are fewer than 5 expected outcomes per cell, Fisher's exact test. Two-sided $p < 0.05$ was considered indicative of statistical significance. Statistical calculations were performed using STATA Statistics Version 12 (StataCorp LP, College Station, Texas).

3. Results

The study population consisted of a total of 269 patients undergoing transcatheter aortic valve replacement at UMMC and MVAHCS between 2012 and 2015. The mean age of the patients ($n = 50$) treated in the new program during the first year was 79 (± 8) and the mean Society of Thoracic Surgeons (STS) risk score was 6.8. Transfemoral (TF) access was used in 70% and alternative access in the remaining 30%. Alternative access included transapical ($n = 8$), transaortic ($n = 2$), and subclavian ($n = 5$) types. Of the TF cases at the established program, 90 were percutaneous and 43 used a cut-down approach. Most cutdowns were used during 2012-2013, with first-generation valves. At the new program, all TF cases were percutaneous. At the established program, general anesthesia was used in all cases but 7 which were done with moderate sedation, and 1 was epidural. All of the cases at the new program were done with general anesthesia. A 12% increase, from 64% to 76%, in TF access was seen in the second half of the year ($p = 0.36$). A balloon-expandable valve (SAPIEN XT or SAPIEN 3, Edwards Life Sciences, Irvine, CA) was used in 80% of cases and a self-expandable valve (Corevalve or Evolut R, Medtronic, Minneapolis, MN) in the remaining 20%. The average valve size was 27.7 (± 2) mm. The mean age of the patients ($n = 219$) treated in the established program was 81.5 (± 9) and the mean STS score was 8. Patients in the established program had a higher prevalence of hypertension, heart failure, and previous myocardial infarction (Table 1). A total of 14 VIV procedures were performed in the established program and 8 in the new program. Other baseline characteristics were similar as outlined in Table 1. Individual operator experience is provided in the Supplementary Appendix in Supplementary Material available online at https://doi.org/10.1155/2017/7524925.

3.1. Procedural Efficiency. Overall procedure time was 158 ± 59 minutes for the new program and 148 ± 62 minutes for the established program ($p = 0.27$) (Table 2). Average procedure time was 20 minutes lower for the last 25 patients treated in the new program relative to the first 25 cases, but these differences were not statistically significant ($p = 0.26$) (Figure 1). Contrast volume was 201 (± 114) mL in the new program and 192 (± 111) mL in the established program ($p = 0.61$) (Table 2). Contrast utilization remained unchanged during the first and second half of the first year of the new program (201 ± 136 mL versus 201 ± 88 mL, $p = 0.5$).

3.2. Procedural Outcomes. Device success was high, 96% for the new program and 87% for the established program ($p = 0.08$) (Table 2). In the established program, 19 device failures occurred including 14 that required a second valve, 2 aborted due to access complication, 2 converted to valvuloplasty, and 1 valve embolization into the left ventricle. In the new program, there were 2 device failures, and both required a second valve (Table 2). Serious procedural complications

TABLE 1: Baseline characteristics.

Parameter	Established program overall ($n = 219$)	New program overall ($n = 50$)	p	New program First half ($n = 25$)	New program Second half ($n = 25$)	p
Clinical characteristics						
Age (years)	81.4 ± 9.1	78.9 ± 8.7	0.08	79 (±8)	78 (±9)	0.47
Male gender	53% (115)	100% (50)	<0.01	100%	100%	NA
STS Score	8.0 ± 4.7	6.8 ± 6.0	0.15	6.2 ± 5	7.4 ± 7	0.25
Height (cm)	167 ± 11	172 ± 7.4	<0.01	171 ± 7.5	173 ± 7.4	0.57
Weight (kg)	81 ± 24	92 ± 25	<0.01	93 ± 31.5	91 ± 17	0.84
Ejection fraction	52.9 ± 12.1	50.3 ± 11.2	0.15	51.7 ± 11.2	48.8 ± 11.2	0.37
Heart failure	33% (73)	12% (6)	<0.01	0% (0)	24% (6)	0.02
Myocardial infarction	28% (61)	15% (7)	<0.01	8% (2)	21% (5)	0.42
PCI	36% (79)	35% (17)	0.86	20% (5)	50% (12)	0.04
Atrial fibrillation	44% (97)	42% (21)	0.77	40% (10)	44% (11)	0.78
Stroke	15% (32)	16% (8)	0.76	4% (1)	29% (7)	0.02
Porcelain aorta	6% (14)	4% (2)	0.74	8% (2)	0% (0)	0.49
Pacemaker	13% (29)	10% (5)	0.64	8% (2)	12% (3)	1.00
Smoker	7% (16)	6% (3)	1.00	4% (1)	8% (2)	1.00
Hypertension	89% (195)	52% (26)	<0.01	52% (13)	52% (13)	1.00
Dialysis	5% (10)	12% (6)	0.05	8% (2)	16% (4)	0.67
PAD	33% (72)	24% (12)	0.25	24% (6)	24% (6)	0.94
Diabetes mellitus	33% (73)	32% (16)	0.31	36% (9)	28% (7)	0.83
Home oxygen	13% (28)	22% (11)	0.10	24% (6)	20% (5)	1.00
Anticoagulant	19% (33)	10% (5)	0.15	8% (2)	12% (3)	1.00
Aortic valve measurements						
Area	0.82 ± 0.52	0.76 ± 0.23	0.43	0.72 ± 0.22	0.80 ± 0.23	0.27
Peak velocity	4.2 ± 0.69	3.9 ± 0.68	0.01	4.1 ± 0.7	3.7 ± 0.6	0.03
Mean gradient	43.9 ± 14	38.2 ± 14.2	0.01	42.2 ± 16.5	34.4 ± 10.6	0.05
Procedural characteristics						
Transfemoral access	61% (138)	70% (35)	0.25	64%	76%	0.36
Alternative access	39% (87)	30% (15)	0.25	36%	24%	0.36
Balloon-expandable	79% (171)	80% (40)	0.61	84%	76%	0.73
Self-expandable	21% (52)	20% (10)	0.61	16%	24%	0.73
Valve size (mm)	26 ± 2.5	27.7 ± 2.2	<0.01	27.5 (±2)	27.9 (±2)	0.40

TABLE 2: Procedural efficiency, device success, and safety.

Parameter	Established program overall ($n = 219$)	New program overall ($n = 50$)	p	First half ($n = 25$)	Second half ($n = 25$)	p
Procedural efficiency						
Contrast (cc)	192.4 ± 111.2	201.3 ± 114.7	0.61	201 (±136)	201 (±88)	0.5
Procedure time (min)	148 ± 62.7	158.9 ± 59.1	0.27	169 ± 62.7	149.6 ± 55.2	0.26
Procedural success and safety						
Device success	87.2%	96%	0.08	96%	96%	0.5
Stroke	4.0% (9)	0% (0)	0.37	0%	0%	—
Vascular complications	6.3% (14)	2% (1)	0.32	0%	1 (4%)	0.29
Paravalvular leak(>mild)	0.4% (1)	2% (1)	0.34	4%	0%	1.00
Pacemaker placement	9.7% (21)	18% (9)	0.10	7 (26%)	2 (8%)	0.08
Length of stay (days)	6.9 ± 7.5	5.42 ± 3.5	0.17	6 (3)	5.3 (3)	0.7
In-hospital mortality	6.7% (15)	4% (2)	0.75	1 (4%)	1 (4%)	0.50

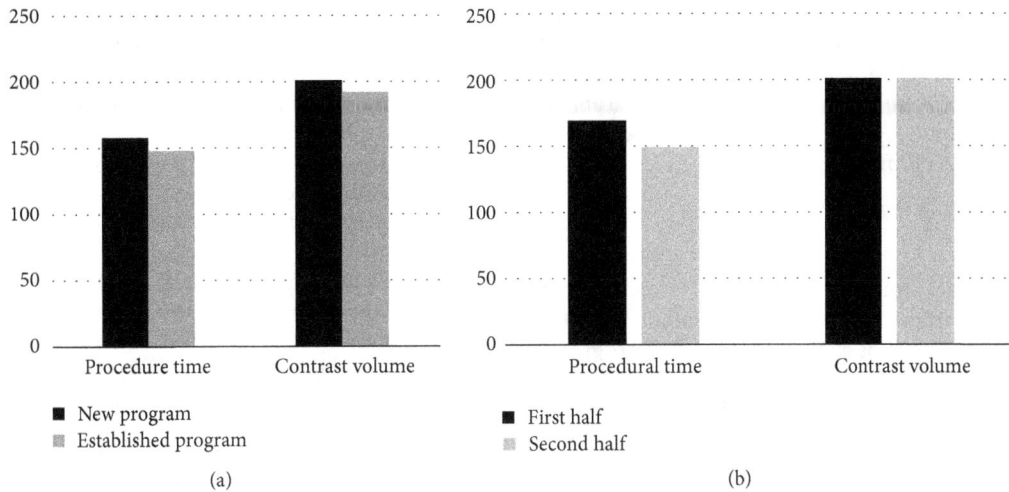

FIGURE 1: Procedural efficiency of new TAVR program relative to established program (a) and comparison of results of first versus second half of the first year of the new TAVR program.

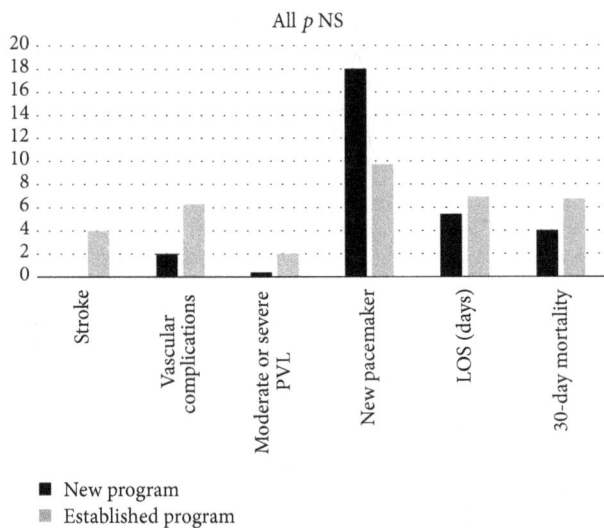

FIGURE 2: Procedural complications, length of stay, and in-hospital mortality.

were infrequent during the first year of the new program: vascular complications 2%, paravalvular leak moderate/severe 2%, and no strokes (Table 2). A permanent pacemaker was required in 18% of patients treated during the first year of the new TAVR program (Table 2). A trend toward reduction in pacemaker requirement was seen in the second half of the year (8%) relative to the first half (26%). In-hospital mortality was 4% and length of stay was 5 ($\pm$3 days) (Table 2). A comparison of procedural outcomes with the established program is presented in Figure 2 (all p = NS).

4. Discussion

There are several significant findings from this study. First, a new TAVR program launched in close collaboration with an existing TAVR program was associated with low complication rates and high device success from its inception. Second, procedural efficiency and length of stay were similar between the existing and the new TAVR programs. Third, mortality at 30 days was low at 4%, which is similar to the most recent STS/ACC TVT registry report [8]. Fourth, a learning curve previously described for TAVR procedures in the PARTNER trial was not observed in our series despite high-procedural complexity (nontransfemoral valve delivery in 30% of cases).

TAVR procedures are highly complex and require a multidisciplinary heart team approach between medical and surgical disciplines to achieve optimal outcomes [9]. A learning curve has been well-documented in the PARTNER trial as well as in single center experience [3, 10, 11]. Alli et al. reported their experience with the first 44 patients treated at the Mayo Clinic using a TF approach [10]. With increased experience, they showed significant reductions in contrast volume and time from valvuloplasty to valve deployment with evidence of plateau after 30 cases. Similarly, in the PARTNER I trial, Minha et al. showed that it took an average of 28 cases to achieve a consistently low risk of 30-day major adverse events for institutions entering the trial early. Interestingly, centers that came into PARTNER late into the trial were able to shorten the learning curve to 26 cases, which suggest they benefited from the experience gained and shared by existing programs [11]. It should be noted that both the Mayo Clinic and PARTNER I trial description of learning curve with TAVR procedures is restricted to TF access. Our series include 30% of patients treated with alternative access, mostly TA but also subclavian and transaortic. The learning curve for TA access is steeper with 30–45 cases required to achieve optimal procedural efficiency [12].

In the United States, the number of TAVR programs enrolled in TVT registry has more than doubled from 156 in 2012 to 348 in 2014 [8]. Given that the majority of surgical aortic valve replacement (SAVR) procedures are performed in lower risk patients [13], it is expected that this trend of growth in the number of TAVR programs will continue or even accelerate in the near future. Our experience of close collaboration with an existing TAVR program demonstrates that the learning curve associated with these procedures can be mitigated by training, proctorship, and sharing of best practices. This model of collaboration could be used as template for other TAVR programs.

5. Limitations

Our study has several limitations. First, we recognize that most VA Medical Centers have an academic affiliation with Universities and this may not be the case for other programs in the private sector. Competition for market share, limited time for physician training, and obtaining hospital privileges in multiple institutions could be important barriers to collaboration. Second, we are not able to identify which aspect of the training was more important. Third, reductions in the size of the delivery system and enhanced valve performance have significantly simplified the procedure as reflected by increased adoption of conscious sedation [14]. Future valve enhancements may reduce the need for intense training and proctorship. Finally, comparator cohort includes historical learning curve with utilization of first-generation valves and low device success rate.

6. Conclusions

We found that establishing a partnership with an existing TAVR program mitigated the learning curve associated with these complex procedures. The new program had similar outcomes to established programs in the US since its inception.

This collaborative model could be used by other institutions planning to become TAVR centers.

Disclosure

All authors listed meet the authorship criteria according to the latest guidelines of the International Committee of Medical Journal Editors and are in agreement with the manuscript.

Competing Interests

The authors declare that they have no competing interests.

References

[1] M. Murzi, A. G. Cerillo, S. Bevilacqua, D. Gilmanov, P. Farneti, and M. Glauber, "Traversing the learning curve in minimally invasive heart valve surgery: a cumulative analysis of an individual surgeon's experience with a right minithoracotomy approach for aortic valve replacement," *European Journal of Cardio-thoracic Surgery*, vol. 41, no. 6, pp. 1242–1246, 2012.

[2] R. Ahmadi, A. Willfort, W. Lang et al., "Carotid artery stenting: effect of learning curve and intermediate-term morphological outcome," *Journal of Endovascular Therapy*, vol. 8, no. 6, pp. 539–546, 2001.

[3] O. Alli, C. S. Rihal, R. M. Suri et al., "Learning curves for transfemoral transcatheter aortic valve replacement in the PARTNER-I trial: technical performance," *Catheterization and Cardiovascular Interventions*, vol. 87, no. 1, pp. 154–162, 2016.

[4] https://www.advisory.com/research/cardiovascular-roundtable cardiovascular-rounds/2014/07/what-can-you-learn-from-fy-2013-tavr-data.

[5] M. B. Leon, C. R. Smith, M. J. Mack et al., "Transcatheter or surgical Aortic-valve replacement in intermediate-risk patients," *The New England Journal of Medicine*, vol. 374, pp. 1609–1620, 2016.

[6] V. H. Thourani, S. Kodali, R. R. Makkar et al., "Transcatheter aortic valve replacement versus surgical valve replacement in intermediate-risk patients: a propensity score analysis," *The Lancet*, vol. 387, no. 10034, pp. 2218–2225, 2016.

[7] M. B. Leon, N. Piazza, E. Nikolsky et al., "Standardized endpoint definitions for transcatheter aortic valve implantation clinical trials: a consensus report from the valve academic research consortium," *Journal of the American College of Cardiology*, vol. 57, no. 3, pp. 253–269, 2011.

[8] D. R. Holmes, R. A. Nishimura, F. L. Grover et al., "Annual outcomes with transcatheter valve therapy: from the STS/ACC TVT registry," *The Annals of thoracic surgery*, vol. 101, no. 2, pp. 789–800, 2016.

[9] C. L. Tommaso, R. M. Bolman III, T. Feldman et al., "Multi-society (AATS, ACCF, SCAI, and STS) expert consensus statement: operator and institutional requirements for transcatheter valve repair and replacement, part 1: transcatheter aortic valve replacement," *Catheterization and Cardiovascular Interventions*, vol. 80, no. 1, pp. 1–17, 2012.

[10] O. O. Alli, J. D. Booker, R. J. Lennon, K. L. Greason, C. S. Rihal, and D. R. Holmes Jr., "Transcatheter aortic valve implantation: assessing the learning curve," *JACC: Cardiovascular Interventions*, vol. 5, no. 1, pp. 72–79, 2012.

[11] S. Minha, R. Waksman, L. P. Satler et al., "Learning curves for transfemoral transcatheter aortic valve replacement in the PARTNER-I trial: success and safety," *Catheterization and Cardiovascular Interventions*, vol. 87, no. 1, pp. 165–175, 2016.

[12] R. M. Suri, S. Minha, O. Alli et al., "Learning curves for transapical transcatheter aortic valve replacement in the PARTNER-I trial: technical performance, success, and safety," *Journal of Thoracic and Cardiovascular Surgery*, vol. 152, no. 3, pp. 773.e14–780.e14, 2016.

[13] V. H. Thourani, R. M. Suri, R. L. Gunter et al., "Contemporary real-world outcomes of surgical aortic valve replacement in 141,905 low-risk, intermediate-risk, and high-risk patients," *Annals of Thoracic Surgery*, vol. 99, no. 1, pp. 55–61, 2015.

[14] D. Dvir, R. Jhaveri, and A. D. Pichard, "The minimalist approach for transcatheter aortic valve replacement in high-risk patients," *JACC: Cardiovascular Interventions*, vol. 5, no. 5, pp. 468–469, 2012.

25

The Concordance between Myocardial Perfusion Imaging and Coronary Angiography in Detecting Coronary Artery Disease: A Retrospective Study in a Tertiary Cardiac Center at King Abdullah Medical City

Fatma Aboul-Enein,[1] **Majed O. Aljuaid,**[2] **Hail T. Alharthi,**[2] **Abdulkarim M. Almudhhi,**[2] **and Mohammad A. Alzahrani**[2]

[1]*Department of Adult Cardiology, KAMC, Makkah 21955, Saudi Arabia*
[2]*Medical College, Taif University, Taif 21974, Saudi Arabia*

Correspondence should be addressed to Majed O. Aljuaid; dr.x-m@outlook.sa

Academic Editor: Robert Chen

Background. Coronary artery disease (CAD) is considered as the leading cause of the cardiovascular fatalities worldwide. CAD is diagnosed by many modalities of imaging such as myocardial perfusion imaging (MPI) and coronary angiography (CAG). *Methods.* A retrospective cross-sectional study was conducted that included all patients referred to the KAMC (King Abdullah Medical City) nuclear cardiology lab from its opening until the end of May 2014 (a period of 17 months). A total of 228 patient reports with a history of conducting either CAG or MPI or both were used in this study and statistically analyzed. *Results.* An analysis of the MPI results revealed that 78.5% of the samples were abnormal. On the other hand, 26.75% of the samples revealed that they were subjected to CAG and MPI. There was a significant and fair agreement between MPI and CAG by using all the agreement coefficients (kappa = 0.237, phi = 0.310, and *P* value = 0.043). The sensitivity, specificity, and accuracy of MPI with reference to CAG were 97.8%, 20%, and 78.69%, respectively. In addition, positive predictive and negative predictive values were 78.95% and 75%, respectively. *Conclusion.* In a tertiary referral center, there was a significant agreement between MPI and CAG and a high accuracy of MPI. MPI was a noninvasive diagnostic test that could be used as a gatekeeper for CAG.

1. Background

Cardiovascular diseases (CVDs), especially the coronary artery diseases (CADs), are among the leading causes of fatalities worldwide [1–3]. CAD caused more than 7 million deaths worldwide in 2001 [2]. It causes more than 4.5 million deaths in the developing countries [3]. About 5.5% of the population in Saudi Arabia is suffering from these diseases [4]. CAD is diagnosed by many modalities of imaging. Although coronary angiography (CAG) is invasive, it is considered as the gold standard for CAD diagnosis [5].

CAG is used to show the patency of the coronary arteries by using a contrast medium and radiographic visualization [6]. Many complications have limited its use, including arrhythmia, aneurysms, arteriovenous fistulas, hemorrhage and hematomas, perforation of the heart or great vessels, allergic reactions, embolisms, infections, and death [6]. One of these modalities that are used to detect CAD other than CAG is myocardial perfusion imaging (MPI), which is a widely available noninvasive test that is indirectly showing how well blood reaches the myocardium by using radiopharmacological agents [7]. Single photon emission computed tomography (SPECT) and positron emission tomography (PET) are the two techniques used for MPI [7]. SPECT was used at the hospital in which this study was done.

In terms of indications and contraindications of MPI and CAG comparatively, CAG is more dangerous compared to MPI. CAG has indications in many cases such as unstable angina, chronic stable angina, and coronary syndrome and when used before a bypass surgery, while MPI is used in the evaluation of myocardial perfusion abnormalities in patients with a low to moderate likelihood of CAD as well as when suggested by the location, extent, and severity of chest pain [6, 7]. CAG is contraindicated in multiple conditions including allergy to dye, hypertension, coagulopathy, and kidney failure. On the other hand, MPI is not used in many cases like recent myocardial infarction, the inability to fulfill the exercise stress test fitness criteria, and contraindication conditions to adenosine stress testing [6, 7].

Patients with chest pain, especially when it is atypical and they have low to intermediate likelihood of CAD, need to show objective evidence of ischemia (ECG/MPI) before being referred for CAG with consideration that exercise ECG had no added prognostic value in the presence of normal findings in stress MPI [8]. Two meta-analyses involving a total of 6972 patients had been conducted to calculate the sensitivity and specificity of MPI in detecting CAD with reference to echocardiography, which found that sensitivity and specificity were ≥87% and ≥73%, respectively [9]. On the other hand, sensitivity and specificity of MPI with reference to CAG for 96 patients were 95% and 83%, respectively [10]. Patients with syndrome X and the perfusion defect with normal coronary angiography were found to be at risk for the development of coronary event (acute coronary syndrome) [11]. Similarly, patients with abnormal MPI and normal CAG were more liable to develop CAD, especially if CAG was after revascularization, as the results of both investigations in this phase will vary throughout this period [12].

MPI is used for detecting ischemia in the myocardium. The utility of the MPI in the CAD is a controversial point from many perspectives such as priority and dependence in the clinical decision. These perspectives had been argued by many researchers who had studied and weighed the anticipated high accuracy, specificity, and sensitivity against the projected risks and as consequences of dependence on its results in a clinical scenario [13–16].

The aim of the current study was to evaluate the relationship between MPI and CAG in a tertiary cardiac center at King Abdullah Medical City (KAMC).

2. Materials and Methods

The current study is a retrospective cross-sectional study that included all patients who were referred to the KAMC (King Abdullah Medical City) nuclear cardiology lab and have available reports from its opening until the end of May 2014 (a period of 17 months). Data was collected from patients' electronic health records and placed into an Excel sheet using a hospital computer in the department, not showing any nominative information. The patients were identified by a serial study code and their initials. These were linked to patients' names and their medical record number (MRN) in a separate identification log sheet, which had been kept in a safe locked place. After verification, data were transferred to the statistical database directly by using SPSS. The reports of MPI and CAG performed for those patients were examined. Files of patients with negative MPI reports were reviewed for

possible subsequent referral to CAG 3 months after receiving a negative MPI to ensure that all the cases where patients took both tests were included in this study in hope to minimize the effect of the referral bias. The duration of follow-up was the mean of interval periods that separate CAG and MPI among patients of KAMC. Since CAG is considered the gold standard for CAD, patients who have been subjected to both tests are statistically investigated. The CAG has to be subsequent to MPI in order to be involved in this study. The IRB of KAMC had approved the waiver of the informed consent as it was a retrospective study.

2.1. Coronary Angiography Protocol. The standard Judkins approach was used in performing the coronary angiography. The angiograms were analyzed specifically for this study by one observer who was unaware of the clinical and scintigraphic data.

2.2. Rest-Stress MPI Protocol. Stress/rest separate acquisition 99mTc-sestamibi MPI was used [17]. Patients who used agents which affected the stress study were instructed to discontinue their use before the stress test was performed such as the consumption of antihypertensives, nitrates, and caffeine products. There are two major types of stress tests that are pharmacological (85.5%) and use coronary vasodilators such as adenosine and exercise stress tests using the Bruce protocol (14.5%). One injection of 99mTc sestamibi at peak stress was given to patients who were subjected to exercise stress [17]. Exercise at high speed and grade was continued for 1 min after injection and for an extra 2 min at lower speed and grade [17]. For adenosine stress, adenosine was given intravenously at a dose of 140 g/kg/min for 6 min. At the end of the second or third minute of infusion 99mTc sestamibi was injected, and approximately 1 h later SPECT was conducted [17]. These two stress protocols are used according to the patient's characteristics; for instance, if the patient was young and had no previous MI, physician could use an exercise protocol, while in the elderly and patients with previous MI he/she must use the pharmacological method [7]. On a separate day, another dose of 99mTc-sestamibi was given at rest and a patient's image was taken after 1 hour.

2.3. MPI Acquisition Protocol. Acquisition was done using Siemens Symbia T-16 SPECT-CT, dual head gamma camera, using standard energy Windows for Tc-99 sestamibi [17]. Image analysis was done using Syngo MI software and a 4 DMSPECT package.

2.4. Image Analysis. The 17-segment model of MPI images was used for scoring. The 5-point scoring system was used to assess each segment: 0: normal; 1: equivocal; 2: moderate; 3: severe reduction of radioisotope uptake; and 4: absence of detectable tracer uptake in a segment (Figure 1). Summed stress score (SSS) is calculated by adding the 17 segment scores of the stress images while summed rest score (SRS) was calculated by adding the 17 segment scores for rest images. Summed difference score (SDS), the difference between stress and rest scores, is measuring the defect induced by stress (Figure 1). MPI results were considered normal if SSS < 3 and abnormal if SSS ≥ 3 [18].

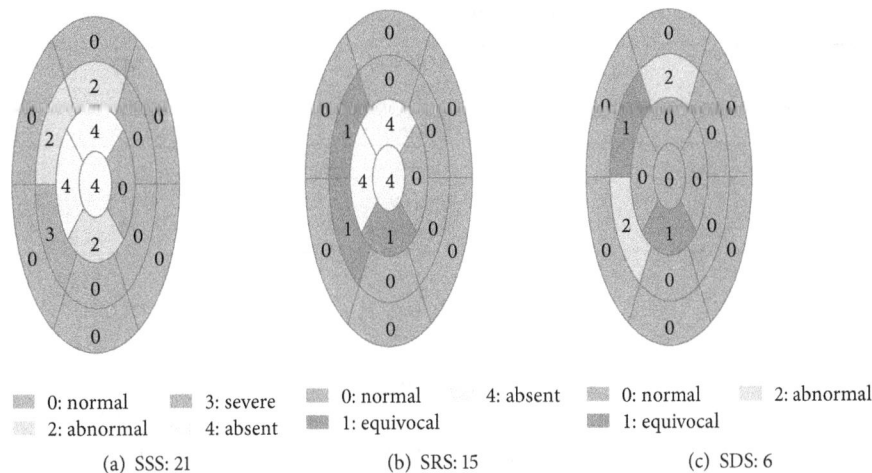

(a) SSS: 21   (b) SRS: 15   (c) SDS: 6

Legend (a): 0: normal, 3: severe, 2: abnormal, 4: absent
Legend (b): 0: normal, 4: absent, 1: equivocal
Legend (c): 0: normal, 2: abnormal, 1: equivocal

FIGURE 1: The 17-segment model with a 5-point scoring system for MPI. Circles (a) and (b) show the MPI images during the stress test and rest, respectively. Circle (c) is the difference between (a) and (b) MPI images. SSS: summed stress score; SRS: summed rest score; SDS: summed difference score.

2.5. Statistical Analysis. Patients who were subjected to MPI and CAG were classified as either an ischemic group or nonischemic group (Table 2). The ischemic group included true positive "TP" and false negative "FN." TP is defined as the patient who was classified as positive in both tests. Also, FN is defined as the patient who was classified as negative by MPI while being classified as positive by CAG. On the other hand, the nonischemic group included the true negative "TN" and the false positive "FP." TN is defined as the patient who was classified as negative in both tests. FP is defined as the patient who was classified as positive by MPI while being classified negative by CAG. MPI's sensitivity, specificity, accuracy, positive predictive value, and negative predictive value were calculated as described by the Altman method which is as follows: sensitivity = TP/(TP + FN), specificity = TN/(FP + TN), accuracy = (TP + TN)/(TP + FP + FN + TN), positive predictive value = TP/(TP + FP), and negative predictive value = TN/(FN + TN) [19, 20]. All continuous variables were expressed as mean ± SD. Categorical variables were compared with the χ^2 test and t-test for comparing the means of continuous variables. The P value 0.05 was considered significant. The chance-corrected (kappa) and chance-independent (phi) coefficients were used to obtain the exact relationship between these two tests [21].

3. Results

A total of 228 patient reports (n = 228) were involved in this retrospective cross-sectional study. These patients ages ranged from 27 years to 89 years with a mean of 59.03 ± 11.03 years. Two-thirds of the samples were male (n = 151) while about one-third were female (n = 77). Clinical characteristics of the two groups according to the results of the MPI are shown in Table 1. No significant differences were observed except for myocardial infarction (MI) and percutaneous coronary intervention (PCI). On the other hand, 26.75% of the samples revealed that they were subjected to CAG and MPI. We analyzed the MPI results and found that 78.5% of

our sample was classified as having abnormal MPI results. By reviewing the means of SSS in relation to the risk factors, we found that there was a significant relationship with the risk factors (DM and HTN). Also, presenting signs and symptoms (atypical chest pain, typical chest pain, shortness of breath, and abnormal ECG) affected the means of SSS significantly.

Agreement between the MPI and CAG in detecting CAD could be assessed by many coefficients such as chance-corrected (kappa), chance-independent (phi), and Cronbach's alpha coefficients. There was a significantly fair agreement between MPI and CAG by using all the agreement coefficients (kappa = 0.237, phi = 0.310). The P value was 0.043 for kappa and phi. The sensitivity, specificity, and accuracy of MPI with reference to CAG were 97.8%, 20%, and 78.69%, respectively. In addition, positive predictive and negative predictive values were 78.95% and 75%. Referral bias was the cause for the increase of the sensitivity and decrease of the specificity by decreasing the number of the true negatives and false negatives. If we did not consider referral bias by including patients who were classified as negative with MPI and without referral to CAG for more than 3 months and considered them as a true negative "TN," the sensitivity, specificity, accuracy, positive predictive value, and negative predictive value of MPI with reference to CAG would be 97.8%, 66.67%, 80.49%, 78.95%, and 96%, respectively. The sensitivity and the positive predictive value were not changed because there were no false negatives detected in those patients.

4. Discussion

By reviewing most of the studies in this field and to the best of our knowledge, there is no similar comparative published study. Yaghoubi and his colleagues [13] have examined the findings of CAG and MPI in cardiac syndrome X (CSX) (which is considered as one of the CAD) and found that 68.75% of MPIs showed an ischemia without a fixed lesion and transient left ventricular (TLV) dilatation. Researchers

TABLE 1: Patients' characteristics according to the MPI results.

Characteristic	MPI +ve (n = 179)	MPI −ve (n = 49)	P value
Age	59.63 ± 10.91	56.86 ± 11.33	0.0001
Gender			
(i) Male	124 (69.3)	27 (55.1)	NS
(ii) Female	55 (30.7)	22 (44.9)	NS
Comorbidity			
(i) Diabetes	119 (66.5)	31 (63.3)	NS
(ii) Hypertension	130 (72.6)	34 (69.4)	NS
(iii) Dyslipidemia	108 (60.3)	27 (55.1)	NS
(iv) Current smoker	32 (17.88)	5 (10.2)	NS
(v) Ex-smoker	18 (10.06)	6 (12.24)	NS
(vi) Nonsmoker	2 (1.12)	1 (2.04)	NS
Presentation			
(i) Atypical chest pain	132 (73.74)	28 (57.14)	NS
(ii) Typical angina	16 (8.93)	4 (8.16)	NS
(iii) Shortness of breath	55 (30.73)	14 (28.57)	NS
Past medical history			
(i) Myocardial infarction (MI)	46 (25.7)	4 (8.2)	0.01
(ii) Coronary angiography (CAG)	39 (21.8)	7 (14.3)	NS
(iii) Percutaneous coronary intervention (PCI)	58 (32.4)	7 (14.3)	0.01
(iv) Coronary artery bypass graft (CABG)	29 (16.2)	3 (6.1)	NS
Result of resting ECG			
(i) Normal	94 (52.5)	30 (61.2)	NS
(ii) Abnormal	85 (47.5)	19 (38.8)	NS
Type of stress test			
(i) Exercise (Bruce protocol)	22 (12.3)	11 (22.4)	NS
(ii) Pharmacological (adenosine stress test)	157 (87.7)	38 (77.6)	NS

NS: not significant; ECG: electrocardiogram.
Data are numerical with percentages in the brackets or mean ± SD.

TABLE 2: Agreement between MPI and CAG.

	MPI +ve	MPI −ve
CAG +ve	45	1
CAG −ve	12	3

TP = 45; TN = 3; FP = 12; FN = 1.
The total number of patients who have been subjected to both tests is 61.

claimed that the results of the myocardial perfusion imaging were not concordant with angiographic findings, which was possibly due to the nature of this disease (nonfixed lesion). In another study, the investigator examined the value of using SPECT-MPI to detect the graft disease after a coronary artery bypass surgery (CABG), and it was claimed that "SPECT-MPI has a good sensitivity and accuracy for detecting graft disease in an unselected patient population 1 year post-CABG under optimal stress conditions" (with the presence of variation in accuracy and sensitivity of SPECT-MPI between the exercise stress test and the pharmacological stress test) [14]. On the other hand, Shelley and his colleagues [15] have attempted to compare SPECT-MPI with multislice computed tomography (MSCT), and it was found that "whenever MSCT was negative, MPI was almost negative." In addition, a study conducted by Delcour et al. [16] included 48 patients with normal CAG and abnormal MPI who were followed up for at least 3 years from the conduction of MPI. It was found that 15 out of the studied patients had cardiovascular events, and 6 of them had coronary events (within a period of 0.5 to 8.67 years). The application of Delour's study methods on the current study was impossible as the nuclear cardiology center in KAMC was established 3 years ago. So, the retrospective follow-up of the patients who were classified as false positives for as long as 15 years is not possible. Also, patients who had a revascularization procedure showed abnormal MPI and normal CAG as MPI is more sensitive to the complex biological process that precedes restenosis earlier than CAG [12]. These results changed without intervention as the period that separates the investigation from the angioplasty changed [12]. So, for that reason it was recommended that MPI has to be before and after revascularization in order to predict the final result of perfusion [12]. Reviewing the data of those who had angioplasty procedures and had MPI and/or CAG was out of the scope of this study as we do not have access to cardiac surgery department patients results and our study was concentrating on patients who presented with a CAD clinical picture and had MPI alone or MPI and CAG as a subsequent investigation.

This significant fair agreement is not expected, but it is most probably due to referral bias, which occurs when patients with abnormal MPI results are referred for CAG at a higher rate than patients with normal MPI. These results were reviewed from a comparative perspective and it was found that a nonnegligible number was classified as a false positive, which could be justified by the high sensitivity of the MPI to minor changes of blood supply to heart muscles as long as the MPI was quantitatively investigating the richness of heart muscles with blood. On the other hand, the false negative was negligible. The very low specificity could be justified by the low number of patients with negative MPI that were subjected to CAG. This scarcity in the number of patients who did both tests was due to the invasivity of the CAG. In a comparative view of other patients' characteristics, there was a significant difference between the two groups, which was the presence or absence of a past history of MI or PCI. In the clinical scenario, patients with a past history of MI and/or PCI were more potential to develop perfusion defects.

5. Study Limitations

Referral bias was the main limitation in this study, as the patients who were included in this study usually were referred for CAG after observing abnormal MPI, which led to a lower number of patients matching the statistical criteria. Clinical characteristics were more liable to be affected by the recall bias from either patients or doctors; the latter was less affecting these characteristics.

6. Recommendation

We recommend that more studies be conducted in many tertiary centers around the country with a larger sample size of patients who had both tests.

7. Conclusion

In a tertiary referral center, there is a significantly fair matching between MPI and CAG results with a higher accuracy of MPI. MPI is a noninvasive diagnostic test that could be used as a gatekeeper for CAG as long as the positive predictive value is quite high compared to the negative predictive value.

Competing Interests

The authors declare that there is no conflict of interests regarding the publication of this paper.

References

[1] S. Mendis, S. Davis, and B. Norrving, "Organizational update: the World Health Organization global status report on noncommunicable diseases 2014; one more landmark step in the combat against stroke and vascular disease," Stroke, vol. 46, no. 5, pp. e121–e122, 2015.

[2] T. A. Gaziano, A. Bitton, S. Anand, S. Abrahams-Gessel, and A. Murphy, "Growing epidemic of coronary heart disease in low- and middle-income countries," Current Problems in Cardiology, vol. 35, no. 2, pp. 72–115, 2010.

[3] K. Okrainec, D. K. Banerjee, and M. J. Eisenberg, "Coronary artery disease in the developing world," American Heart Journal, vol. 148, no. 1, pp. 7–15, 2004.

[4] M. M. Al-Nozha, M. R. Arafah, Y. Y. Al-Mazrou et al., "Coronary artery disease in Saudi Arabia," Saudi Medical Journal, vol. 25, no. 9, pp. 1165–1171, 2004.

[5] S. Kohsaka and A. N. Makaryus, "Coronary angiography using noninvasive imaging techniques of cardiac CT and MRI," Current Cardiology Reviews, vol. 4, no. 4, pp. 323–330, 2008.

[6] P. J. Scanlon, D. P. Faxon, A. M. Audet et al., "ACC/AHA guidelines for coronary angiography: executive summary and recommendations. A report of the American College of Cardiology/American Heart Association Task Force on Practice Guidelines (Committee on Coronary Angiography) developed in collaboration with the Society for Cardiac Angiography and Interventions," Circulation, vol. 99, no. 17, pp. 2345–2357, 1999.

[7] H. W. Strauss, D. D. Miller, M. D. Wittry et al., "Procedure guideline for myocardial perfusion imaging 3.3," Journal of Nuclear Medicine Technology, vol. 36, no. 3, pp. 155–161, 2008.

[8] N. K. Sabharwal and A. Lahiri, "Role of myocardial perfusion imaging for risk stratification in suspected or known coronary artery disease," Heart, vol. 89, no. 11, pp. 1291–1297, 2003.

[9] M. Salerno and G. A. Beller, "Noninvasive assessment of myocardial perfusion," Circulation, vol. 2, no. 5, pp. 412–424, 2009.

[10] S. Koumna, C. Yiannakkaras, P. Avraamides, and O. Demetriadou, "Specificity and sensitivity of SPECT myocardial perfusion studies at the Nuclear Medicine Department of the Limassol General Hospital in Cyprus," Journal of Physics: Conference Series, vol. 317, no. 1, Article ID 012024, 2011.

[11] E. Jones, W. Eteiba, and N. B. Merz, "Cardiac syndrome X and microvascular coronary dysfunction," Trends in Cardiovascular Medicine, vol. 22, no. 6, pp. 161–168, 2012.

[12] D. D. Miller and M. S. Verani, "Current status of myocardial perfusion imaging after percutaneous transluminal coronary angioplasty," The Journal of the American College of Cardiology, vol. 24, no. 1, pp. 260–266, 1994.

[13] M. Yaghoubi, S. H. Arefi, and M. Assadi, "Comparison of angiographic with myocardial perfusion scintigraphy findings in cardiac syndrome X (CSX)," European Review for Medical and Pharmacological Sciences, vol. 15, no. 12, pp. 1385–1388, 2011.

[14] B. Al Aloul, M. Mbai, S. Adabag et al., "Utility of nuclear stress imaging for detecting coronary artery bypass graft disease," BMC Cardiovascular Disorders, vol. 12, article no. 62, 2012.

[15] S. Shelley, M. Indirani, I. Sathyamurthy et al., "Correlation of myocardial perfusion SPECT with invasive and computed tomography coronary angiogram," Indian Heart Journal, vol. 64, no. 1, pp. 43–49, 2012.

[16] K. S. Delcour, A. Khaja, A. Chockalingam, S. Kuppuswamy, and T. Dresser, "Outcomes in patients with abnormal myocardial perfusion imaging and normal coronary angiogram," Angiology, vol. 60, no. 3, pp. 318–321, 2009.

[17] F. Aboul-Enein, S. Kar, S. W. Hayes et al., "Influence of angiographic collateral circulation on myocardial perfusion in patients with chronic total occlusion of a single coronary artery and no prior myocardial infarction," Journal of Nuclear Medicine, vol. 45, no. 6, pp. 950–955, 2004.

[18] W. A. Al Jaroudi, M. C. Alraies, O. Wazni, M. D. Cerqueira, and W. A. Jaber, "Yield and diagnostic value of stress myocardial perfusion imaging in patients without known coronary artery disease presenting with syncope," *Circulation: Cardiovascular Imaging*, vol. 6, no. 3, pp. 384–391, 2013.

[19] D. G. Altman and J. M. Bland, "Statistics notes: diagnostic tests 1: sensitivity and specificity," *British Medical Journal*, vol. 308, no. 6943, p. 1552, 1994.

[20] D. G. Altman and J. M. Bland, "Diagnostic tests 2: predictive values," *British Medical Journal*, vol. 309, no. 6947, p. 102, 1994.

[21] G. Guyatt, *JAMA's Users' Guides to the Medical Literature*, McGraw-Hill Medical, New York, NY, USA, 1st edition, 2008.

26

Pediatric Heart Failure, Lagging, and Sagging of Care in Low Income Settings: A Hospital Based Review of Cases in Ethiopia

Solmon Gebremariam[1] and Tamirat Moges[2]

[1]Department of Pediatrics and child Health, Mekelle University, Mek'ele, Ethiopia
[2]Department of Pediatrics and Child Health, School of Medicine, Addis Ababa University, Addis Ababa, Ethiopia

Correspondence should be addressed to Tamirat Moges; tamirataklilu09@gmail.com

Academic Editor: Mariantonietta Cicoira

Introduction. Causes of acute heart failure in children range from simple myocarditis complicating chest infection to complex structural heart diseases. *Objective.* To describe patterns, predictors of mortality, and management outcomes of acute heart failure in children. *Methods.* In retrospective review, between February 2012 and October 2015 at a tertiary center, 106 admitted cases were selected consecutively from discharge records. Data were extracted from patients chart and analyzed using SPSS software package. t-test and statistical significance at P value < 0.05 with 95% CI were used. *Result.* Acute heart failure accounted for 2.9% of the total pediatric admissions. The age ranged from 2 months up to 14 years with mean age of 8 years. Male to female ratio is 1 : 2.1. Rheumatic heart disease accounted for 53.7%; pneumonia, anemia, infective endocarditis, and recurrence of acute rheumatic fever were the main precipitating causes. Death occurred in 19% of cases. Younger age at presentation, low hemoglobin concentration, and undernutrition were associated with death with P value of 0.00, 0.01, and 0.02, respectively. *Conclusions and Recommendation.* Pediatric heart failure in our settings is diagnosed mainly in older age groups and mostly precipitated due to preventable causes. Significant mortality is observed in relation to factors that can be preventable in children with underlying structural heart disease. Early suspicion and diagnosis of cases may reduce the observed high mortality.

1. Introduction

Heart failure is a clinical entity where the heart does not function to its level best as it does in its healthy state [1]. Heart failure is a common cause of morbidity and mortality in pediatric patients in the third world [2]. Change in the prevalence, pattern, and etiologies among the different ages, geographic area, and social classes creates difficulties to come up with formidable research in pediatrics. Compared with adult patients, where heart failure resulted from an insult to the myocardium, heart failure in children occurs due to heart lesions that cause volume overload as in large ventricular septal defect or due to lesions that causes obstruction to flow as in aortic stenosis [3]. Often it is hard to diagnose heart failure in children as the clinical manifestations have significantly overlap with other pathologic conditions. Pediatric heart failure has significant consequences: it is associated with

increased mortality, prolonged hospital stay, and increased economic and social burden to the family [2]. Acute heart failure in children in the developed communities is often due to cardiomyopathic causes or palliated congenital heart disease as opposed to developing countries where unoperated congenital heart disease and acquired heart disease are more prevalent [4]. There is also great need for evidence based management guidelines in pediatric heart failure, because the current guidelines in pediatric heart failure management are mainly derived from adult studies [5]. Clinical profiles of heart failure are not well described in the sub-Saharan Africa, though few countries reported childhood heart failure [6, 7]. In Ethiopia although few reports on the patterns of heart disease in children are available, studies on topic of childhood heart failure are nonexistent to our knowledge [8, 9]. Therefore, we sought to describe acute heart failure in children at a tertiary hospital in Addis Ababa, Ethiopia.

Objective. The objective of this paper is to describe patterns, association for mortality, and management outcomes of acute heart failure in children. Method: it includes study design which was a hospital based retrospective review of admitted cases and setting which is Tikur Anbessa Specialized Hospital (TASH), a tertiary referral center in Ethiopia in the pediatric medicine. The hospital is located in the center of Addis Ababa the capital city; Department of Pediatrics has eight different service units to which these patient groups can be referred. The hospital has an average of 170 pediatric beds where 25–30 beds are occupied by pediatric cardiac admissions. Patients were coming from all corners of Ethiopia as the hospital is the biggest tertiary referral center.

Sample. Patients' chart review was performed on 106 consecutive discharged patients with acute heart failure from February 2012 to October 2015. Patients under the age of 15 years from pediatric wards and emergency care unit with the discharge diagnosis of acute heart failure were included.

Inclusion Criteria. The clinical criteria for heart failure in a pediatric patient were made if any three of the following were fulfilled: (1) significant tachycardia for age (heart rate > 160 bpm in infancy, >140 bpm at the age of 2 years, >120 bpm at the age of 4 years, and >100 bpm above 6 years of age); (2) significant tachypnoea for age (respiratory rate > 60/min in newborn, >40/min in <24 months of age, >30/min in 2–5 years of age, >28/min in 5–10 years of age, and >25/min >10 years of age); (3) cardiomegaly (displaced apical beat with a central trachea or cardiothoracic ratio >60% in <1 year of age, >55% in 1–5 years of age, and >50% in >5 years of age); (4) tender hepatomegaly of at least 3 cm size below the right costal margin [10].

Independent variables included age, sex, duration of symptoms, underlying heart disease, precipitating cause, left ventricular systolic function (LV EF), right ventricular systolic function, date of start of treatment, type of treatment, and noncardiac treatment. Outcome variables included total pediatric admissions during study period, prevalence and etiology of heart failure, severity of heart failure, growth failure, pulmonary hypertension, recurrent chest infections (pneumonia), length of hospital stay, number of patients with improvement on discharge, mortality rate, and being defaulted.

Cases with incomplete information and age above 14 years were excluded from the study. Sample size was determined based on the prevalence of heart failure in sub-Saharan African countries using a single population sample size calculation method. Questionnaires were developed based on desired information. Each query was appropriately pretested to determine appropriate information. Based on available data, information about the onset of illness, the presenting complaint, duration of illness, treatments received, and other pertinent clinical features were obtained. The type and severity of cardiac lesions were ascertained on the basis of physical examination and radiologic and electrocardiographic data, including echocardiography. The cardiac unit is equipped with 4 modern echocardiographic machines with pediatric probes, ECG machines, pulse oximeter devices.

All cases were classified according to etiology, age, and clinical characteristics. Congenital and rheumatic heart diseases were defined according to the specific criteria available for their classifications [11, 12]. Diagnosis of congenital as well as acquired heart disease is confirmed by echocardiographic examination (2D, M-mode, and color-doppler mode imaging).

Data were extracted from the patient charts and were filled into the questionnaire format by the investigators. Data quality was checked for its completeness, corrected on the spot for information that appeared inconsistent. To ensure consistency, double data entry was used. Data concerning number of pediatric visits, pediatric admissions, and cardiac cases during the study period were obtained from the record office.

Data were entered into SPSS version 20, IBM, USA, and Excel 2013. Categorical data were presented as percentages or proportions. A chi-square test is used to determine whether an association between two categorical variables is significant or not. Continuous variables were analyzed using mean, median, and standard deviations. Student's t-test was used to compare mean values. Statistical significance was considered when P value falls below 0.05 at 95% confidence interval. Results were presented in tables and figures.

Operational Definition. Congenital heart disease (CHD) is a problem with the heart structure and function that is present at birth. Rheumatic valvular heart disease (RVHD) is active or inactive disease of the heart that results from rheumatic fever and is characterized by reduced functional capacity caused by inflammatory changes in the myocardium or scarring of the valves. Mild anemia is defined as a hemoglobin concentration in the range of 9.5–11 gm/dL. Moderate anemia is defined as hemoglobin in the range of 8–9.5 gm/dL. Severe anemia is defined as hemoglobin concentration < 8 gm/dL [13]. Treatment is defined in this particular case as medical treatments given excluding surgery and/or catheter intervention of the cardiac lesions. Left ventricular systolic dysfunction is considered when the left ventricular ejection fraction falls below 55% as determined by 2D-echocardiography [14, 15]. Pneumonia in a child with congestive heart failure is diagnosed in the presence of fever, increased in chest X-ray evidence of lung parenchymal infiltrates and elevated white blood cell count in the presence of evidence for acute heart failure. Severe acute heart failure for children 0–5 years of age is considered if symptoms occurred at rest with tachypnea, retractions, grunting, or diaphoresis. For children above the age of 5 years, severe acute heart failure is referred to as NYHA classes III and IV [10, 16]. Management outcome refers to the discharge outcome. Malnutrition is classified based on weight for height percentile of the median: (1) adequate weight for height measurement is defined when the percentile falls between 90 and 120%; (2) mild wasting is considered when the percentile value falls between 80 and 89% of the median value; (3) moderate wasting is considered when the percentile value falls between 70 and 79% of the median value; (4) severe wasting is considered when the percentile value < 70% of the median value [17, 18]. The study was approved by the department research and promotion committee.

TABLE 1: Patient characteristics of childhood heart failure at Tikur Anbessa Specialized Hospital, 2016.

	Male	Female	Total
Age			
0–36 months	5 (14.7%)	16 (22.2%)	21 (19.8%)
37–72 months	4 (11.8%)	12 (16.7%)	16 (15.1%)
73–108 months	4 (11.8%)	16 (16.7%)	20 (19.0%)
109–168 months	21 (61.8%)	28 (38.9%)	49 (46.0%)
Type of heart disease			
CHD	12 (41.7%)	30 (35.3%)	42 (39.6%)
RVHD	19 (52.8%)	38 (55.9%)	57 (53.7%)
Other causes	3 (5.6%)	4 (8.8%)	7 (6.6%)
RVSD	3 (2.8%)	6 (5.7%)	9 (8.5%)
LVSD	8 (7.5%)	18 (17%)	26 (24.5%)

CHD: congenital heart disease, RVHD: rheumatic valvular heart disease, RVSD: right ventricular systolic dysfunction, and LVSD: left ventricular systolic dysfunction.

TABLE 2: Predictors of mortality based on outcome; childhood heart failure at Tikur Anbessa Specialized Hospital, Addis Ababa, Ethiopia, 2016.

variable	Outcome		P value
	Death	Discharged	
Mean age at presentation in years	5.9	9.4	0.001
Mean duration of symptoms (days)	15.2	19.3	0.5
Mean duration of hospital stay (days)	16.7	24.8	0.05
Mean weight (Kg)	16.4	20.5	0.02
LV ejection fraction% (mean)	39.0	36.8	0.64
Mean hemoglobin level (gm/dl)	8.7	10.3	0.01
Mean furosemide dose in mg/kg	1.1	1.0	0.97
Mean digoxin dose/kg	0.006	0.007	0.36
Mean spironolactone dose/kg	0.9	0.9	0.70
Mean dose of captopril/kg	0.4	0.4	0.35

2. Result

During the study period, 3672 pediatric admissions were registered to the different pediatric units. Out of these, there were 106 cases of acute heart failure. The prevalence of acute heart failure was 2.9% of all pediatric admissions. The mean age at presentation was 8 years. All cases were classified in New York Heart Association (NYHA) or Rose functional class IV severity grade. Table 1 shows the distribution of different age categories. Over 65% of the cases were above the age of 6 years. Children below the age of 3 years accounted only for 20% of the cases. Female sex predominates in all age categories. From the same table, one can see that rheumatic heart disease accounted for over half of the cases. Mitral and aortic valves were involved in 100% and 31% of the cases, respectively. Congenital plus acquired nonrheumatic heart diseases cases accounted for the remainder of the cases. Systolic dysfunction was observed in 8.5% and 24.5% of the right and the left ventricular muscles, respectively. Earlier age at presentation, low body weight (kg), and low hemoglobin concentration were shown to be predictors of mortality as seen in Table 2.

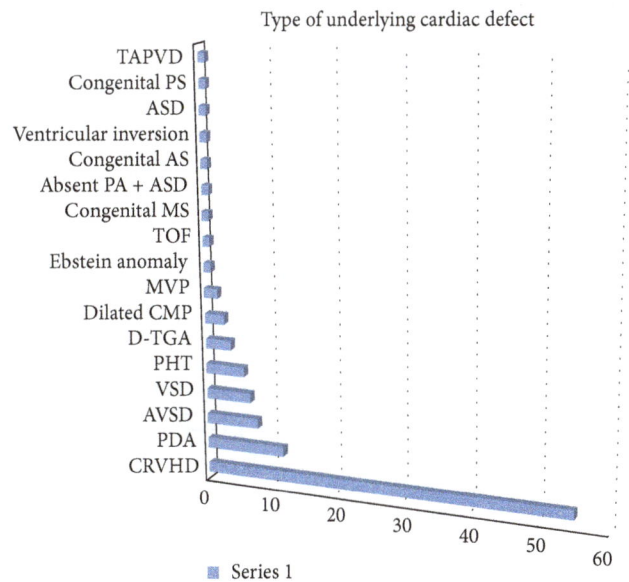

FIGURE 1: Frequency of underlying cardiac lesions; childhood heart failure at Tikur Anbessa Specialized Hospital, 2016. ASD: atrial septal defect, As: aortic stenosis, PA: pulmonary artery, MS: mitral stenosis, TOF: tetralogy of Fallot, MVP: mitral valve prolapse, CMP: cardiomyopathy, D-TGA: D-type transposition of the great arteries, PHT: pulmonary hypertension, VSD: ventricular septal defect, AVSD: atrioventricular septal defect, PDA: patent ductus arteriosus, CRVHD: chronic valvular heart disease, TAPVD: total anomalous pulmonary venous drainage, and PS: pulmonary stenosis.

Figure 1 shows frequency of underlying cardiac conditions that predisposes to acute heart failure. Heart failure was precipitated by the list of factors displayed in Figure 2. Pneumonia, infective endocarditis, and rheumatic fever recurrence were the most common causes of heart failure in decreasing order. Weight for height status is also shown in Figure 3 with mild, moderate, and severe wasting observed in 53.8%, 17.9%, and 7.5% of cases, respectively.

Medication profile of cases is displayed in Figure 4. Furosemide was prescribed for all cases at the time of

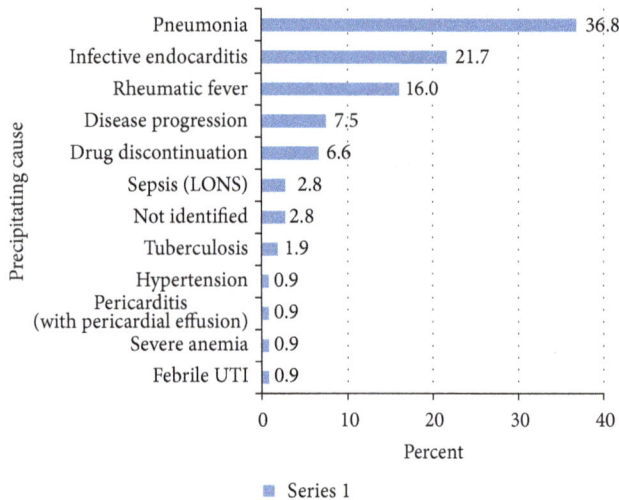

FIGURE 2: Precipitating causes of childhood heart failure at Tikur Anbessa Specialized Hospital, 2016. LONS: late onset neonatal sepsis and UTI: urinary tract infection.

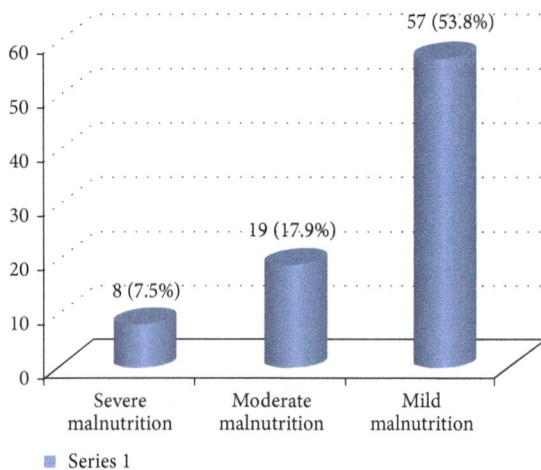

FIGURE 3: Weight for height status of cases of childhood heart failure at Tikur Anbessa Specialized Hospital, 2016. y-axis: percentage of patients.

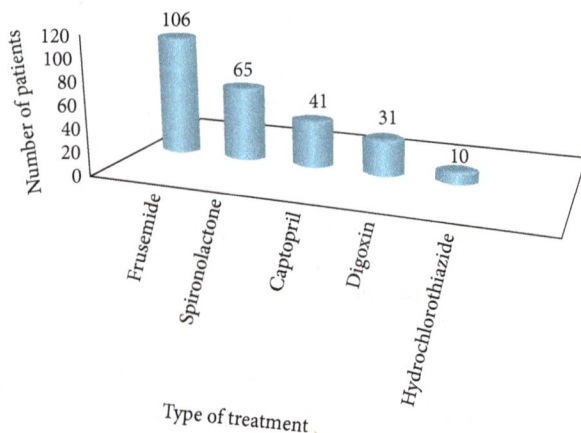

FIGURE 4: Drug treatment profile of cases in TASH 2016. y-axis: number of patients.

admission, whereas spironolactone, captopril, digoxin, and hydrochlorothiazide were prescribed in 65%, 41%, 31%, and 10%, respectively. Beta blockers were not part of the medication lists. Seventy-five percent of the cases were discharged improved, 19% died, and the rest of them were either defaulted or returned back to their original institution to complete their medications.

3. Discussion

This hospital based retrospective chart review represented the general population of patients that sought care at Tikur Anbessa Hospital from all regions of Ethiopia. Data collection was reliable as the investigators coded all the diagnoses. The mean age at first presentation was low for mortality cases. This may have to do with the severity of underlying cardiac disease. Some of the findings were unique in our setting compared to reports from international sources. For example, infants and young children accounted for low proportion of the cases in this review. Massin et al. reported in one review that 58.1% of their study subjects were infants [19] In another study, 75.7% of deaths due to acute heart failure occurred in patients younger than 1 year of age [4, 20]. In a report of pediatric acute heart failure from Kenya, the reported mean age was 4.7 years, with a peak at 1–3 years. In another report of childhood heart failure from Calabar, Nigeria, 69% percent of the patients were aged between 1 and 5 years [6]. One possible explanation for this observation in our settings may be the challenge of diagnosing heart failure in small children. Other clinical conditions may have a similar clinical presentation, for example, respiratory tract infections. In many occasions, an infant may present with both heart failure and pneumonia. Thus, there is a tendency among the staff to record pneumonia as final diagnosis and omit heart failure because health providers are not confident enough in the diagnosis of acute heart failure in small children. Hyperactive air way disease can also be confused with heart failure in infants. The study subjects in the current study were the unoperated cases of cardiac structural problems. Therefore, those patients with severe structural cardiac disease may have died early, with only those with less severe structural disease presenting later in life. This is suggested in Table 2.

In this review, female sex appears to be more commonly reported at all age groups. It appears from many studies that female sex has higher risk of developing cardiovascular disease compared to male sex [21]. It has been reported that sex disparities in cardiovascular health exist among women of all ages, socioeconomic backgrounds, and racial subgroups. According to Singh, parental preference for male children exists in many societies, where girls with heart disease are not provided with the same treatment opportunities as boys. Based on suggestion of Navin and Nanda, there may also be an underlying biological sex difference [22] However, Julius A Ogeng'o et al. from Kenya reported male preponderance in their report of 158 cases [23]. Other studies suggest that there is increased female preponderance for mitral stenosis in patient with known rheumatic heart disease [22, 24]. All these factors may explain our findings of female predominance. Yet more evidence is required to explain these observations.

One of the prevailing findings in the current review is coexisting infections. Several studies reported respiratory infections to be common with acute heart failure particularly in children with structural heart disease [7, 25]. The mechanism by which recurrent chest infections cause heart failure has been postulated by Sadoh. It was suggested that, with pulmonary overcirculation and pulmonary edema associated with large left to right shunting of blood, pulmonary congestion ultimately becomes a focus of infection in the lower respiratory tract [26].

Children with rheumatic heart disease in Ethiopia are at risk of developing recurrence of rheumatic fever, as many of them are not receiving appropriate secondary prophylaxis with penicillin [8]. It is reported that the risk of rheumatic fever recurrence is significantly high if a patient is taking less than 80% of the prescribed doses [27]. On the other hand, dental health and dental hygiene are often compromised among communities. It is also known that children with congenital and/or acquired valvular heart lesions are at high risk of developing infective endocarditis, especially if they are not covered with subacute bacterial endocarditis prophylaxis during certain invasive procedures. This problem is well reflected in our previous report [9]. Over half the cases in our current study had laboratory evidence of anemia. A similar observation was made in adult patients with heart failure by Tang et al. They reported that up to one-fifth to one-third of heart failure cases had developed anemia. Accordingly, the prevalence of anemia increases with severity of the heart failure [28]. On the other hand, Worens Luiz reported the prevalence of anemia in the study population to be 41.0% [29]; Lindenfeld reported that anemia is consistently associated with poorer survival in all patient populations [30]. The high prevalence of anemia in our current study may be related to NYHA or Ross class IV severity grading. Plasma volume expansion that occurs in congestive heart failure may also contribute to anemia by a process of hemodilution. Chronic kidney disease is common comorbidity in heart failure and is strong independent predictor of anemia [31]. According to Tang, any abnormality that reduces renal secretion or bone marrow responses to erythropoietin may result in anemia. We were unable to collect this information in our current report. We would like to emphasize the importance of kidney evaluation in all patients admitted with heart failure. It was also reported that patients with cardiac cachexia are at increased risk for anemia. Reports suggest that serum level of proinflammatory cytokines is increased in cachexic patients with congestive heart failure and may contribute to development of anemia by several mechanisms [32]. Significant weight differences correlated with increased mortality in the current study. Seventy-nine percent of the patients had malnutrition based on weight for height measurements. According to a report of heart failure patients in adults by Amare et al. from Jimma University, in South-West Ethiopia, 77.8% of the these patients were malnourished [33]. It has been reported that the risk of death associated with heart failure is significantly increased in patients at risk of malnutrition or with concomitant malnutrition [34]. Coatsa followed the one-year mortality rate of patients in a prospective study, who were classified as malnourished according to the "Mini Nutritional Assessment score." A one-year mortality rate was found to be 56% in malnourished patients, compared to 23.5% in patients at risk of malnutrition and 11.3% in those patients with an adequate nutritional status [35].

Malnutrition in heart failure has been ascribed to neurohormonal alterations, especially anabolic/catabolic imbalance and increased cytokine release. Anorexia becomes worse, particularly during acute decompensation of heart failure [32]. Hormonal factors related to heart failure can affect appetite, further interfering with nutrition. According to the discussion by Niya Jones, chronic heart failure interferes with the absorption of fats and protein in particular; diminished blood flow to the intestines and fluid accumulation, called gut edema, contribute to malabsorption and likely promote the development of cardiac cachexia [36]. In general, children with acute heart failure have increased work of breathing and increased cardiac activity to compensate for the low cardiac function. This exposes them to high energy expenditure in the face of limited intake leading to cardiac cachexia.

The number of cases who died in the current study is relatively higher compared to most reports in the sub-Saharan African countries and most others outside the region. We already discussed the role of malnutrition and anemia in increasing risk of death in heart failure. However, studies from other sub-Saharan African countries did not report the role of malnutrition in their reviews. In adult studies, the rate of malnutrition was not as high as seen in our current report. The high prevalence of undernutrition, anemia and coinfection in our context may explain the high mortality rate observed [6, 23].

We observed in our study that captopril treatment was initiated with the lowest starting dose of 0.1 to 0.3 mg/kg/dose once (OD) daily up to three times daily (TID); however, escalation of dose was not subsequently done. Therefore, angiotensin converting enzyme inhibitor (ACE-inhibitor) therapy was, in general, suboptimal in our setting. However, literature recommends that, following a starting dose, a tittered dose as high as 0.5–2 mg/kg every 8 hours can be used in pediatric heart failure [37, 38]. The observed treatment disparity in comparison to the standard practice is, we believe, a call to prepare management protocols for our interns and residents. Therapy with beta blockers was not used in any of our patients. Our result differs from the Kenyan and Nigerian study in the mean age and gender of cases described. Surprisingly our result is similar to most reports in adult patients. This may be due to the fact that we have described older patients in contrast to the Kenyan or the Nigerian patients groups [6, 7].

4. Conclusion

Age distribution of pediatric heart failure in our setting is dominated by older age population. Acute heart failure in infants and small children may have been underreported, due to misdiagnosis or early death of patients. Female sex predominance observed in adult reports is also noted in the current study. Underlying cardiac defects predisposing patients to heart failure were dominated by rheumatic heart disease in this review. This highlights the importance of national mobilization against this preventable condition. Undernutrition, anemia and infections were also important preventable comorbid conditions predisposing to death of cases.

Additional Points

Recommendation. Presence of undernutrition, anemia and infections should be evaluated in all cardiac patients and should be treated early. Delayed suspicion and detection of congenital heart disease may be prevented by careful auscultation of the heart during medical evaluation of every child by a primary care physician. Primary and secondary prophylaxis of acute rheumatic fever should be a national agenda.

Competing Interests

The authors do not have any conflict of interests.

Acknowledgments

The authors' ardent feeling goes to Dr. Michelle Yates from Soddo Christian Hospital who did major review on their paper. It is also their joy to thank their faculty members who gave them constructive feedback during both departmental dissertation and conference presentation of the paper. Finally, their families who were patient with them and always understood them during their absence and silence for the sake of accomplishing the work were also acknowledged.

References

[1] E. Madriago and M. Silberbach, "Heart failure in infants and children," *Pediatrics in Review*, vol. 31, no. 1, pp. 4–12, 2010.

[2] P. Bondi and F. Jaiyesimi, "Heart failure in an emergency room setting," *Nigerian Journal of Paediatrics*, vol. 17, no. 1-2, pp. 1–6, 1990.

[3] V. Chaturvedi and A. Saxena, "Heart failure in children: clinical aspect and management," *Indian Journal of Pediatrics*, vol. 76, no. 2, pp. 195–205, 2009.

[4] E. Morell, J. Wolfe, M. Scheurer et al., "Patterns of care at end of life in children with advanced heart disease," *Archives of Pediatrics and Adolescent Medicine*, vol. 166, no. 8, pp. 745–748, 2012.

[5] A. Damasceno, B. M. Mayosi, M. Sani et al., "The causes, treatment, and outcome of acute heart failure in 1006 Africans from 9 countries: results of the Sub-Saharan Africa survey of heart failure," *Archives of Internal Medicine*, vol. 172, no. 18, pp. 1386–1394, 2012.

[6] M. U. Anah, O. E. Antia-Obong, C. O. Odigwe, and V. O. Ansa, "Heart failure among paediatric emergencies in Calabar, South Eastern Nigeria," *Mary Slessor Journal of Medicine*, vol. 4, no. 1, pp. 58–62, 2004.

[7] I. A. Lagunju and S. I. Omokhodion, "Childhood heart failure in Ibadan," *West African Journal of Medicine*, vol. 22, no. 1, pp. 42–45, 2003.

[8] K. Oli and J. Porteous, "Rheumatic heart disease among school children in Addis Ababa City: awareness and adequacy of its prophylaxis," *Ethiopian Medical Journal*, vol. 37, no. 3, pp. 155–161, 1999.

[9] T. Moges, E. Gedlu, P. Isaakidis et al., "Infective endocarditis in Ethiopian children: a hospital based review of cases in Addis Ababa," *Pan African Medical Journal*, vol. 20, article 75, 2015.

[10] R. D. Ross, R. O. Bollinger, and W. W. Pinsky, "Grading the severity of congestive heart failure in infants," *Pediatric Cardiology*, vol. 13, no. 2, pp. 72–75, 1992.

[11] MedicineNet, Definition of Rheumatic heart disease, 2016, http://www.medicinenet.com/script/main/art.asp?articlekey= 11964.

[12] B. M. C. Staff, *Congenital Heart Disease in Adults*, 2016, http://www.mayoclinic.org/diseases-conditions/congenital-heart-disease/basics/definition/con-20034800.

[13] A. Carley, "Anemia: when is it not iron deficiency?" *Pediatric Nursing*, vol. 29, no. 3, pp. 205–211, 2003.

[14] ECHOpEDIA.oRG, "Up todate list of echocardiographic normal values," 2015, http://www.cardionetworks.org/.

[15] G. K. Singh and M. R. Holland, "Diastolic dysfunction in pediatric cardiac patients: evaluation and management," *Current Treatment Options in Cardiovascular Medicine*, vol. 12, no. 5, pp. 503–517, 2010.

[16] American Heart Association, *Little, Nomenclature and Criteria for Diagnosis of Diseases of the Heart and Great Vesseis*, American Heart Association, 9th edition, 1994.

[17] London School of Hygiene and Tropical Medicine, "The use of epidemiological tools in conflict-affected populations: open-access educational resources for policy-makers," 2009.

[18] Unicef/Unu/Who, "Measuring and interpreting malnutrition and mortality," http://www.unhcr.org/45f6abc92.pdf.

[19] M. M. Massin, I. Astadicko, and H. Dessy, "Epidemiology of heart failure in a tertiary pediatric center," *Clinical Cardiology*, vol. 31, no. 8, pp. 388–391, 2008.

[20] C. Morin, R. Hiram, E. Rousseau, P. U. Blier, and S. Fortin, "Docosapentaenoic acid monoacylglyceride reduces inflammation and vascular remodeling in experimental pulmonary hypertension," *American Journal of Physiology—Heart and Circulatory Physiology*, vol. 307, no. 4, pp. H574–H586, 2014.

[21] D. Singh, G. S. Wander, and R. J. Singh, "Gender equality in India for children with congenital heart disease: looking for answers," *Heart*, vol. 97, no. 23, pp. 1897–1898, 2011.

[22] C. Navin and N. K. Nanda, *Heart Disease in Women Circulation*, 2016.

[23] J. A. Ogeng'o, P. M. Gatonga, B. O. Olabu, D. K. Nyamweya, and D. Ong'era, "Pattern of congestive heart failure in a Kenyan paediatric population," *Cardiovascular Journal of Africa*, vol. 24, no. 4, pp. 117–120, 2013.

[24] C. N. Manjunath, P. Srinivas, K. S. Ravindranath, and C. Dhanalakshmi, "Distribution of Mitral Stenosis cases according to etiology and gender," *Indian Heart Journal*, vol. 66, no. 3, pp. 320–326, 2014.

[25] S. Andres, G. Bauer, S. Rodríguez, L. Novali, D. Micheli, and D. Fariña, "Hospitalization due to respiratory syncytial virus infection in patients under 2 years of age with hemodynamically significant congenital heart disease," *Jornal de Pediatria*, vol. 88, no. 3, pp. 246–252, 2012.

[26] W. E. Sadoh and W. O. Osarogiagbon, "Underlying congenital heart disease in Nigerian children with pneumonia," *African Health Sciences*, vol. 13, no. 3, pp. 607–612, 2013.

[27] F. O. W. Heart, *Diagnosis and Mangagement of Acute Rheumatic Fever and Rheumatic Heart Disease*, 2007.

[28] W. H. W. Tang and P. S. D. Yeo, "Epidemiology of anemia in heart failure," *Heart Failure Clinics*, vol. 6, no. 3, pp. 271–278, 2010.

[29] W. L. Cavalini, N. Ceulemans, R. B. Correa, P. W. Padoani, E. F. Delfrate, and E. M. Maluf, "Prevalence of anemia in patients with heart failure," *International Journal of Cardiovascular Sciences*, vol. 29, no. 1, 2016.

[30] J. Lindenfeld, "Prevalence of anemia and effects on mortality in patients with heart failure," *American Heart Journal*, vol. 149, no. 3, pp. 391–401, 2005.

[31] Y. D. Tang and S. D. Katz, "Anemia in chronic heart failure: prevalence, etiology, clinical correlates, and treatment options," *Circulation*, vol. 13, no. 20, pp. 2454–2461, 2006.

[32] I. Bourdel-Marchasson and J.-P. Emeriau, "Nutritional strategy in the management of heart failure in adults," *American Journal of Cardiovascular Drugs*, vol. 1, no. 5, pp. 363–373, 2001.

[33] H. Amare, L. Hamza, and H. Asefa, "Malnutrition and associated factors among heart failure patients on follow up at Jimma university specialized hospital, Ethiopia," *BMC Cardiovascular Disorders*, vol. 15, no. 1, article 128, 2015.

[34] J. L. Bonilla-Palomas, A. L. Gámez-López, M. P. Anguita-Sánchez et al., "Impact of malnutrition on long-term mortality in hospitalized patients with heart failure," *Revista Espanola de Cardiologia*, vol. 64, no. 9, pp. 752–758, 2011.

[35] A. J. S. Coatsa, "Chronic heart failure, nutritional status and survival," *Revista Española de Cardiología*, vol. 64, no. 9, pp. 743–744, 2011.

[36] D. M. Niya Jones, "Malnutrition in Patients With Chronic Heart Failure," http://livehealthy.chron.com/malnutrition-patients-chronic-heart-failure-8495.html.

[37] F. Shann, *Drug Dose*, Collective P/L, Melbourne, Australia, 15th edition, 2010.

[38] K. Momma, "ACE inhibitors in pediatric patients with heart failure," *Pediatric Drugs*, vol. 8, no. 1, pp. 55–69, 2006.

Permissions

List of Contributors

Suprakash Chaudhury
Department of Psychiatry, Pravara Institute of Medical Sciences (Deemed University), Loni, Maharashtra 413736, India

Rajiv Saini
Department of Psychiatry, AFMC, Pune, Maharashtra 411040, India

Ajay Kumar Bakhla
Department of Psychiatry, Rajendra Institute ofMedical Sciences, Ranchi, Jharkhand 834009, India

Jaswinder Singh
Department of Cardiothoracic Surgery, MH CTC, Pune, Maharashtra 411040, India

Sergio Conti, Massimo Moltrasio, Gaetano Fassini, Fabrizio Tundo, Stefania Riva, Antonio Dello Russo, Michela Casella, Benedetta Majocchi, VittoriaMarino,Valentina Catto, Salvatore Pala and Claudio Tondo
Cardiac Arrhythmia Research Centre, Centro Cardiologico Monzino IRCCS, Via Carlo Parea 4, 20138 Milan, Italy

Pasquale De Iuliis
St. Jude Medical, Agrate Brianza, Italy

Sylvia Marie Biso, Marvin Lu, Toni Anne De Venecia, Supakanya Wongrakpanich, Mary Rodriguez-Ziccardi, Sujani Yadlapati and Marina Kishlyansky
Department of Medicine, Einstein Medical Center, 5401 Old York Road, Suite 363, Philadelphia, PA 19141, USA

Harish Seetha Rammohan
Bassett Medical Center, Bassett Healthcare Network, Cooperstown, NY, USA
CUMC, College of Physicians & Surgeons, Columbia University, New York, NY, USA

Vincent M. Figueredo
Einstein Institute for Heart and Vascular Health, Einstein Medical Center, Philadelphia, PA, USA
Sidney Kimmel Medical College,Thomas Jefferson University, Philadelphia, PA, USA

Manoucher Manoucheri, Junhong Gui, Divyanshu Malhotra, Jason D'souza, Fnu Virkram, Aditya Chada and Haibing Jiang
Internal Medicine Residency Program, Department of Medicine, Florida Hospital Orlando, Orlando, FL, USA

Shengchuan Dai
Internal Medicine Residency Program, Department of Medicine, Florida Hospital Orlando, Orlando, FL, USA
Division of Cardiology, University of Illinois at Chicago, Chicago, IL, USA

Xiang Zhu
Center for Interventional Endoscopy, Florida Hospital Orlando, Orlando, FL, USA

Shenjing Li
Division of Cardiology, University of South Dakota, Vermillion, SD, USA

Amin Daoulah
Section of Adult Cardiology, Cardiovascular Department, King Faisal Specialist Hospital & Research Center,Jeddah, Saudi Arabia

Mushabab Al-Murayeh
Cardiovascular Department, Armed Forces Hospital Southern Region, Khamis Mushayt, Saudi Arabia

Salem Al-kaabi
Cardiology Department, Zayed Military Hospital, Abu Dhabi, UAE

Ali Youssef
Suez Canal University, Ismailia, Egypt

Alawi A. Alsheikh-Ali
College of Medicine, Mohammed Bin Rashid University of Medicine and Health Sciences, Dubai, UAE
Institute of Cardiac Sciences, Sheikh Khalifa Medical City, Abu Dhabi, UAE

Alessio Galli and Federico Lombardi
Cardiovascular Diseases Unit, Fondazione IRCCS Ca' Granda Ospedale Maggiore Policlinico, Department of Clinical and Community Sciences, University of Milan, Via F. Sforza 35, 20122 Milan, Italy

Marco Antonio Peña-Duque, Marco Antonio Martínez-Ríos, Leslie Quintanar-Trejo,Gad Aptilon-Duque, Mirthala Flores-García, David Cruz-Robles and Guillermo Cardoso-Saldaña
Instituto Nacional de Cardiología Ignacio Chávez, Grupo Genética Intervencionista, Departamentos de Biología Molecular, Hemodinámica, Endocrinología, 14080 México City, Mexico

Benjamin Valente-Acosta and Aurora de la Peña-Díaz
Instituto Nacional de Cardiología Ignacio Chávez, Grupo Genética Intervencionista, Departamentos de Biología Molecular, Hemodinámica, Endocrinología, 14080 México City, Mexico
Departamento de Farmacología, Facultad de Medicina, Universidad Nacional Autónoma de México, 04510 México City, Mexico

Manuel Alfonso Baños-González
Instituto Nacional de Cardiología Ignacio Chávez, Grupo Genética Intervencionista, Departamentos de Biología Molecular, Hemodinámica, Endocrinología, 14080 México City, Mexico
Divisi´on Académica de Ciencias de la Salud, Universidad Juárez Autónoma de Tabasco, Hospital Regional de Alta Especialidad "Dr. Juan Graham Casasús", 86126 Villahermosa, TAB, Mexico

Georgia Audi, Aggeliki Korologou, Ioannis Koutelekos, Georgios Vasilopoulos and Maria Polikandrioti
Faculty of Health and Caring Professions, Department of Nursing, Technological Educational Institute of Athens, Athens, Greece

Kostas Karakostas
Thriasio General Hospital, Elefsina, Athens, Greece

Kleanthi Makrygianaki
Alexandra General Hospital, Athens, Greece

Courtney E. Bennett
Mayo Clinic, 200 First Street SW, Rochester, MN 55902, USA

Ronald Freudenberger
Lehigh Valley Health Network, 1250 S Cedar Crest Boulevard, Allentown, PA 18103, USA

Yoga Yuniadi, Dicky A. Hanafy, R. W. M. Kaligis, Manoefris Kasim and Ganesja M. Harimurti
Department of Cardiology and Vascular Medicine, Faculty of Medicine, University of Indonesia and National Cardiovascular Center Harapan Kita, Jakarta 11420, Indonesia

Yuyus Kusnadi, Lakshmi Sandhow, Rendra Erika and Caroline Sardjono
Stem Cell and Cancer Institute, Jakarta 13210, Indonesia

M. J. Pearson and N. A. Smart
School of Science and Technology, University of New England, Armidale, NSW2351, Australia

Hussain Ibrahim and Jubran Rind
Grand Rapids Medical Education Partners, Michigan State University, Grand Rapids, MI 49503, USA

Bohuslav Finta
Spectrum Health Medical Group Cardiovascular Services, Grand Rapids, MI 49503, USA

Apirak Sribhutorn
Ph.D. Program in Clinical Epidemiology, Faculty of Medicine, Chiang Mai University, Chiang Mai 50200,Thailand
Department of Pharmacy Practice, School of Pharmaceutical Sciences, University of Phayao, Phayao 56000, Thailand

Arintaya Phrommintikul, Wanwarang Wongcharoen and Apichard Sukonthasarn
Cardiology Division, Department of Internal Medicine, Faculty of Medicine, Chiang Mai University, Chiang Mai 50200,Thailand

Usa Chaikledkaew
Social and Administrative Pharmacy Excellence Research (SAPER) Unit, Department of Pharmacy, Faculty of Pharmacy,Mahidol University, Bangkok 10400,Thailand

Suntara Eakanunkul
Department of Pharmaceutical Sciences, Faculty of Pharmacy, Chiang Mai University, Chiang Mai 50200, Thailand

Francesca Galati and Sera ina Massari
Department of Biological and Environmental Sciences and Technologies, University of Salento, 73100 Lecce, Italy

Antonio Galati
Department of Cardiology, "Card. G. Panico" Hospital, Tricase, 73039 Lecce, Italy

Ephraim B. Winzer, Robert Höllriegel, Tina Fischer, Axel Linke, Gerhard Schuler, Volker Adams and Sandra Erbs
Leipzig Heart Center, Department of Cardiology, Leipzig University, 04289 Leipzig, Germany

Pauline Gaida
Saechsisches Krankenhaus Altscherbitz, 04435 Leipzig,
Germany

Daniel R. Bayzigitov and Elena V. Dementyeva
Federal Research Center, Institute of Cytology and
Genetics, Siberian Branch of the Russian Academy of
Sciences, Academy Lavrentyev Avenue 10,
Novosibirsk 630090, Russia
Institute of Chemical Biology and Fundamental
Medicine, Siberian Branch of the Russian Academy of
Sciences, Academy Lavrentyev Avenue 8,
Novosibirsk 630090, Russia
State Research Institute of Circulation Pathology,
Rechkunovskaya Street 15, Novosibirsk 630055, Russia

Sergey P. Medvedev and Suren M. Zakian
Federal Research Center, Institute of Cytology and
Genetics, Siberian Branch of the Russian Academy of
Sciences, Academy Lavrentyev Avenue 10,
Novosibirsk 630090, Russia
Institute of Chemical Biology and Fundamental
Medicine, Siberian Branch of the Russian Academy of
Sciences, Academy Lavrentyev Avenue 8, Novosibirsk
630090, Russia
State Research Institute of Circulation Pathology,
Rechkunovskaya Street 15, Novosibirsk 630055, Russia
Novosibirsk State University, Pirogova Street 2,
Novosibirsk 630090, Russia

**Sevda A. Bayramova, Evgeny A. Pokushalov and
Alexander M. Karaskov**
State Research Institute of Circulation Pathology,
Rechkunovskaya Street 15, Novosibirsk 630055, Russia

Anne B. Gregory and Kendra K. Lester
Department of Clinical Epidemiology, Faculty of
Medicine, Memorial University of Newfoundland, St.
John's, NL, Canada A1B 3V6

Deborah M. Gregory and William K. Midodzi
Department of Clinical Epidemiology, Faculty of
Medicine, Memorial University of Newfoundland, St.
John's, NL, Canada A1B 3V6
Department of Medicine, Faculty of Medicine,
Memorial University of Newfoundland, St. John's, NL,
Canada A1B 3V6

Laurie K. Twells
Department of Clinical Epidemiology, Faculty of
Medicine, Memorial University of Newfoundland, St.
John's, NL, Canada A1B 3V6
School of Pharmacy, Memorial University of
Newfoundland, St. John's, NL, Canada A1B 3V6

Neil J. Pearce
Department of Medicine, Faculty of Medicine,
Memorial University of Newfoundland, St. John's, NL,
Canada A1B 3V6
Eastern Health, St. John's, NL, Canada A1B 3V6

**Om Prakash Yadava, Vikas Ahlawat, Anirban Kundu
and Bikram K. Mohanty**
Department of Cardiothoracic Surgery, National Heart
Institute, 49-50 Community Centre, East of Kailash,
New Delhi 110065, India

Vinod Sharma and Rekha Mishra
Department of Cardiology, National Heart Institute,
49-50 Community Centre, East of Kailash, New Delhi
110065, India

Arvind Prakash
Department of Cardiac Anesthesiology, National Heart
Institute, 49-50 Community Centre, East of Kailash,
New Delhi 110065, India

Amit K. Dinda
Department of Pathology, All India Institute of Medical
Sciences, New Delhi 110029, India

Chikahiko Koeda
Division of Cardioangiology, Department of Internal
Medicine, Iwate Medical University, Iwate, Japan

Shohei Yamaya and Maiko Hozawa
Department of Cardiology, Iwate Prefectural Kuji
Hospital, Iwate, Japan

**Masayuki Sato, Kazuhiro Nasu, Tomohiro Takahashi
and Katsutoshi Terui**
Department of Emergency, Iwate Medical University,
Iwate, Japan

Anne B. Gregory
Eastern Health, St. John's, NL, Canada A1B 3V6
Department of Clinical Epidemiology, Faculty of
Medicine, Memorial University of Newfoundland, St.
John's, NL, Canada A1B 3V6

Neil J. Pearce
Eastern Health, St. John's, NL, Canada A1B 3V6
Department of Medicine, Faculty of Medicine,
Memorial University of Newfoundland, St. John's, NL,
Canada A1B 3V6

Kendra K. Lester and William K. Midodzi
Department of Clinical Epidemiology, Faculty of
Medicine, Memorial University of Newfoundland, St.
John's, NL, Canada A1B 3V6

Deborah M. Gregory
Department of Clinical Epidemiology, Faculty of Medicine, Memorial University of Newfoundland, St. John's, NL, Canada A1B 3V6
Department of Medicine, Faculty of Medicine, Memorial University of Newfoundland, St. John's, NL, Canada A1B 3V6

Laurie K. Twells
Department of Clinical Epidemiology, Faculty of Medicine, Memorial University of Newfoundland, St. John's, NL, Canada A1B 3V6
School of Pharmacy, Memorial University of Newfoundland, St. John's, NL, Canada A1B 3V6

Kaneez Fatima, Mohammad Yousuf-ul-Islam, Mehreen Ansari, Faizan Imran Bawany, Muhammad Shahzeb Khan and Akash Khetpal
MBBS-Dow University of Health Sciences (DUHS), Karachi 74100, Pakistan

Neelam Khetpal
Kharadar General Hospital, Karachi, Pakistan

Muhammad Nawaz Lashari
Cardiology, Civil Hospital, DUHS, Karachi 74100, Pakistan

Mohammad Hussham Arshad
Aga Khan University of Health Sciences, Karachi 74800, Pakistan

Raamish Bin Amir, Hoshang Rustom Kakalia, Qaiser Hasan Zaidi and Sharmeen Kamran Mian
Department of Biological Sciences, The Lyceum, Karachi 75600, Pakistan

Bahram Kazani
The Karachi Grammar School, Karachi 75600, Pakistan

Xiangming Wang, Chuanwei Zhou, Deeraj Mungun, Zakaria Iyan and Yan Guo
Department of Geriatric Cardiology, The First Affiliated Hospital of Nanjing Medical University, Nanjing, China

Na Kong
Reproductive Medicine Center, The Affiliated Drum Tower Hospital of Nanjing University, Nanjing, China

Zhijian Yang
Department of Cardiology, The First Affiliated Hospital of Nanjing Medical University, Nanjing, China

Anjala Chelvanathan, David Allen, John Ducas, Kunal Minhas, Minh Vo, Malek Kass, James W. Tam and Farrukh Hussain
Section of Cardiology, Department of Internal Medicine, University of Manitoba, Winnipeg, MB, Canada R2H 2A6

Amir Ravandi
Section of Cardiology, Department of Internal Medicine, University of Manitoba, Winnipeg, MB, Canada R2H 2A6
Institute of Cardiovascular Sciences, St. Boniface Research Centre, University of Manitoba, Winnipeg, MB, Canada R2H 2A6

Davinder S. Jassal
Section of Cardiology, Department of Internal Medicine, University of Manitoba,Winnipeg, MB, Canada R2H 2A6
Institute of Cardiovascular Sciences, St. Boniface Research Centre, University of Manitoba, Winnipeg, MB, Canada R2H 2A6
Section of Oncology, Department of Internal Medicine, University of Manitoba, Winnipeg, MB, Canada R2H 2A6
Department of Radiology, University of Manitoba, Winnipeg, MB, Canada R2H 2A6

Hilary Bews
Institute of Cardiovascular Sciences, St. Boniface Research Centre, University of Manitoba, Winnipeg, MB, Canada R2H 2A6

Sergey Gurevich, Ranjit John, Rosemary F. Kelly, Ganesh Raveendran, Gregory Helmer, Demetris Yannopoulos, Timinder Biring and Brett Oestreich
University of Minnesota-Fairview Medical Center, Minneapolis, MN, USA

Santiago Garcia
University of Minnesota-Fairview Medical Center, Minneapolis, MN, USA
Minneapolis VA Healthcare System, Minneapolis, MN, USA

Fatma Aboul-Enein
Department of Adult Cardiology, KAMC, Makkah 21955, Saudi Arabia

Majed O. Aljuaid, Hail T. Alharthi, Abdulkarim M. Almudhhi and Mohammad A. Alzahrani
Medical College, Taif University, Taif 21974, Saudi Arabia

Solmon Gebremariam
Department of Pediatrics and child Health, Mekelle University, Mekéle, Ethiopia

Tamirat Moges
Department of Pediatrics and Child Health, School of Medicine, Addis Ababa University, Addis Ababa, Ethiopia

Index